The
PSYCHIATRIC
HOSPITAL
and the
FAMILY

Edited by

Henry T. Harbin, M.D.
Maryland Mental Hygiene Administration
 and
Institute of Psychiatry and Human Behavior
University of Maryland School of Medicine
Baltimore, Maryland

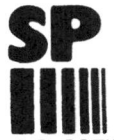

SP MEDICAL & SCIENTIFIC BOOKS
a division of Spectrum Publications, Inc.
New York • London

To My Parents

SPECTRUM PUBLICATIONS, INC.
175-20 Wexford Terrace, Jamaica, N.Y. 11432

Library of Congress Cataloging in Publication Data
Main entry under title:

The Psychiatric hospital and the family

    Bibliography: p.
    Includes index.
1. Psychiatric hospital care — Addresses, essays, lectures. 2. Family psychotherapy — Addresses, essays, lectures. 3. Mentally ill — Family relationships — Addresses, essays, lectures. — I. Harbin, Henry T.
[D.N.L.M.: 1. Family Therapy 2. Hospitals, Psychiatric. 3. Mental disorders — Therapy WM 27.1 P974]
RC 488.5.P77 1982   616.89'156   82-5971
                                AACR2

ISBN 978-94-011-9818-9   ISBN 978-94-011-9816-5 (eBook)
DOI 10.1007/978-94-011-9816-5

Contributors

Carol M. Anderson, M.S.W.
Associate Professor
Department of Psychiatry
Director of Family Therapy
Western Psychiatric Institute and Clinic
University of Pittsburgh
Pittsburgh, Pennsylvania

John E. Bell, Ed.D
Associate Professor
Clinical Psychiatry and Behavioral
  Sciences
Stanford University
Stanford, California

Peter Bruggen, M.D.
Consultant Psychiatrist
Hill End Hospital
Adolescent Unit
St. Albans, Herts
Great Britain

John F. Clarkin, Ph.D.
Associate Professor of Clinical
  Psychology in Psychiatry
Cornell University Medical College
Director of Psychology
The New York Hospital–Westchester
  Division
New York, New York

MarJeanne Collins, M.D.
Assistant Professor of Pediatrics
Department of Pediatrics
University of Pennsylvania School of
  Medicine
Philadelphia, Pennsylvania

Ira D. Glick, M.D.
Professor of Psychiatry
Department of Psychiatry
Cornell University Medical College
Associate Medical Director for Inpatient
  Services
Payne Whitney Clinic
The New York Hospital–Cornell Medical
  Center
New York, New York

James R. Greenley, Ph.D.
Associate Professor of Psychiatry and
  Sociology
Department of Psychiatry
Clinical Sciences Center
University of Wisconsin
Madison, Wisconsin

Jay Haley
Director, Family Therapy Institute of
  Washington D.C.
Professor, Clinical Institute of Psychiatry
  and Human Behavior
University of Maryland School of
  Medicine
Baltimore, Maryland

Henry T. Harbin, M.D.
Assistant Director, Maryland Mental
  Hygiene Administration
Associate Professor of Psychiatry,
  Clinical
Institute of Psychiatry and Human
  Behavior
University of Maryland School of
  Medicine
Baltimore, Maryland

Gordon Hodas, M.D.
Assistant Professor, Clinical
Department of Psychiatry
University of Pennsylvania School of
  Medicine
Associate Director, Pediatric Liaison
  with Children's Hospital of
  Philadelphia
Associate Director of Child Psychiatry
  Training
Philadelphia Child Guidance Clinic
Philadelphia, Pennsylvania

E. Raymond Kidwell, M.D.
Chief Resident, Department of
  Behavioral Medicine and Psychiatry
West Virginia University Medical Center
Morgantown, West Virginia

Thomas Krajewski, M.D.
Superintendent, Springfield State
  Hospital Center
Sykesville, Maryland
Assistant Professor, Clinical
Institute of Psychiatry and Human
  Behavior
University of Maryland School of
  Medicine
Baltimore, Maryland

Ronald Liebman, M.D.
Psychiatrist-in-Chief
Children's Hospital of Philadelphia
Director, Philadelphia Child Guidance
  Clinic
Associate Professor of Child Psychiatry
  and Pediatrics
University of Pennsylvania School of
  Medicine
Philadelphia, Pennsylvania

Cloe Madanes
Co-Director, Family Therapy Institute of
  Washington D.C.
Associate Professor, Adjunct
Institute of Psychiatry and Human
  Behavior
University of Maryland School of
  Medicine
Baltimore, Maryland

William R. McFarlane, M.D.
Assistant Professor, Clinical
Department of Psychiatry
Albert Einstein College of Medicine
Bronx, New York
Associate Director, Fellowship Program
  in Public Psychiatry
New York State Psychiatric Institute
New York, New York
Senior Faculty, Family Institute of
  Westchester
White Plains, New York

Herbert L. Nelson, M.D.
Professor of Psychiatry
Department of Psychiatry
University of Iowa
Iowa City, Iowa

Charles O'Brian
Senior Social Worker
Hill End Hospital
Adolescent Unit
St. Albans, Herts
Great Britain

Douglas J. Reiss, Ph.D.
Coordinator, Family Treatment of
  Schizophrenia Research
Western Psychiatric Institute and Clinic
University of Pittsburgh
Pittsburgh, Pennsylvania

Joan M. Scratton, M.S.W.
Associate Professor
Director, Family Clinic
Coordinator, Family Therapy Training
Institute of Psychiatry and Human
  Behavior
University of Maryland School of
  Medicine
Baltimore, Maryland

Patti M. Seman, M.S.W.
Assistant Professor, Clinical
Family Therapy Supervisor
Institute of Psychiatry and Human
  Behavior
University of Maryland School of
  Medicine
Baltimore, Maryland

Stephan P. Spitzer, Ph.D.
Associate Professor of Sociology
Department of Sociology
University of Minnesota
Minneapolis, Minnesota

Marvin B. Sussman, Ph.D.
UNIDEL Professor of Human Behavior
University of Delaware
Newark, Delaware

Raymond M. Weinstein, Ph.D.
Associate Professor, Department of
  Sociology
University of South Carolina at Aiken
Aiken, South Carolina

Stanley E. Weinstein, M.S.W., Ph.D.
Director, Mental Health Manpower
  Development Project
Maryland Mental Hygiene
  Administration
Assistant Professor, Clinical
Institute of Psychiatry and Human
  Behavior
University of Maryland School of
  Medicine
Baltimore, Maryland

David J. Withersty, M.D.
Professor, Clinical
Department of Psychiatry
West Virginia University School of
  Medicine
Private Practice Psychiatry
Morgantown, West Virginia

Preface

In 1977 there were an estimated 1,846,090 patient care episodes in psychiatric hospitals across the United States. The number of patient care episodes in inpatient facilities continues to increase from that measured in 1955 despite the national emphasis on "deinstitutionalization." Yet the nature and focus of psychiatric hospitals, both public and private, have changed dramatically in the past fifty years. No longer are all mentally ill patients placed in distant hospitals that encourage separation from family and community. Many hospitals now work to include the patient's natural support system, and families are increasingly vocal about their right to stay involved with their hospitalized family member.

As hospital stays have become briefer, the need to incorporate the family in the treatment process has been recognized. We are witnessing the development of new roles for families with the psychiatric hospital and novel treatment strategies offered by inpatient staff to families. These exciting changes have led to an alteration in the attitudes of mental health professionals as well as an expansion of our knowledge and skills regarding the family of the hospitalized psychiatric patient. This book brings together the works of many of those professionals who have developed innovative and pragmatic clinical and research strategies for these families.

As the patients in the psychiatric hospital represent those with the most severe problems, then by necessity family-oriented research and clinical programs in the hospital must be tailored to meet the needs of these special groups. Consequently the authors of the various chapters are describing family approaches for a distinctly underserved group in our mental health system: the seriously disturbed patient. By the editor's design, a number of chapters emphasize strategies for working with the families of schizophrenics as well as those with other difficult problems.

The book is divided into three major sections: Clinical Strategies for the Family of the Hospitalized Patient, Research Studies, and Special Topics. Clinicians will be particularly interested in the first section, which includes chapters that focus on creative, practical approaches to help families and patients change. Topics range from the prevention of admission and readmission to hospitals, to the design of inpatient programs specific for families. Of particular note are those ideas presented about how to work with the families of chronic schizophrenics, a most challenging and difficult population.

The research chapters cover a variety of studies that have attempted to quantify different aspects of family-hospital involvement. Included are reviews of all major outcome studies in addition to measures of how family attitudes and reactions effect patients' readmission rates and length of hospitalization.

The final section contains a group of chapters that cover a wide range of topics. Information is presented to explain how hospitals in other countries involve families for medical and psychiatric care. Also included are chapters with a theoretical focus; e.g., how theories of schizophrenia effect utilization of hospitals in addition to ones that look at training issues. Professionals and consumers alike will be interested in the chapter in this section that looks at the growth of the family/consumer movement and how it has diverged from the goals of professionals. Readers of this book will quickly realize the exciting potential that exists for families and hospitals when they form effective alliances for the goal of improved patient care.

Henry T. Harbin

Contents

**Part III
Special Topics**

PART I

Clinical Strategies for the Family of the Hospitalized Patient

1

Family Treatment of the Psychiatric Inpatient

HENRY T. HARBIN

This chapter focuses on family therapy techniques useful for the hospitalized psychiatric patient in contrast to other chapters in this book that look at family therapy during the preadmission and discharge phases of hospitalization. In addition to a review of pertinent literature, I summarize the development of a special family-oriented psychiatric inpatient unit [21,22]. The treatment techniques developed on this ward have now been applied to a wide variety of inpatient settings, for example, state hospitals, private psychiatric hospitals, and psychiatric units in general hospitals. Family-oriented treatment in these hospitals does not refer to the admission of whole families; rather it means the application of a social system conceptual model and family therapeutic modalities when one family member is hospitalized. Several broad parameters have influenced the type of treatment suggestions that have evolved from these inpatient settings. The first and foremost is the need for a pragmatic, flexible family orientation which can be integrated with other hospital treatment programs, and that will transcend inherent limitations to family involvement existing within the psychiatric hospital. Another important guideline is the necessity of utilizing a type of family therapy appropriate for the more severely disturbed patients who are the most frequent inhabitants of modern psychiatric wards.

The motivation behind this chapter and indeed the whole book is to address the lack of extensive application of family treatment modalities within psychiatric hospitals. This is in marked contrast to the widespread utilization of family therapy approaches in outpatient settings. Most hospitals involve families during the early or late stages primarily to gather information and plan discharge. Rarely are attempts made to alter the organization or interaction of family members. Families are usually not included in any integral manner in the treatment program and primary therapists are frequently not trained to handle families. The following literature review will attempt to place this chapter in a historical context and to outline the evolution of family therapy approaches in the psychiatric hospital.

LITERATURE REVIEW

Mental hospitals have had a peculiar development that include radical oscillations even within the past few decades. Historically, the sequestering of mentally ill persons has taken place in a variety of settings, beginning with jails and almhouses [2,33]. The 19th century ushered in an era that saw the advent of "moral" treatment of hospitalized psychiatric patients, particularly in Europe [14]. However, these humanistic efforts were defeated by the vast numbers of patients and the inadequate public facilities available, leading to the phenomenon of custodial warehousing of persons with a variety of psychiatric and neurological problems. One consequence of long-term psychiatric hospitalization, whether by intent (e.g., when one's treatment philosophy is that severely ill patients "need" 24-hour-care) or by default (e.g., when insufficient public resources prevent early placement of poor patients), is the increased separation of the inpatient from his or her family. This contributes to the family's difficulty in allowing reintegration of the patient upon discharge. The combined efforts of modern psychopharmacologic treatment and the push to keep patients in their community has led to a reduction in the population of most public hospitals with a concomitant rise in the number of brief-stay admissions. These trends have also led to an increase in psychiatric inpatient units connected with general hospitals and community mental health centers. However, the basic assumption underlying the hospital treatment approach, no matter what the particular historical stage of development, has been an individually oriented (either biological or psychological) etiological model of madness. Yet most people are placed in the hospital because their family or the community is unable to tolerate their disturbing behavior, no matter what the etiology of the illness happens to be. Families have been excluded from the hospital often because of their own wishes and the ignorance of the hospital staff.

Most people are familiar with the development of family therapy as a potent treatment alternative used in outpatient and clinic settings. It is interesting that many of the earliest observations about problem families were made by professionals treating hospitalized schizophrenics [4,15,26,43]. Additionally, some of the early research and treatment efforts with disturbed families were made when mental health professionals hospitalized whole families [1,7,8,44].

However, most of this work has been discontinued, probably for economic and practical reasons. Several projects have demonstrated the efficacy of admitting mothers and infants together, and others have hospitalized marital couples in order to treat both more intensively [18,32,42]. Presently, most of the practitioners and theoreticians in the field of family therapy use outpatient populations as their base of information. Furthermore, little attention has been paid to the administrative and structural development of hospitals that do attempt to treat families, even though a few articles address the types of clinical approaches needed for the families of psychiatric inpatients.

During the past two decades, a variety of mental health professionals have presented data concerning family therapy with psychiatric inpatients [10,16,17,28,36,12,38,41]. The largest number focused on the use of conjoint family therapy with selected inpatients. Other articles have presented information concerning the involvement of families of hospitalized adolescents and also within day hospital programs [37,47]. Gralnick, in particular, has written about the important place that family therapy holds within the overall hospital treatment plan and has stated, "I believe I can say that given a fair therapeutic risk, and ample time, we never accomplish a good therapeutic result without simultaneously achieving a positive change in the family, or some significant member of it [16]." However, it is clear from much of this work that family treatment is often a secondary consideration and may only be initiated if some pressing family conflict is identified during individual treatment sessions. In fact, several authors have stated that a general rule was not to begin conjoint family therapy at the onset of hospitalization but to wait until the acute crisis settles down [3,38]. Often, family therapy is only initiated because one member of the team is interested in this approach or is assigned it, but there may be no systematic application. This fragmentation of services is usually representative of the ideological conflicts that are rampant among hospital staff, with some professionals viewing mental problems as chiefly biological or intrapsychic in origin, and others seeing the causes as coming from dysfunctions in the larger social structure.

There have been two recent articles that have specifically focused on family treatment of inpatients. Lansky has presented his experiences in establishing a family-oriented inpatient ward in a Veterans Administration psychiatric unit [27]. There are some similarities in the structure of this unit and the one described in my earlier paper, such as (1) family-oriented intake meeting, (2) frequent use of family therapy, (3) multifamily groups, and (4) changes in the milieu caused by a family approach. Lansky focuses on the overall administrative structure of the staff and milieu and how that has been changed by the inclusion of a family-oriented approach. However, there is little discussion about the type of family therapeutic approaches or procedures that would be specific and most helpful for inpatients. In the little discussion there is about these matters, there seems to be a trend toward helping the families become more effective custodians of the chronically ill person, rather than initiating changes within the family system.

Anderson speaks more directly about specific procedures that can be used to involve families of psychiatric inpatients including: contact at admission, appointment of a family representative, and creation of an accepting milieu for the family [3]. Her article stresses the importance of integrating other treatment modalities with the family approach and emphasizes "patient"-oriented family therapy using supportive methods and task assignments. It is unclear from this article which member of the team does the family therapy; it appears that this role is split off from the inpatient's primary therapist.

In addition to some of the direct clinical experiences of working with families of hospitalized patients, there is a great deal of indirect data that points to the need for inclusion of families in the hospital treatment process. Moore and McCrary have highlighted some of the ways family members can prolong the hospital stay for the identified patient and they have demonstrated how a family-focused treatment could overcome this problem [35]. Other workers have shown how the exclusion of families from the inpatient treatment process can lead to a crisis in discharge planning and, consequently, an increased possibility of therapeutic failure [29]. Davies and Hansen have demonstrated the same problem of family exclusion with physically ill patients [11]. In their article and in one by Bell, a transitional type of family-oriented care for physically ill patients is described [5]. John Bell has also reported much information on how other cultures include families in the care of physically and mentally ill patients [6]. He has also shown some of the ways in which the administrative structure of hospitals worked to discourage family-patient contact, such as maintaining inconvenient visiting hours (or no visiting hours) and lack of privacy. Additionally, data have been accumulating that repeated hospitalizations are very much influenced by familial factors [9,39,45,40].

In reviewing this literature, I conclude that practitioners who have utilized this approach have found it helpful even though outcome data are sparse. Chapters in this book by Glick and Withersty summarize the research literature regarding outcome with family treatment and family involvement respectively. However, the paucity of attention paid to this subject and the inconsistency with which family treatments are implemented is remarkable. Families are often used only as sources of historical information about the identified patient; or are referred to an ancillary psychotherapist, not the primary therapist of the identified patient. Some hospitals may only involve the family at the end of hospitalization, and even this approach may be applied only to selective inpatients.

A SPECIAL FAMILY-ORIENTED
PSYCHIATRIC INPATIENT WARD

In 1975, I began to develop a unique family-oriented psychiatric ward at the University of Maryland Medical School [21]. During the three years that I directed this unit, families of over 80 percent of the inpatients were involved in regular family therapy sessions. The specialized therapeutic approaches developed there were utilized within a short period of time in the other inpatient wards at the same hospital éven though they were not managed by psychiatrists with a family orientation. Further, along with several psychiatrists trained in this unit and other professionals, I have applied these concepts and techniques to a variety of other inpatient settings including: (1) state hospital acute and chronic wards, (2) adolescent units, and (3) nonuniversity-connected general hospital psychiatric admitting units. Even though I have left this particular inpatient unit and the subsequent ward directors have not always had an orientation toward families, the majority of the inpatients are still treated with family therapy. There are a number of reasons for this, not all of which are discussed in this paper. One of the more important factors is that the family approaches that were developed were pragmatic, flexible, able to be integrated with other treatment modalities, and did not require additional manpower. Even though well-designed outcome studies were never performed in this unit, the primary therapists were often struck with how the individual patient's progress seemed to be significantly enhanced when the families were integrally involved.

Brief Description of the Unit

The actual ward is a fifteen-bed admitting unit located within a large university-connected general hospital. A wide range of patients were admitted; at any one time approximately 25 percent of the patients were under 18. All major diagnostic groups were represented, with the majority having a diagnosis of a major affective disorder or schizophrenia. No involuntary patients were admitted and this excluded a number of difficult forensic cases. Techniques for handling families with a member who is court or involuntarily committed have now been developed at several public hospitals in Maryland. The unit is well staffed with all disciplines represented. The psychiatric residents are the primary therapists and rarely have more than five patients. Multiple therapeutic modalities were utilized on this ward and the family treatment approaches were introduced as additional therapies not totally replacing any other psychotherapeutic technique. Patients were admitted randomly to this unit or to two other psychiatric wards. During the first year of management of this family-oriented unit, 85 percent of the 112 patients admitted were treated with regular conjoint family sessions; approximately 630 family therapy interviews were completed. During the second and third years of operation 90 to 95 of families were involved in regular family treatment modalities. When contemplating the establishment of this type of unit, many therapists raise the question about the difficulty of engaging the majority of families. These statistics highlight the fact that it is possible to involve a wide variety of families in this type of hospital treatment program.

Families were involved in multiple ways, including

(1) family admission interviews, (2) conjoint family therapy sessions, (3) multi-family groups, (4) family oriented therapeutic leave of absences, (5) a constant review, via staff meetings and conferences, as to how the family is affecting the hospitalized patient's behavior and vice versa, and (6) administrative policies that encourage the inclusion of families into the ward life [21].

The involvement of the family held a high priority in this unit and a great deal of effort was made toward engagement. Often the frequency of individual psychotherapeutic sessions was reduced to allow time for family work. Additionally, the group and milieu approaches, although still utilized, became less important for some patients. The emphasis in the ward meetings shifted away from a focus on how the patients related to each other, to how the patients were relating to their families on the weekend home visits.

The term *family* was defined loosely; any important person who had frequent contact with the patient, or was viewed as significant in the present, such as lovers, friends, and landlords, in addition to parents, spouses, siblings, and children, would be included as family. Those few patients who had no family were treated by traditional means; however, some attempt was made to involve anyone in the natural support system that existed outside the hospital. More of these patients reside in the public mental health system, especially chronic schizophrenics. With this population it becomes necessary to involve anyone who has contact with the patient, particularly foster parents, guardians, landlords, and so on. The family techniques for working with this nonfamilial group are often similar because many of the conflicts that these patients had with their families of origin are re-created in their present social network.

RESISTANCE TO THE DEVELOPMENT OF
FAMILY TREATMENT IN THE HOSPITAL

Resistance to the establishment of a family-oriented psychiatric hospital can come from a variety of sources: (1) the consumer himself or herself, i.e., the patient or family; (2) the hospital as an organizational entity; and (3) the clinical staff. In this section I focus primarily upon staff resistance. If a clinician sets out to change a traditional inpatient unit to a family-oriented one, he or she will need to use the manpower resources existing in that unit. The discipline of the change agent will be a major factor influencing the type of problem encountered, as will the administrative position of the change agent. Obviously the situation will be easiest if the change agent is a psychiatrist who is director of the unit or hospital. Unfortunately, this is rarely the case and even when it is, a number of problems arise.

Psychiatrists

In most hospitals, psychiatrists have the greatest amount of authority over clinical programs. A key variable is their openness to a new theoretical and technical framework. Most psychiatrists have had little training or experience in family therapy and often feel threatened when this modality is introduced[23]. Their understanding of mental illness is based upon either biological or psychological factors; rarely upon interpersonal variables. However, many psychiatrists are willing to tolerate other treatment modalities if they construe them as nonconflictive with their individual therapy sessions or the psychopharmacological regimen. Consequently., conflicts are inevitable as these treatment approaches are always affected by family treatment modalities. Some clinicians have attempted to conduct family therapy with inpatients only to find that the psychiatrist, without consulting the family therapist, has: (1) changed the medications, hence altering the clinical picture; (2) made a decision about discharge; or (3) gave advice in the individual session contrary to the treatment suggestions given in the family treatment. Naturally, any of these maneuvers can lead to an undermining of both family *and individual* treatment.

Nurses

The nursing staff (including paraprofessional nursing aids) have historically been in the position that makes them most competitive with families. The work schedule and routines of the nursing staff are often responsible for the exclusion of family members from the ward. For example, visiting hours may be reduced because visitors disrupt nursing activities, or families may be excluded when patients are on special precautions of some kind because they complicate the nursing work. The nursing staff often becomes a substitute family for the patient, encouraging them to blame or reject the real family. The attitudes and work patterns of the nursing staff must be addressed if a family-oriented ward is to be successful. Nurses are the group that is most consistently responsible for patients. They have the most frequent contact with patients and also with visiting families. Nurses, both at the professional and paraprofessional level, rarely have any training that helps them to conceptualize the role of the family with psychiatric illnesses, or how to intervene with families.

Social Workers

Social workers have long been the professional group advocating the involvement of families in all psychiatric service settings. In many traditional inpatient units, the social worker initially evaluates the family, serves as a liaison between the hospital and the family, and helps prepare the family for discharge. Usually he or she carries out these functions without having much real clinical authority over the case; having to check with the psychiatrist or team at every turn, for instance, when conjoint family therapy is indicated for a particular patient. Of course, the major problem is that the psychiatrist or other team member may not have the experience or training to know whether family therapy is indicated or contraindicated. Ironically, the social work staff can sometimes be very resistant to moving a traditional inpatient unit to a family-oriented one. Precisely because they have adjusted to the situation as it is they may feel threatened when change is suggested. This may happen even though the changes introduced may be in a direction consistent with their therapeutic philosophy. An important reason for social worker resistance to the family-oriented word is that they have to share the function of conducting family therapy with other disciplines. This becomes a particular threat if some of the other professionals begin to be seen as "experts" in this area, thus challenging one of the traditional social work territorial preogatives. The organizational change agent who expects to establish a family-oriented ward should not look blindly to the social work staff for total support.

Psychologists

My experience with psychologists in inpatient settings has been limited because many of the wards for which I have consulted relegated psychologists to a rather peripheral clinical role. In those units where they function more centrally, they often have the same problems with family therapy that psychiatrists do: they have been trained to think in monadic terms. Psychologists, of course, usually have less of a problem adjusting to a behaviorally oriented family approach than the traditionally trained psychoanalytically oriented psychiatrist.

Strategies for Overcoming Staff Resistance

Retraining the present staff remains the most useful mechanism for changing the therapeutic direction of an inpatient facility. There rarely exists the ideal situation where one can hire new staff to run an innovative program. Psychiatrists, nursing staff, and psychologists are, of course, most in need of training in the basics of family treatment techniques and the conceptualization of psychiatric problems within an interpersonal systems model.

The nursing staff, who usually have the least amount of formal education in any mental health area, are often the most motivated to learn new methods. In the special family unit described earlier:

the nurses were involved in numerous ways: (a) seminars were given specifically for them; (b) they were encouraged to read and attend lectures on family therapy; (c) they were trained to do the family historical questionnaire; (d) several nurses led the multifamily group sessions, which were supervised; and (e) occasionally nurses with more experience acted as the primary family therapist. [21]

Social workers naturally have to be handled differently depending upon their previous experience and training; some may be willing allies, others may resent intrusion. A helpful strategy is to involve the social worker as a teacher for the other staff about family treatment programs; it is important however that the social worker be skilled in this area. Many social workers have had little experience in family therapy with severely disturbed patients, particularly new M.S.W.s. They often have had a great deal of formal classroom instruction in the area of normal family functioning and values, systems theory, and other topics. However, if their clinical experience has been limited to the traditional role of most hospital social workers, then they might not have developed sufficient experience and expertise in the handling of full clinical responsibility for intensive family work. They, like the other professionals, may need further training or experience. However, the social work group usually has the most resources of any of the professionals to help bring about change in this direction.

CLINICAL STRATEGIES

In the following section I discuss some of the family treatment strategies that have proved most helpful with hospitalized patients, and illustrate strategies with case examples. The presentation of particular techniques is clustered around the usual stages of inpatient treatment: admission, middle or consolidation phase, and discharge.

Admission, Evaluation, and Engagement

For the purpose of this chapter, the first stage begins after admission of the patient to the hospital, with the expectation that the person will stay for a period of time. The chapter by Bruggen and O'Brian focuses on the preadmission phase with a greater emphasis on using the initial family work to prevent admission. If the family has been involved prior to hospitalization, all the better. If not, the first day of admission is the time to include them and if this is impossible, then they should be involved as soon as possible thereafter. The more rapid the engagement, the more accurate the evaluation, and consequently, the more appropriate the choice and direction of the therapy. If the family is with the patient on admission, they should be given a tour of the facility and a similar orientation as the patient. This is the time to inform the family of the staff's expectation of their participation in the hospital treatment program, for example, in conjoint family therapy, if indicated, or multifamily group therapy. Since the primary therapist is not usually the person conducting the orientation, then the admitting staff members need to be trained in orientation techniques. Every patient may not receive regular family therapy sessions or multifamily group therapy; the primary therapist needs to keep his or her options open. In the ward I developed and administered, I formulated a letter to be given to each family member inviting them to participate in the weekly multifamily meetings and to generally inform them that they were expected to be a part of the treatment program. The nursing staff member who orients the patient should also extend a verbal invitation. If it is not possible for the primary therapist to conduct a family interview on the first day, or within a few days of admission, then another staff member may be designated to interview the family for an introductory assessment and history taking. The primary therapist can then make use of this information when he or she first sees the family.

Some inpatient units split the role of the primary individual therapist from that of the primary family therapist. Although this division of roles has some advantages, in my opinion it usually does not work, particularly with a short-term hospitalization. With a long-term inpatient stay of six months or more, there may be some rationale for this split because the patient's relationship with the individual therapist may take on a more important role in creating change. However, in short-term hospitalization, the family therapist needs to be in control of the whole treatment process, including privileges in the milieu, discharge decisions, and so on, in order to be effective. So much happens so quickly in a four- to eight-week hospitalization that it usually reduces therapist confusion for one person to be in charge of individual treatment, milieu decisions, and family therapy.

The hospital's admission process needs to be examined for its effects on the family's first exposure to the ward. The financial aspect of the intake procedure may be of crucial importance; sometimes the person who performs this role may be a secretary or clerk who presents the treatment philosophy of the hospital in such a way as to discourage the family's participation, or to close off certain therapeutic strategies. For example, one secretary who served as the admissions officer routinely gave the message to adolescents admitted by their parents that they should also sign themselves in (even though this was not necessary) because she felt that the parents should not have that much authority over the teenager. In another hospital one of the signs at the entrance stated clearly that children under 12 were not allowed to visit. Certainly this policy did not encourage the inclusion of the family. The chances of engaging the family in a positive therapeutic alliance will be considerably enhanced if all hospital personnel, from the cleaning staff to the medical director, give a consistent message.

Problem Identification and Formulation

The first family interview by the primary therapist is of crucial importance both for the purpose of obtaining an accurate assessment of the situation and to induce change. For some families this might be the first time they have sat down together to discuss the problem directly and overtly. This is usually an anxiety-laden interview and it requires great skill by the therapist. Many family members, especially parents, but also spouses and even children, may expect to be blamed in some indirect fashion. Indeed, family theories have unfortunately been used by some naive professionals to imply family responsibility for the causation of an illness. At this time the etiology of the major mental illnesses is not known. Most therapists would agree that a supportive and consistent family atmosphere will help restore a person's health, be it physical or mental, irrespective of the original cause of the illness. Indeed, it is hard to argue with such a commonsense notion. Some families may be interested in indepth information about the latest research on the causes of mental illness. Particularly some families of chronic schizophrenics, who have struggled for many years and have become quite expert in their own fashion on how to cope with their family member, may want to know more. Certainly this information should be provided with some assessment by the clinician about the prevailing philosophies of treatment, validity of the research, and so on. The therapist's stance should be at all times to reassure the family he or she is not present to blame anyone, including the patient, but that the purpose of the therapy is to look to the present and the future. The past can offer some clues about what has been tried, but hope lies in handling the problems of the patient in a different and possibly more productive manner in the future. If the family members launch into blaming each other this should be stopped because it will be counterproductive to later engagement.

Once the therapist has set up a positive and nonjudgmental atmosphere he or she can proceed toward helping the family and patient define the problem more clearly. The aim here is to help the patient and family identify preferably behavioral, but at least quantifiable, attitudinal or cognitive problems. The emphasis is on action, not on subjective distress, even though the skilled therapist will be empathic to each family member's experience of the situation. Most families will speak at length about how they have felt about the problem or will analyze why things went wrong. These statements should be listened to by the therapist but the subject matter of the conversation should be tactfully guided toward a behavioral/task-oriented one. I emphasize the need for empathy and tact because some inexperienced family therapists who have a problem-solving orientation will cut off patients prematurely when they are ventilating. If this is done brusquely and the family does not feel understood, it can block further engagement and heighten resistance to change.

The therapist's role is to help the family orient themselves toward a new definition of the problem. For example, in a hypothetical but typical case, a 35-year-old woman was hospitalized for a suicide attempt after several months of depression. The husband, while being interviewed for the first time in the hospital, states that his wife has been "depressed": "She feels worthless, not interested in anything. I don't know why she feels this way, maybe the kids are getting to her." The wife says, "I don't feel motivated to do anything, nobody cares for me, etc." It is a mistake to leave the definition of the problem here. The next set of questions for the therapist could be: "What does your wife *do* when she gets depressed?" "How does she act?" "When she isn't interested in doing anything what does she do?" "What responsibilities does she presently carry out even though she is depressed?" All of these questions are designed to elicit the behavioral consequences of the depressed state. Based upon this information, the therapist can then begin to formulate a directive/task-oriented intervention. For example, the husband might say, with his wife's agreement, that she sits in her room all day and does not do any housework, only occasionally taking care of the kids. The therapist will then focus upon what the husband *does* when his wife is *acting* this way. For instance, he might have taken over most of the household responsibilities because of the popular hypothesis that depression is the kind of illness best treated by rest and a reduction in obligations or responsibilities. Indeed, this may have been the reason why the family or the referring professional sought psychiatric hospitalization. After the therapist identifies this pattern of behavioral communication, he or she can begin to think of a family directive that might address this imbalance, for example, suggesting that the wife begin to clean the house again, and the husband should not help because this kind of activity will assist his wife in overcoming her depression.

In a recent paper, Krajewski has presented some of the common difficulties that arise when a hospitalized psychiatric patient's problem is reframed in this manner [25]. It does not matter whether the pathology is of a psychotic nature; the eventual goal · is translation into a more concrete, specific, and quantifiable terminology. Schizophrenia may become auditory hallucinations; this may be translated into becoming distracted by internal voices in certain social situations, finally becoming an example of how the patient is impolitely not paying attention to his or her family when they are talking about important issues. The therapist is helping the family reframe the psychopathology into: (1) a language that everyone and not just the professionals can understand, and (2) a guide toward options and solutions for how to *act*. If one leaves the definition of the problem purely on an affective/cognitive/diagnostic level, then the options for therapeutic suggestions will be narrowed, often leading to solutions that promote understanding and insight or pharmacological prescriptions. Of crucial importance is the therapist's assistance in defining in behavioral terms the family's own reactions to the problems of the patient; thus looking for certain sequences of communication in the family that incorporate the pathology. The clinician looks for how the symptomatic behavior fits into the family system as a whole; particularly as to whether the pathology has become part of a homeostatic mechanism for the family. I am placing a greater emphasis in this discussion upon the elicitation of behavioral definitions because this is often not done by mental health professionals. This does not mean that a therapist will ignore cognitive or affective distortions and patterns within and among family members. However, in short-term, crisis-oriented inpatient treatment, a major focus needs to be upon the behavioral components of the illness.

Families have a diversity of reactions to hospitalization. Some see this as a helpful intervention and are happy to work closely with the staff. Others see the hospital as a way to get rid of an irritating person temporarily and, unfortunately at times, some wish for a permanent separation. Still others see the hospitalization as an unwelcome intrusion, forced on them by outside professionals. Some feel relief at being included in the therapy, for others their inclusion evokes guilt. The chapter in this book by Spitzer et al. gives an interesting typology of family reactions to mental patients and how this influences rehospitalization. Spitzer focuses particularly on the expected level of performance for the patient and the family's tolerance for deviance. These are useful concepts and the clinician can assess how various families handle this set of issues. These various reactions of the families impart a great deal of diagnostic information; the therapist should try to learn the family's style and work as much as possible within their framework of understanding.

Engagement as Therapy

Gerald Zuk has clearly identified how much change can occur during the engagement process in outpatient family therapy [46]. This same assumption can be made about the first one or two family interviews in the hospital when the therapist is attempting to clarify the problem and engage the family. Hospitalization for psychiatric problems often galvanizes the family or support system into action because no one can deny the seriousness of the issue any longer. During the crisis time the family is often willing to try different ways to define and deal with pathological behavior. The family therapist will have to move rapidly during the first few interviews as the family and patient try to define the issues. These struggles will often involve the hospitalization and treatment process itself: whether admission is necessary, when to leave, whether the staff or family will be responsible for the patient's behavior, and so forth.

A major difference between outpatient and inpatient family work is related to this engagement struggle. When the family brings the patient to the hospital they often feel a reduction in anxiety; sometimes this decreases their motivation for change. Even though this is a crisis time and everyone is upset, the family may feel that their solution to the crisis is now at hand, that is, the hospital staff will be responsible for the problem. Undoubtedly, at times, a reduction in the family's anxiety level and the provision of a brief respite from the struggle can be helpful. This will be a positive step only if it does not lead to a giving up or an enhancement of resistance to change on the family's part. One of the major tasks for inpatient family work is to keep the family engaged and in continuous contact with the patient in order to maintain their motivation; while, at the same time, supporting them so that they feel some sense of relief from their own considerable stress. This maintenance of contact can be accomplished in numerous ways: frequent and convenient visiting hours, leaves of absence, multifamily groups, conjoint family therapy, and so on. The following case demonstrates some of these engagement issues and how powerful a first family interview can be.

Case 1   Betty is a 56-year-old woman who was admitted to a state psychiatric hospital for the first time. She had been psychotic for several months; precipitating events included a recent move to a new community and her husband's retirement from his job. She presented extreme paranoid and depressive symptoms, and had persecutory delusions about her husband. Her diagnosis waivered between an acute paranoid reaction and a major depressive disorder. She was placed on a neuroleptic and a tricyclic anti-depressant. Her anger at her husband, her feeling that he was trying to kill her, and her bizarre reactions to these thoughts were the predominant symptoms that led to her hospitalization. About one month prior to coming to the hospital, she attacked her husband with a knife and cut several tendons in his wrist. She claimed that her husband had beaten her on numerous occasions; describing these events in strange and extreme terms. She had called the police but no evidence from friends and neighbors could corroborate her accusations. In fact, the neighbors complained about her reclusive, bizarre actions. The husband tolerated his wife's aggression and psychotic behavior for months. When he finally moved to have her evaluated he was frustrated by the byzantine and inadequate emergency forensic procedures that existed in his county (and seem to exist in most regions). Nevertheless, with much guilt and ambivalence, he had her committed. The first conjoint family interview took place about two weeks after admission; the husband had been interviewed alone prior to this as the wife refused to talk with him or see him. I conducted the first interview with the couple accompanied by a psychiatric resident who was the primary therapist for the patient and family. The wife was still acutely psychotic at the time of the interview, and the session began with the wife making long rambling accusations about the husband. Her thought processes were fragmented and loose. She switched topics at random and ended up appearing confused and unreliable. The husband weakly denied her accusations and appeared rather helpless, looking to the therapist for an intervention. Certainly an intervention was necessary to correct what must have been a typical communicational sequence for this couple; the wife's escalating, irrational aggression and the husband's helpless, passive response. The husband would defend himself on the merits of certain accusations, but never confronted his wife with her style of communication, that is, her gross irrationality and peculiar style of thought. The absence of a confrontation led to his providing some affirmation of her persistent self-disqualifications.

The general thrust of the therapeutic intervention was to first empathize and form an alliance with both husband and wife. This was easy in one sense as they had both suffered considerably; in another sense this was difficult with the wife because she demanded agreement with her paranoid position, and any supportive comments to her were seen in this light. Nevertheless, after establishing some empathic base, I moved quickly to block the psychotic rambling of the wife by asking her close-ended, highly structured questions, pushing her to be more organized. These maneuvers calmed her down quickly. I then pointed out that she seemed very unhappy in the marriage but that she was presenting herself as confused and irrational. Further, this made it difficult for anyone to believe all of her story. (Additionally, friends and neighbors had stated that there didn't seem to be any truth to her statements of persecution.) Betty was confronted, politely, with the fact that she had seriously hurt her husband physically and there was no discernible justification for this. Before giving the wife a chance to respond, the husband was asked about his views of his wife's behavior, encouraging him to be more assertive. He began to deal with his wife in a more structured manner, mimicking the therapist. I then confronted the husband for not having protected himself or his wife sooner, and that it was clear from this interview that his wife needed help. He became somewhat defensive but agreed that he should have stood up to his wife's irrational behavior. As the session went on, I put the husband increasingly in charge of helping to structure his wife's verbal behaviors. Interestingly, the wife who had been angry and unreasonable throughout the beginning of the session began behaving much more cooperatively and logically with her husband. She agreed to continue talking to him and to begin working more constructively on their problems. This proved to be a key therapeutic experience for the wife who was nondelusional within a few days. She later stated that her husband had never beaten her, and eventually some of the covert marital problems surfaced.

This example demonstrates several key issues: (1) it is possible to successfully conduct a highly directive, structured family session with a psychotic person; (2) the positive potential for using the presenting symptoms to change dysfunctional interpersonal patterns that then lead to a change of the presenting problems; and (3) the importance of involving and supporting the nonhospitalized family members early on before they retreat. Although most of the couple's therapy dealt with marital problems, the first step in the treatment was to decrease the power of the wife's symptomatology and to place the husband more clearly in charge while the wife was acting "crazy." Cloe Madanes has clearly articulated some of the hierarchical issues involved in couple's therapy when one spouse is symptomatic [30].

Middle Phase or Consolidation

The middle phase of hospital family treatment begins when engagement has been established. However, in a three- to four-week hospital stay there may be only an admission and discharge stage. Certainly the goals for discharge should be raised and kept in mind from the first interview through the consolidation phase. As the family treatment moves into the middle stage, most of the work in the conjoint sessions revolves around the patient's therapeutic leave of absence at home.

This is a good place to describe briefly the general type of conjoint family therapy used in these inpatient settings. I have attempted to synthesize several schools of family therapy, borrowing what is appropriate from each, attempting not to be tied to particularly rigid technical or theoretical frameworks [31]. The major technical principles are that the family therapy should be: (1) directive, (2) symptom-oriented, (3) primarily behavior- and secondarily insight-oriented, (4) emphasizing the present and future, (5) aimed at changing the organization of the family, (6) pragmatic, and (7) flexible. Minuchin and Haley have written extensively about the types of family therapy that have formed the basis for these approaches [19,20,34]. It should be clear from the previous discussion that the patient is not "descapegoated" immediately. Instead, the presenting symptoms are made the focus of the therapy and are used as a leverage to create change in the family structure. Once the presenting problems have diminished or disappeared, other family issues might be addressed; usually this will take place after discharge.

Although insight into a problem is considered helpful, it is clearly not enough to help seriously disturbed patients change. Too often the inpatient team will spend hours suggesting to a patient and family that "talking out their problems" and "understanding what has happened" will bring about change.

This is rarely enough, and the patient and family will frequently wonder what to do next, particularly after they have achieved some understanding. To the patient's and family's query, "What do I *do* when I feel or act this way?" the staff is often silent. The therapeutic void is usually filled with a prescription for medication. A word here about pharmacological treatment. No clinician working with seriously ill patients can or should avoid the judicious use of psychotropic medications for some patients at some point during their illness. But these drugs cannot be considered a panacea as has happened all too often, especially in modern psychiatric hospitals. The creativity of the hospital staff is often blocked by an over-reliance on medication. These drugs have serious and dangerous side effects and do not readily effect change in major areas of the patient's functioning, e.g., social isolation and vocational performance. Although they are enormously effective in the reduction of acute symptomatology, they should be seen as adjuncts to other psychotherapeutic modalities, particularly family treatment. Family treatment has a wider scope and perspective; individual, group, and pharmacological approaches should be considered a part of the overall family assessment and intervention. When these treatments are used, their impact on the patient's family has to be considered.

Once the patient and family have identified specific concrete problems and have engaged with the hospital staff, then a therapeutic weekend leave of absence should be planned. One hopes this will happen within one or two weeks but it depends upon the clinical condition of the patient and the cooperativeness of the family. If the patient is too suicidal, homicidal, or grossly disturbed to be sent home under family supervision within a few weeks, then the family should be encouraged to visit the hospital for longer periods of time, perhaps taking the patient around the hospital grounds for a few hours. A prolonged period of separation without family-patient contact outside of the hospital is to be avoided. Unfortunately an increasing number of external constraints, such as judicial restrictions or third party payment exclusions for leaves of absence, may severely diminish the clinician's flexibility and in the long run decrease therapeutic effectiveness.

I have observed several cases in which the hospital staff and patient have engaged in an escalating struggle for control as the patient becomes increasingly self- or other-destructive and the staff becomes increasingly restrictive, controlling, and intrusive. Some examples have included patients with diagnoses of psychotic depression, anorexia nervosa, and schizophrenia. Often the first maneuver that a staff will use to gain control of the patient is to forbid the family to visit, or to stop weekend visits with the family. I do not point this out to question the motives of the staff or the patient. The staff usually acts on what they consider to be the best interest of the patient and family. They view the patient as too fragile to be with the family and worry that family members will be hurt, or that they will be unable to properly supervise the patient. Often, in this situation, the patient spends increasing amounts of time in the seclusion room (increasing his or her social isolation) and receives large doses of major tranquilizers. It was rarely clear to me in these cases why this happens, but such a pattern, once established, is extremely difficult to break. Often one has to take a risk and try a different approach with the hope that the runaway escalation will reverse. This may mean having the family spend time with the patient in the seclusion room: in the case of an anorectic, it may mean having the family take responsibility for some forced feedings at meal time, or to risk a brief, highly structured, supervised visit home even though the patient does not seem to be prepared. I have seen these techniques help break a destructive cycle that has developed between patient and hospital staff. The introduction of a different response that enlisted the family's aid in helping the patient with his or her loss of control seemed in these instances to have positive consequences.

A common pattern on inpatient units is for the team to use the restriction of the right to go home on the weekend as a way of negatively rewarding (punishing) a patient for breaking ward rules. I am not against using negative reinforcement techniques but one that prohibits home visits is rarely necessary and should be avoided if at all possible. This course of action is often a convenient one for the staff but it has other unintended destructive consequences for family treatment. Often the family therapist will work on a planned leave of absence only to find that another staff member has restricted the patient for the weekend. Again, the family therapist needs to be in control of milieu decisions.

An enormous amount of time in conjoint family sessions is spent assigning tasks to realign the family's interaction surrounding the presenting problem. These tasks can only be accomplished during the weekend leave of absence when the family is a separate unit from the hospital and they are clearly in charge. Although the University of Maryland is experimenting with a program that places the family in charge of the hospital milieu program for selected patients, this is still to be considered a basically untested procedure for most patients [13]. The biggest difficulty is in implementation because of the amount of communication that is required between the family members and the nursing staff. Thus the weekend leave of absence becomes a cornerstone for family treatment; a time for the patient and family to try new approaches to solving their problems, with the hospital in the background. The following case illuminates the usefulness of a carefully planned leave of absence.

Case 2   A 19-year-old boy, Gene, was admitted to University Hospital for repetitive violent episodes primarily directed at his mother and sisters. He had been arrested because of an attempt to steal a newspaper vending machine; after testimony by the mother about his previous assaultive behavior he was sent to the hospital. In the first family interview, which was quite stormy, the therapist made a firm alliance with the mother. Her husband had died about one and a half years prior to hospitalization and she was struggling to be a single parent to four children. Gene was living at home but was clearly disrespectful to his mother's authority; the most obvious example of this were his physical attacks upon her when she attempted to correct him. Family therapy was the major treatment modality in this eight-week hospitalization that ended successfully from the symptomatic point of view, that is, Gene stopped being violent. This major problem had been identified in the first session and formulated as a problem for the whole family.

In the second and third family interviews, the major focus was upon planning a leave of absense. Gene had not demonstrated any physically violent behavior in the hospital and was sent home under the supervision of his mother within two weeks. The therapist spent most of the second interview asking the mother about what she planned to do if her son became violent at home. She repeatedly responded in a helpless and passive manner; prior to the hospitalization she had never called the police or sought any outside intervention even though the son had called the police on himself twice. The planning process was tied to: 1) the presenting symptom, and 2) the immediate future. It forced a change in the family's structure by supporting and pushing the mother to clarify the authority hierarchy in the family. Mother finally agreed that she had to take some positive action and decided to first notify the hospital and then call the police to have them bring back her son if he became physically aggressive. The therapist strongly supported this course of action. Gene was indignant that the therapist and his mother considered the possibility that he would lose his temper again. Several weekends passed uneventfully, finally a violent episode occurred at home and the mother managed to call the police. To our knowledge this was the last such episode for Gene in a two-year follow-up period after hospitalization. It should be noted that the follow-up outpatient treatment was based primarily on family therapy.

This case clearly demonstrates the necessity of the family being at home, rather than in the hospital, when it is attempting to change. When the mother tried to handle Gene in the family session or in the ward she usually deferred to the authority of the staff; this was appropriate for the beginning phase of treatment. At home she was on her own. Any number of "acting out" problems can be handled in this manner, such as delinquent acts and suicidal behavior, among others. The family can receive support from the hospital as it attempts to gradually handle its problems in a different manner.

Resistant Families

Some families will absolutely refuse to participate in the family treatment program or will continuously break appointments. In a short-term hospitalization it takes only two or three broken appointments to undermine the therapy. These cases present a special challenge and can evoke creative responses from the inpatient team. Each case should be reviewed for the importance of including the family. If the conclusion is that family treatment will be crucial for a positive outcome, then the family should be directly confronted with their resistance. If rational persuasion is not productive the threat of possible discharge should be raised. A note of caution is necessary. Some inexperienced or impatient therapist will too easily look to premature discharge for resistant patients or families (they usually go together) without trying other methods first. This is a technique of last resort. Nevertheless a threat can be extremely effective in motivating some resistant families; in the three years that I was managing the special family-oriented inpatient unit, only one patient was ever discharged for family noncompliance. Dozens, however, were threatened with this. Naturally this maneuver can not be implemented if the patient is so clinically unstable that discharge would equate with medical abandonment. Also, the patient and family should be referred to another hospital or therapist upon discharge. Some families do not respond to this technique because they do not care whether the patient is discharged. With these families other types of leverage must be sought. One possible technique is raising the question of ending the patient's disability payments (assuming that he or she has them) for family and/or patient noncompliance. Of course, a professional cannot do this unless he or she sincerely feels the patient is capable of working. Many families have become quite dependent upon the disability payments and the mere suggestion that they will be ended will motivate them to take a more active role in treatment. Again, this is a technique to be used with extreme caution and only after more straightforward methods have been utilized.

Discharge Phase

Planning for discharge should begin on the first day of hospitalization and the family should be integrally involved. The decision as to when the patient will be ready for discharge can be viewed as a tripartite one involving the primary therapist, the family, and the patient. Ideally, the primary therapist for the family in the hospital should be the outpatient therapist. Since this is rarely possible, the involvement of the outpatient therapist during the final week of the hospital stay is necessary; this person should preferably meet with the family prior to discharge. It is best if the inpatient therapist can refer the patient and family to a person who has a family treatment method similar to that described in this chapter. This may be difficult depending upon the training resources in a particular region. In Maryland, an intensive effort has been made in the past three years to train large numbers of outpatient community mental health center staff (85 persons to date) in a problem solving/strategic mode of family therapy. Since these skills are also being developed by staff in some of the public hospitals, this should accelerate the development of continuous care for families as the patient moves from home to hospital to home.

CONCLUSION

Presented in this chapter is a summary of pertinent literature and a description of a specific inpatient unit and specialized family engagement and treatment techniques for psychiatrically hospitalized patients. Professionals interested in moving a traditional inpatient unit in the direction of a family-oriented one can learn about some strategies for bringing this about. Much work remains to be done to further refine the ideas presented here. Some patients do not respond even when their families are intimately involved, and it is not always clear why this is so. If inpatient units are going to fully realize their therapeutic potential for the patient and the family, they need to become even more oriented toward involving the family and other natural support systems. When an individual is experiencing or causing enough distress to necessitate hospitalization, this is a signal that the natural, interpersonal support system should be thoroughly examined and possibly changed. For the family this may mean evaluating all members thoroughly both individually and as a unit, moving toward a true family psychiatry [24]. The therapeutic treatment program outlined above is a major step in that direction but it is clearly not enough. Naturally, if the hospital staff were able to adopt a comprehensive family treatment orientation a great deal of preventive work would be done. One hopes this would lead in the long run to a reduction in the use of psychiatric hospitals themselves for patients and their families.

REFERENCES

1. Abroms, G.; Fellner, C.; Whitaker, C. "Admission of whole families." *American Journal of Psychiatry* 127 : 1363–1369, 1971.
2. Alexander, F. and Selesnick, S.T. *The History of Psychiatry*. New York: Harper and Row, 1966.
3. Anderson, C.M. "Family intervention with severely disturbed inpatients." *Archives of General Psychiatry* 34 : 697–702, 1977.
4. Arieti, S. *Interpretation of Schizophrenia*. New York: Basic Books, Inc., 1974, pp. 9–29.
5. Bell, J.E. *Family Therapy*. New York: Jason Aranson, 1975.
6. Bell, J.E. "Family in medical and psychiatric treatment: selected clinical approaches." *J Oper Psychiatry* 8 : 57–65, 1977.
7. Bowen, M. "Family psychotherapy with schizophrenia in the hospital and in private practice." In: I. Boszormenyi-Nagy and J.L. Framo (eds). *Intensive Family Therapy*. Hagerstown, MD: Harper and Row, 1965, pp. 213–245.
8. Brodey, W. "Some family operations and schizophrenia." *Archives of General Psychiatry* 1 : 379–402, 1959.
9. Brown, G.W.; Birley, J.L.T.; Wing, J.K. "Influence of family life on the courses of schizophrenic disorders: a replication." *British Journal of Psychiatry* 121 : 241–258, 1972.

10. Burks, H. and Serrano, A. "The uses of family therapy and brief hospitalization." *Diseases of the Nervous System* 26 : 804–806, 1965.
11. Davies, N.H. and Hansen, E. "Family focus: a transitional cottage in an acute care hospital." *Family Process* 13 : 481–488, 1975.
12. Fleck, S.; Cornelison, A.R.; Norton, N. et al. "II interaction between hospital staff and families." *Psychiatry* 20 : 343–350, 1957.
13. Fox, M. Personal communication.
14. Freedman, A.M.; Kaplan, H.I.; and Sadock, B.J. (eds) *Comprehensive Textbook of Psychiatry,* Vol I. Baltimore: Williams and Wilkins Co., pp. 43–48.
15. Fromm-Reichmann, F. "Notes on the development of treatment of schizophrenia by psychoanalytic psychotherapy." *Psychiatry* 11 : 267–277, 1948.
16. Gralnick, A. "Conjoint family therapy: its role in rehabilitation of the inpatient and family." *Journal of Nervous and Mental Disease* 136 : 500–506, 1963.
17. Gralnick, A. "Family psychotherapy: general and specific considerations." *The Psychiatric Hospital as a Therapeutic Instrument.* New York: Brunner/Mazel, 1969, p. 158.
18. Grunebaum, H.U.; Weiss, J.L.; Gallant, O.H. et al. "Mentally ill mothers: in the hospital and at home." *The New Hospital Psychiatry.* New York: Academic Press, 1971, pp. 159–174.
19. Haley, J. *Uncommon Therapy.* New York: Ballentine Books, 1973.
20. Haley, J. *Problem Solving Therapy.* New York: Jossey-Bass, 1976.
21. Harbin, H.T. "A family oriented psychiatric inpatient unit." *Family Process* 18 : 281–292, 1979.
22. Harbin, H.T. "Families and hospitals: collusion or cooperation?" *American Journal of Psychiatry* 12 : 1496–1499, 1978.
23. Harbin, H.T. "Family therapy training for psychiatric residents." *American Journal of Psychiatry* 137 : 1595–1598, 1980.
24. Howell, J. *Principles of Family Psychiatry.* New York: Brunner/Mazel, 1975.
25. Krajewski, T. "Inpatient family therapy." *International Journal of Family Psychiatry.* In press.
26. Laing, R.D. and Esterson, A. *Sanity, Madness and the Family.* New York: Basic Books, 1965.
27. Lansky. "Establishing a family oriented inpatient unit." *J Oper Psychiatry* 8 : 66–74, 1977.
28. Laqueur, H.P. and LaBurt, H.A. "Family organization on a modern state hospital ward." *Mental Hygiene* 48 : 544–551, 1964.
29. Leavitt, M. "The discharge crisis: the experience of families of psychiatric patients." *Nurs Reg* 24 : 33–40, 1975.
30. Madanes, C. "Marital therapy when a symptom is presented by a spouse." *International Journal of Family Therapy* 2 : 120–136, 1980.
31. Madanes, C. and Haley, J. "Dimensions of family therapy." *Journal of Nervous and Mental Disease* 165 : 88–98, 1977.
32. Main, T.F. "Mothers with children in a psychiatric hospital." *Lancet* II : 845–847, 1958.
33. Maxmen, J.S.; Tucker, G.J.; and Lebow, M. *Rational Hospital Psychiatry.* New York: Brunner/Mazel, 1974.
34. Minuchin, S. *Families and Family Therapy.* Cambridge, MA: Harvard University Press, 1974.
35. Moore, K.B. and McCravy, N. "Family interaction as a factor in prolonging hospitalization." *Journal of Nervous and Mental Disease* 136 : 485–491, 1963.
36. Norton, N.M.; Detre, T.P.; and Jarecki, H.G. "Psychiatric services in general hospitals: a family oriented redefinition." *Journal of Nervous and Mental Disease* 136 : 475–484, 1963.
37. Orvin, G.H. "Intensive treatment of the adolescent and his family." *Archives of General Psychiatry* 31 : 801–806, 1974.
38. Rabiner, E.L.; Molinski, H.; and Gralnick, A. Conjoint family therapy in the inpatient setting. *American Journal of Psychiatry* 16 : 618–631, 1962.
39. Richart, R.H. and Millner, L.M. "Factors influencing admission to a community mental health center." *Community Mental Health* 4 : 27–35, 1962.

40. Rose, C.L. "Relative's attitudes and mental hospitalization." *Mental Hygiene* 43 : 194–203, 1959.
41. Schween, P.H. and Gralnick, A. "Factors affecting family therapy in the hospital setting." *Community Psychiatry* 7 : 424–431, 1966.
42. Steinglass, P.; Davis, D.I.; and Berenson, D. "Observations of conjointly hospitalized alcoholic couples during sobriety and intoxication: implications for theory and therapy." *Family Process* 16 : 1–16, 1977.
43. Sullivan, H.S. *Clinical Studies in Psychiatry.* New York: W.W. Norton, 1956.
44. White, N. and Molnar, G. "Admissions of married couples." *Canadian Psychiatry Journal* 17 : 449–454, 1972.
45. Wood, E.C.; Rakuson, J.M.; and Morse, E. "Interpersonal aspects of psychiatric hospitalization." *Archives of General Psychiatry* 3 : 632–641, 1960.
46. Zuk, G. *Family Therapy: A Triadic Based Approach.* New York: Behavioral Publications, 1971, pp. 102–128.
47. Zwerling, I. and Mendelsohn, M. "Initial family reactions to a day hospitalization." *Family Process* 4 : 50–63, 1965.

2

An Adolescent Unit's Focus on Family Admission Decisions

PETER BRUGGEN AND CHARLES O'BRIAN

1. A young woman threatened to jump from the fourteenth floor of an office building today. She sat on a ledge while police talked to her for several hours. Eventually they persuaded her to come down and she was taken to the hospital. Later in the day she was allowed to leave.

2. A woman was admitted to the hospital for observation after she broke out in a rash. Just before the doctor's morning ward rounds, she learned that her husband had been taken seriously ill. She informed the doctor that she would be leaving later that day.

Specialist: I am afraid you can't do that because you need to stay for a few more days. I am not going to let you leave.
Woman: How are you going to stop me?
Specialist: Well, of course I can't stop you, but my advice is that you should stay.
Woman: Thank you for your advice, Doctor, but I have to care for my husband and so I am leaving today.

3. A woman is in the hospital with terminal cancer and her 14-year-old son wants to visit her.

Ward Nurse: I am afraid your mother is too ill to be visited today so you will have to go home.

The boy rushed past the nurse and reached his mother's bedside just in time to see the cardiac monitoring machine stop.

4. A British Hospital Management Committee Meeting is in progress:

Consultant Physician: Of course, you will all agree, that doctors are the only persons who have the right to discharge patients.

Committee Member: No, you are not.
Consultant Physician: Then who else?
Committee Member: The patient.

INTRODUCTION

In the wave of philanthropy of the 18th century, financiers gave expression to their altruistic feelings by building hospitals. In the ensuing 125 years, 150 new hospitals and dispensaries were established in Britain [15]. "Lying in hospitals" in the principal towns, county hospitals, and some of the major metropolitan teaching hospitals were founded during this time.

In this same period, the medical mandate over persons who seemed to be acting oddly began in earnest. Problems of behavior were reclassified as illness and madhouses were retitled "asylums for the insane," and retitled yet again as, "mental hospitals." Psychiatric hospitals and Departments of Psychological Medicine came in the 20th century. Inmates were referred to as patients, staff were trained as nurses and doctors, files became medical records.

Persons staffing these institutions developed into the "tinkering" professionals [6]. Their growth ran parallel with that of other "service" industries, such as plumbing and car mechanics. As all of these services have become more elaborate, the site of their delivery has changed from the house to the workshop. The workshop complex took over from the house call in providing large-scale specialist services, but there was still a simple relationship between client and server.

The State then started to intervene and introduced legislation with the intent of safeguarding the rights and well-being of individuals. This complicated the relationship between client and server. In legal services, laws now govern many aspects of the client/lawyer relationship. So, too, in the field of medical care. What drugs can be prescribed and who can prescribe them, are both restricted by the State. Who can practice medical care is restricted to those legally sanctioned to do so. In language much used by family therapists, the relationship, when one seeks medical help, is no longer a dyadic and linear one, but is triadic and circular.

A major difference between the car mechanic and the doctor is that the car mechanic can work without the presence of the owner: It is not the owner's presence that helps or hinders the work. In the client-doctor relationship, a body cannot be left under the care of the server while the client goes about his business. The client remains very interested in what is happening to his body, aware of it, and in an excellent position to see what is being done.

One solution which enables the doctor to get on with his work without being interfered with by the client or patient is to use general anesthesia. A psychic solution is for the physician to separate, in his mind, the illness from the social person of the client. The illness is seen as an independent entity and he can make decisions about treatment without consultation with the patient. This is what happened in example two above. However, when confronted with his inability to enforce his decision, the doctor moved into another relationship with his client—he stopped making decisions and offered advice.

Can a dying woman be too ill to be visited? Caught in the trap of unresolved thinking, we, in the "tinkering" professions, are often unrealistic and pompous. Therefore, when a child asks to say goodbye to his dying parent, we respond as in the third example. Why do nurses and doctors have to feel that they are in charge and why does society want them to seem so?

One view held by both tinkerers and clients is that the hospital establishment in which we work is beyond question. Another commonly held view is that this establishment is terrible and should be pulled down. These two views are held by groups both in our profession and in society. We are still potential patients and yet are often the last to go into the hospital if we can possibly help it. When we do, as a last resort, go into the hospital, many of the processes of "closure," [14] seem to apply to us just as they do to others. We hand over our responsibility to ourselves to the specialists, we accept advice as if it is an order, we collude with the idea that the best is always being done for us, and we become quietly institutionalized. The most that we ever do is to be uncooperative or write an article for the popular professional press about our experience. Rarely, if ever, do we take an active part in changing the patient's role to that of a participant—decision maker. High-principled thinking about confidentiality has helped to obscure and muddle everything even further, but family therapy with its emphasis on opening and clarifying communications, has helped.

SOME EARLY IMPORTANT RESEARCH WORK ON ADMISSION RATES

Some clearly definable medical conditions are generally accepted as being uniformly distributed among the general population, and yet admissions for, for example, pharyngitis, tonsillitis, and appendicitis vary among localities by as much as 10 to 30 times [13]. Even in supposedly uncomplicated physical conditions, concensus differs among physicians. Shifting the emphasis to a psychiatric service, an elderly man who had cut himself and swallowed poison was helped by a psychiatrist to understand that his suicidal behavior made people anxious and that this was why he was in a psychiatric ward [1,10]. Here is an important early example that acknowledges how anxiety in others is the reason for psychiatric admissions.

A second important study [9] showed that general psychiatric hospital admission was no better than outpatient family crisis therapy which was cheaper and quicker. In a controlled sample of 150, the admission decision was reversed. The only factors which influenced the decision were: (1) the designated patient had to live within an hour's travelling distance of the hospital, (2) the patient had to have a family, and (3) be between 15 and 65 years of age. The only other requirement was the team's ability and confidence to offer family crisis therapy which they had decided to do for the period of the research study.

Important as these examples are, both depended upon medically made decisions. The first was to admit for reasons of community anxiety; the second was to admit as part of research strategy. This chapter investigates the decision-making process itself, and its use as a therapeutic force in its own right.

DECISION MAKING [4]

For choices to be real, alternatives must be clear and the consequences of each potential choice must be known. There is no point (or reality) in looking for ideal placements which are not available and may not even exist. No matter how loaded they are in terms of possible benefit, there is always the likelihood that institutions will also damage.

Power and Stability in the Decision-Making Structure

Who carries the authority for making the decision? Does that person have sufficient support to carry out the decision and to carry out revisions of it in the future? If someone else can—at any moment and without consultation—change the decision, then power lies with that person and not with the original decision maker. This is an entirely different way to view decision making.

The capacity to make decisions is altered in families when one of their members is disturbed. When a member of a family is referred for admission, the whole family may be in such a state that they do not know what is happening or what to do. They may also be caught in an uncomfortable ambivalence about the issue of admission. They wish for the problem member to be separated from them by going to the hospital, but may also wish the family to stay together. Traditionally, this issue is resolved by a tinkerer (a mental health professional), who makes the decision while the person's role is limited to accepting or rejecting the specialist's advice.

Handing over the decision making to a tinkerer, and then going along with the decision to admit, successfully deals with a number of family tensions. The need for separation is met, anxiety is reduced without hostility. ("You only have to leave home because we want the best treatment for you.") Admission is then seen as an act of love without uncomfortable feelings of rejection. The pain of having to make decisions within the family is avoided. Any sense of responsibility on behalf of the family, or especially the parents, is shifted. It is now shared between the psychiatrist, who makes the decision, and the designated patient, who is labelled as a problem. The heat is taken off everybody who may be wondering what to do next. The professional people also feel less anxious because they do not have to wonder about what to do next, and all problems to do with finding placements can be shelved with a great big sigh of relief. Changes are so dramatic and so rapid that it is easy to see how any of the people involved, if faced with a similar set of circumstances in the future, will look for the same solution. The readmission rates of the control group mentioned above confirmed this sort of learning and development of a particular maladaptive response to difficulties.

Crisis Theory

The potential for learning is great during periods of crisis since these are times of change. Lasting from a few hours to a few weeks, they end with the individual or family finding some solution [5]. The solution, either adaptive or maladaptive, will become the pattern for dealing with future crises. Therefore working intensely on problem solving is especially important during the crisis itself. Confirmation of this comes from the family therapy research study [9]. Members of the control group, admitted routinely to a psychiatric hospital, were more likely on discharge to be *readmitted* to the hospital than were experimental group members to be *admitted for the first time* in the follow-up period. The experimental control group had learned a nonhospital method of coping. Examples of nonhospital crisis intervention are to be seen in some psychiatric services and a lead on this method was given in England's Dingleton Hospital Area Service [7,8].

Language

The therapist's language should be similar to that used by the client [2] and should not be littered with medical and treatment terminology. For alternatives to be clear, the words used to describe them must be understandable to those concerned. By choosing words that often only he understands, the psychiatrist consolidates the decrease in the family's skill and ability to make decisions, while increasing the idea of some mysterious knowledge and skill in himself. The venue of the decision making is shifted from the family living arrangements and interactions to the mind of the psychiatrist in the institution. This skill is to be practiced on that person who is identified as the patient. The psychiatrist does all of this, it is important to stress, even if the decision is not to admit.

Reason for Referral to the Hospital

We know about the lasting power of the professional referral. Even when family or individual circumstances have radically changed, the referral request is paramount, as the following examples illustrate.

1. A 15-year-old boy, lacking confidence and with anxieties about schoolwork or future employment, was referred for inpatient treatment. Because of his intelligence and apparently great motivation, his name was placed on the waiting list. Some months later, as his turn came up, a standard letter offering him a place on the following Monday was sent to him. He arrived for admission and proved a willing and cooperative patient. He joined passively and obediently in all therapeutic functions and stayed many months.

What was not known until near his discharge was that since the point of referral, his circumstances had changed. He had obtained a place in a special hostel and a job. He gave up both of these in order to come into the hospital. This he did quite willingly, never questioning that he should take the place offered from the waiting list.

2. A 15-year-old girl, quiet and withdrawn at school, was diagnosed as an elective mute by the psychiatrist who referred her for admission to a psychiatric inpatient unit for adolescents. This diagnosis was readily confirmed by the persistent silence of the girl at the assessment interviews. Some time after admission, the parents of the girl also stopped talking, but the social worker who was seeing them would not put up with it. As interest in family therapy was developing, a family meeting was called. At this meeting a determined attempt was made by the professional staff to withdraw from the earlier assumed role of sage and decision maker, and the parents were asked what they wanted. They said they wanted the girl home. Casually, diffidently, and without expectation of an answer, one of the professional staff said that she wondered what the daughter thought. To their surprise, she spoke, saying that she too wished to leave. This girl visited the unit socially on several occasions over the next few years, demonstrating on each visit such an increased social poise and verbal ability that would have made the staff feel very proud of their treatment, if she had been in it.

ADMISSION PROCEDURE: THE FIRST STAGE

Referrals to Hill End Adolescent Unit are usually made by telephone and are dealt with by a social worker [3]. If they are made by letter, the referrer is telephoned. Referrals come from social workers in Social Service Departments; Child and Family Psychiatric Clinics; doctors in general or psychiatric practice and, less commonly, from probation officers, teachers, or others. The first information sought is the age of the adolescent, where he or she lives, who holds parental authority and whether there is a court case outstanding. Our criteria for involvement are:

1. that parental authority is held by a person living in our catchment area—that of a Regional Health Authority responsible for services in one quarter of London and two counties (the population is about 4 million);

2. that the adolescent is under 16 years old (From the 16th birthday, according to the British Mental Health Act, people may negotiate their own treatment and other legal rights are given.);

3. there must be no court case pending for offenses. If there is, then we will not be involved. We do not like Juvenile Courts to have their deliberations interfered with by the notion that a child is psychiatrically ill or disturbed and therefore needs "special disposal." Also, we do not wish the adolescent to assume that we are a "soft option." This may make it more difficult for him or her to develop a sense of responsibility and to acknowledge that actions have consequences.

In discussing the case, we concentrate on the present crisis—what has led to the problem being referred to us—and we try to clarify what the referrer wants of us. We also ask who it is who wants the adolescent to be admitted to the hospital, why, and what view is held by the person who has legal authority. Emphasis is placed on clarifying the site of legal authority, which, in this age group, must rest with one or more of the adults concerned. Various ways are discussed in which parental authority could be supported other than by admission to the hospital. If other placements are available, we advise that they should be looked into.

We resist the use of words, "suitable," or "appropriate," but do express a belief that admission to a psychiatric unit should be a last resort since adolescence is a time of identity formation and we should try to prevent placement during this stage of development. Spending part of one's life in a psychiatric institution is often a stigmatizing experience. That stigma of psychiatric treatment can last a long time was tragically shown when Senator Thomas Eagleton was proposed for the office of Vice-President.

During the telephone call, emphasis is placed on the availability of a bed if the person in authroity, not the referrer, should decide that he or she can no longer cope with the adolescent in the community. Such a telephone call, which may last from two minutes to one hour, may be all the work we do on a case.

The Second Stage

If the referrer still feels that he or she wants to involve us, we offer a consultation at their place of work and the possibility of meeting with the family as well, after we have met with the referrer. We ask the referrer to invite to the meeting any other professionals who may be significantly involved, so that we may pool our ideas, develop new ones as to the use of shared resources, and have the opportunity to open any covert conflicts which might be hampering our efficiency.

We do not ask for notes or reports. These may make us wiser about the past, but the transaction will deflect those with the problem from the task of problem solving. Seeing ourselves as consultants to other people with a problem, rather than as trouble-shooters who are going to sort everything out, has another advantage. If we are kept waiting by our professional hosts, we are not insulted but see this as their way of using us. We always have something else to do. We send a multidisciplinary team and each professional supervises the other in work with the family.

Since the responsibility for these meetings is not ours, they take differing forms. Usually one or more of the other professionals present wishes to summarize reports, give opinions, or share information. We accept this process and pay attention to such details as the age of the documents and whether they are written by people who have actually seen the subject of the report. We aim to present ourselves, not as coming from a rival or more sophisticated institution, but from a complementary one. Our professional backgrounds and our trainings are similar to those of the other people in the room. The essential difference is that we come from a psychiatric facility which is residential. We have beds.

When an individual comes into our unit, we cannot be sure that they will make use of our skills, or that we will be particularly skillful during the time that they are with us. Nor can we be sure that the process will do the adolescent any good at all. However, there are two significant implications of the adolescent being with us as opposed to being somewhere else. The first of these is best seen in terms of professional anxiety. Certain forms of behavior—that is, crazy behavior (meaning that which we find difficult to understand) and self-destructive behavior—make professional people very anxious. Psychiatric institutions are one of society's means of dealing with that anxiety. Therefore, if an adolescent presenting that sort of behavior is in our unit and not in a children's home, special boarding school, or with their family, then certain professional people will be less anxious. It is important to emphasize that this lessened anxiety may result regardless of how effective we are expected to be and whether the behavior (the symptom) subsides. Second, the adolescent not being in a children's home, special boarding school, or with his or her family, means that those who were looking after him will not have to do so. They will have a break from anxiety (about the sort of symptoms referred to previously), from fatigue (as, for example, comes from dealing with a particularly demanding child), or from receiving the consequence of a symptom (e.g., being hit).

Pressed for an opinion, we return to one of our central notions, namely, that we never know what is best, nor do we know how to find out what is best. All we can say is that it is helpful for adults to state clearly what they want or feel they need for themselves; and that the people who hold parental authority have to make decisions about where, out of the choices that are available, the adolescent lives.

Again, such a discussion may be the end of our involvement with a case. The professional workers may decide to continue as before or they may decide to implement an old plan or a new plan. Their new confidence is often based on the assurance that, should things break down and the caretakers be unable to cope, then we would, if asked by whoever is legally in charge, be prepared to quickly admit.

The Third Stage

The referring professionals may wish more from us and ask us to meet with the family if there is one. Some adolescents are orphans in the care of the local authority—such work is somewhat different. In these meetings, we exploit our status and the seriousness of our involvement: We are a Regional Adolescent Unit and often travel a long way. Often we find that our requests to meet with the whole family are acceded to, when previously our colleagues' requests have been rejected. This seriousness and status is transferred to the meeting. Family members may not only be more willing to attend, they may also be more willing to share information, to engage emotionally, or to make a commitment.

When we meet the family we ask them what the problem is, while emphasizing (in words, or simply in how we approach the interview) that we see things in family terms. As "for the best treatment," as is so often embodied in the reason for admission, we go to some pains to keep them separate. Treatment is available in the community. Most of us, when we want treatment, do not go straight into the hospital. The difference about treatment in our setting is that it involves separation. Why is separation being considered? Who wants it and for what reason? Again, we emphasize how little we can be sure of by agreeing to admission. The metaphor of the theater ticket is sometimes helpful here. The ticket entitles one to a seat at a certain time and for a particular length of time. It does not guarantee enjoyment, emotional fulfillment, or cultural enrichment—

these are extras. So too with admission. The place is guaranteed (unless we find that we cannot cope) but treatment, benefit, growth, saving lives, and reintegration are extras that they may or may not be available.

Family therapy in this session may focus on authority, coping and decision making within the family, or we may give a positive connotation to the symptoms and paradoxically prescribe no change [11,12]. They are offered a handout about our institution to take away with them.

The Fourth Stage

At the meeting at the Unit, the client group is shown around the building and then given a few minutes by themselves to discuss things alone. We professionals use this time to meet briefly to see if there are any professional issues for us to sort out so as to avoid pushing onto our clients the consequences of our inadequately worked-out problem.

In the family meeting, the crisis is explored again. Things may have changed. The family may, possibly because of the previous intervention, have found a new way of dealing with their difficulties. They may be so reassured, or so appalled, by our building, the other adolescents, or ourselves, that they wish to go away without using us. If that is to be their decision, we emphasize that as far as we are concerned, that is fine. We are happy to be employed in this way and see it as a valid use of our resources. We are also happy for them to contact us again, through the referrer, anytime before the 16th birthday of the adolescent child.

The Fifth Stage

If things have not changed and the parents are still wanting a break, then they will be encouraged to make a final decision in the meeting and we will make a formal, verbal agreement with them. This decision and agreement must be made by both parents if both share legal parental authority, or by parent or parents and social worker, if authority is shared between the family and the local authority agency. If a full Care Order made by the Juvenile Court is in operation, we emphasize to the parents, if they are present, that they are there because they care but that they no longer have authority. The verbal agreement includes:

1. The reason for admission.
2. On whose authority the decision is made.
3. The changes required before discharge—we emphasize that these may be in the environment, (the parents may become less anxious), or in the adolescent—(the adolescent may be less violent).
4. A commitment not to alter the arrangements, except at another meeting, is made by adults on all sides.

Another meeting within a few weeks is always fixed at the end of any meeting dealing with an adolescent coming into or residing in the Unit, unless they are being discharged. That meeting is usually held within two or three weeks and an additional meeting may be called by either side. The Unit also makes a commitment not to alter the arrangements, that is not to discharge, except through such a meeting. Explanation for admission is usually presented in the following manner: "Julie, you are being admitted here because your parents can no longer cope with your behavior. They need a break because things are unbearable at home for all of them and there is no other place that is willing to have you." In subsequent meetings with the adolescent and parents, they are again confronted with the reason for admission and are given an opportunity to work toward discharge. Although the Unit does have the right and power to discharge an adolescent, we only do so when we are at the end of our tether and can no longer cope. It is a prerogative which we rarely use.

EXAMPLES

Case 1—The Manager's Anxiety

A senior administrator from a Regional Health Authority wrote to the psychiatrist of its Adolescent Unit, saying that the top man of the Health Authority wished the unit to admit a 13-year-old girl who was at present residing in a private institution. The letter was written with some authority and clearly carried with it an expectation of action.

Since the Adolescent Unit in question had not heard about this girl, and the case had not been brought up at a "difficult-to-place" meeting that week in which representatives of the local county authority were present, the Unit could claim to be as puzzled as the Health Authority. The Unit declined to institute admission procedures but reassured the Health Authroity that if the professional person on the county-level was to make a referral, then the case would be discussed.

What seemed to have happened was this. A psychiatrist recommended that this girl's needs could best be obtained in a particular private institution. The county Social Services Department was content with such an arrangement, but asked the local Health Authority if it would share the cost. The Health Authority declined and the local Authority agreed to continue to pay the bill which was not, by its standards, particularly large. However, one of the county doctors asked the original psychiatrist what it was all about. In reply, the psychiatrist sent a letter to the county medical administration; the county doctor sent a copy of that letter to the Regional Health Authority. At least two officers of the Regional Health Authority saw the letter and one sent a copy to their Regional Adolescent

Unit asking for explanation and action. A copy of that correspondence was also sent to the county authority in whose area the Adolescent Unit lay—a different county authority from that one originally invited to contribute to the cost. Four administrative bodies, the institution looking after the child, the original psychiatrist, and the Adolescent Unit which had not been asked directly to admit the child, were all now involved and ready to tread on each other's toes. The anxiety of the administrators would have been removed by the Adolescent Unit's agreement to admit the girl.

Case 2

Jennifer and her divorced parents had not been getting along for many years, but it was only through her disturbance that her parents came together at all. She ran away from whichever one she was staying with, abused them both, had tantrums in the street, and wet herself. They had been through a few professional agencies and always saw the next as the best. Although she was in an adolescent unit for a long time, she was always struggling toward some further understanding of her problems and resisted long-term institutionalization.

Particularly painful issues were being worked through during family therapy when, over a weekend, she was again disturbing the peace of one of the households. Rather than just drive her back to the psychiatric unit from which she was on temporary leave, one of the parents heard of a new agency and brought in the local Authority services.

Apparently alarmed at the plight of the family as seen on that Sunday morning and hostile already toward psychiatric services where were genuinely felt to be unhelpful, the Social Services Department personnel took over parental powers by way of a "Place of Safety" order. The girl was transferred to a Social Services Assessment Center for children.

In the assessment center her behavior became more disturbing. Her screams, violence, and incontinence were unacceptable and their psychiatrist was called in. This psychiatrist was unwilling to transfer the girl to an adult ward and the Adolescent Unit was asked to take her back a few days later. This they did willingly because she was still nominally on their books.

Not surprisingly, the transactions, moves, and interventions of the local authority and other psychiatric unit had its toll on the girl. She became much more difficult for the adolescent unit to handle and she ran away frequently. This, of course, confirmed the Social Service Department's and the parents' impression that the psychiatric unit was incompetent. A few days later the Social Services Department decided to discharge her from the psychiatric unit and place her again in their own Assessment Center.

Yet again, she became too difficult for them to manage in the Assessment Center. This time they called in a third psychiatric institution which was prepared to admit her, lock her up, demand no family therapy, and keep her for a long time.

Meanwhile the senior officials of the Social Services Department had heard about the case. Negative feelings toward the psychiatric services in the region were communicated by a strong letter of complaint addressed neither to the psychiatrists, the psychiatric institutions, the medical administrators of the districts, the area administration, nor the officers of the Regional Health Authority. Rather, the complaint was sent directly to the lay chairman of the Regional Health Authority. It was the cause of considerable consternation and debate among administrators and clinicians. Some complained about being complained about; some complained about the bypass of their authority; some complained about inadequate services; and some complained about being let down. Scapegoating began in earnest.

This state of disarray and claim of incompetence in the local psychiatric service and the offer to lock up the girl were just the impetus to stop the girl's personal growth which was required by the forces for institutionalism. Most of the professionals were seen as incompetent, the family was absolved, and the girl's career as a mental patient was confirmed.

Case 3—Demystifying the Image of the Expert

A social worker asked us to see a family consisting of a divorced mother with three children; she was having problems with her eldest son. He refused to do as she asked and would not go to school. She worried about the company he kept and was anxious that he might start to take drugs. The social worker felt quite strongly that this boy would need to come into the unit since a case conference that had been called the previous week recommended that what this family needed was a resource which would offer them expert family therapy. The social services department did not feel that they could handle the case and asked us, as expert family therapists and experts in dealing with difficult adolescents, to meet with them to discuss the admission of this boy.

We met first with the social worker in his office and discussed his difficulties with the case. He had only recently qualified and had just returned to the department from his training period. He had read much about family therapy in his course but had little chance of putting it into practice. Therefore, he said, he felt inadequate in working with this family. He asked us if he could work with us while the boy was admitted to the unit so that his practical skills would grow and improve. He said that if the boy was admitted it would give him the opportunity to do this and he would be in a better position to help the family. Here was another reason for admission: to increase the social worker's professional skill.

We then met the family and used our usual model of supervision: one joined the social worker interviewing the family and the other sat outside the circle in a supervisor/consultant role. Under our direction, the family started talking with each other seriously. In particular, we supported the mother in telling her son clearly that she would not accept his behavior. The younger children, hitherto silent, appeared to have important contributions to make, and told their mother and their brother what they felt about the battles. The mother did not want admission but said that as a family, they still needed someone to be able to help them talk more with each other. We inquired if this could be provided by the social worker. He confirmed that it could and before we left, the social worker and the family had arranged an appointment to meet. Some months later we received a letter from the social worker telling us that he had seen them for family therapy. He added that his own confidence in the practice of family therapy had increased and he looked forward to working with other families.

Case 4—The Professional Referrer's Anxiety

A 13-year-old girl was referred for admission by a teaching hospital psychiatrist. She was not going to school, was violent toward her cousins, and destructive in the home of the aunt who looked after her on behalf of her parents who were senior members of a foreign diplomatic service. The psychiatrist who referred the case had been asked to take responsibility for her by a colleague who was a senior member of UNICEF. The aunt, who had been looking after the girl for several years and handled all the financial and boarding school arrangements, said she could no longer cope with the girl. A team from the Adolescent Unit went to the hospital to meet the consultant psychiatrist, the psychologist, and the social worker from the Department of Psychological Medicine. The consultant psychiatrist said that he felt responsible for the girl and wished to arrange for her inpatient treatment. Since the aunt could no longer cope, our criteria was met.

The Unit team has differing views on the case. They said that they appreciated how a colleague could *feel* responsible for a patient or client and how the aunt could have authority to make a number of decisions about her, but neither was really *responsible* for the child. In fact, there was nobody legally responsible for the girl in this country. Her symptoms, her pain, her suffering, and her behavior were the responsibility of, if anybody, herself. Where she lived, where she was educated, and where she had treatment were the responsibilities of those in parental authority over her. Those people were her parents, who lived abroad.

The hospital psychiatrist and colleagues looked incredulously at the Unit team as they spelt out the options as they saw them. The psychiatrist could say to the aunt that he could no longer provide treatment for the girl. The aunt could send the girl back to her parents or change the authority position in this country by adopting her, or going to a social services department who had the power and authority to take a "Place of Safety Order." The psychiatrist called the suggestions preposterous and said forcefully that he had promised his colleague, who worked for the United Nations, that he would look after her and see that she got the treatment she needed. "I am not going to let him down," he added.

The important issue here was maintaining the relationship between the United Nations official and the British psychiatrist. That was the reason for the referral. The needs of the adolescent were not really primary.

The psychiatrist and the social worker did see the aunt again and explained the Unit's point of view. They approached the Social Services Department, a "Place of Safety" order was made, the child was admitted to the Unit and, some months later, went back to join her family in her own country.

Case 5

The police physician telephoned the Adolescent Unit in the middle of the night to arrange the admission of David, a "disturbed and probably psychotic" 14-year-old boy who had refused to go home. The physician found it difficult to listen when the Adolescent Unit psychiatrist asked what was wanted by the parents. (They had been to the police station but had left when the boy had refused to go with them or speak to them.) The Unit psychiatrist also asked why the boy could not stay all night in the police station. The police had called in their physician because they thought the child was ill and should not be there. The physician said that he was now in charge of the boy and demanded that he be admitted. The Unit pointed out that this was not so because the boy's parents were in charge, and offered to meet with him and them the next day. The physician felt that this was an inadequate response. In desperation he then used compulsory powers to admit the boy to another hospital.

But the other hospital was no less pleased. Reinforcing the thought of "probably psychotic" by psychological tests, their spokesman (a psychiatrist) again requested transfer to the Adolescent Unit—this time on the grounds of the unsuitability of the adult ward and the "need for further assessment." Again, immediate transfer was refused and a meeting was offered.

"What is the most useful thing you want from us?" asked the hospital psychologist and psychiatrist, carrying reports and notes, as they met up with the community health visitor and Unit team. "The most useful thing would be, if you really do not want this boy in your ward, is for you to say so and to give a date by which he must go." This sentence takes little time to read, but tact and discussion took longer to convey the sense of it. The hospital did not want him to go, but the health visitor appeared to be the "key" worker. She had been involved with the family for many years in helping them cope with a severely handicapped child, now aged 15. She had known the designated patient for a long time, too, and was as surprised as anyone at the turn of events. She saw no objection to bringing up, with the family present, the subject of what one child felt about the other.

Despite preparation, the Unit team was surprised by the appearance of Jane, the 15-year-old sister. She was small, fat, simple-faced, clean, breathless, and blue. Attention to the younger child's (the designated psychiatric patient) symptomatology was deflected into enquiry as to what was happening in the whole family and inevitably some issues centered on Jane. "She doesn't understand" was the response to our statement that we believed everyone understood something and that included Jane. Jane nodded. "A thing which we all find difficult to understand," the Unit psychiatrist continued, "but a thing which affects all of us, is dying. And a thing which is difficult to talk about is that we all die when we stop living; when I look at you, Jane, I wonder just how long you will live."

Jane's mother burst into tears. Her father looked angry. Her brother looked perplexed. Jane smiled. After a few minutes, her father told us that despite several heart operations, there was no improvement in Jane's physical condition. They had always been told that she would not live beyond 15. The Unit psychiatrist broke the taboo: "And you are 15 now, Jane."

The family acknowledged the link between Jane's 15th birthday (non-death) and her brother's disturbed behavior. The health visitor who had not heard of this 15th birthday death prognosis before, agreed to work with them in further discussions about these anxieties.

There still remained the problem of David, and his parents had to make the decision. The hospital staff did say that he had to leave and the compulsory powers had expired. David said he would not go home and the parents were reminded that he was still of an age when parents decided where he would live. Beseechingly, the parents looked to the experts from the Adolescent Unit for advice. The Unit's offer was to admit either of the children for a time if the parents found it too difficult to cope with their anxiety about the rebelliousness of the one or the dying of the other. The parents took both children home and continued to work with the health visitor.

Case 6—Working With the Family's Anxieties

The disturbance in Ian's behavior had been a problem for his family, his school, and the clinic for a number of years. The terrible violence in the marital relationship led to his mother being badly bruised, physical damage to the home, the father leaving, and the mother obtaining a court injunction against his coming back. It also caused a further deterioration in Ian's behavior. His mother, distressed out of her wits, could no longer cope with his increasing demands, his insomnia, his threats, and his twice taking a drink of household ammonia. She asked for him to be taken into the care of the local authority.

The children's home found Ian difficult and finally, impossible. He attacked other children, disrupted the slightest equilibrium in the institution, and lit a fire.

The Adolescent Unit was asked to admit him and we insisted on meeting not only his mother, but also his father. (A high court judge had told us previously that even in cases in which a divorce court has firmly put custody, care, and control in one parents' hands, the other parent must be consulted about hospital admission.)

The meeting took place in the children's home. It was the first meeting between the three members of the family since the father's last episode of drunken violence. He had been living with a number of different friends since then. Ian, dressed in swastika-decorated jeans and denim jacket complained that the problems arose because he was not given a "Saturday job." Heated discussions about these difficulties were interrupted by the Unit therapist suggesting that resources be examined. The children's home confirmed that it was not prepared to have Ian for more than one night. His mother confirmed that she could not cope with him at home again. His father confirmed that he had no where where they could both live. The Unit therapist pointed out that the use Ian made of whatever opportunity (the "Saturday job" market, life at home with his mother, life in the children's home) was his responsibility. The meeting was adjourned for 24 hours, to be reconvened in the Unit itself.

To this second meeting a new idea was brought. Ian might be able to stay with his father's half-brother and common-law wife in East London. No one admitted knowing who had first made the suggestion. The pros and cons of this plan were written on the blackboard from the point of view of each of the participants.

Table 2-1.

Participant	Pro	Con
Ian	East End of London, not a loony bin	Can't be bothered.
Mother	Nothing	Not a good idea. Annie (common-law aunt) at work all day. She would feel just as anxious.
Father	In a family and with a cousin	My half-brother is easy going and his own boy doesn't go to school much.
Social Worker	Nothing	Anxiety about schooling and worried he might get into trouble with the people he associated with.

In discussion it was pointed out that valid comparisons were not among living with this relative, being in the children's home, or being with his mother because none of those was available; the valid comparison was with the thought of what it would be like if Ian lived in the Adolescent Unit. In the Adolescent Unit there would also be anxieties about the company with whom he would associate.

The father, at this point, showed signs of becoming increasingly distressed and said passionately that he was not prepared to have his son here. He would take him out of the Unit if he was admitted. Ian's mother was asked how far she was prepared to go. She and her husband found great difficulty in communicating. She already had an injunction against his coming into the home. Was she prepared to try to stop her husband taking Ian away now to live with his half-brother? She was not. Despite the mother's and social worker's anxieties, Ian was, in effect, taken out of care and went off with his father. He was not re-referred.

Comment

Admission to the unit would have given the satisfaction of activity. We feel better when we do or prescribe something. Here a solution was proposed by a relative, the father. It did not seem to be a "good" solution, but it did not involve separation from all relatives, psychiatric labelling, and association with people known to be disturbed—all of which would have happened if he had been admitted to the adolescent unit.

Case 7—Admission for the Family's Anxieties

The teachers at Tom's school were worried by his repeated questions about homosexuality. He was referred to a local Child Psychiatric Clinic were he began psychotherapy. His parents had started divorce proceedings. Tom lived with his sister and his mother in one fairground caravan; his father lived in another. One night he climbed to the top of a ferris wheel and when retrieved was obviously terrified, moaning that his father's eyes were turning him into a "queer" and that he must die. He was compulsorily admitted to a mental hospital where he was forcibly sedated because he became violent.

The Adolescent Unit was called in but would not see him without his father and his mother both present on the following morning. In the admission meeting at the Unit he moaned in terror at the top of his voice and attacked his father, confirming both his parents' conviction that they could not cope. At the end of this meeting he attacked staff and was sedated to deal with their anxieties.

At the first family meeting Tom, who had not been sedated that day, slipped in and out of apparent stupor. His parents argued and one of his half-brothers, whom we were meeting for the first time, turned fiercely on his father. We decided to reframe Tom's behavior positively. It was a means of bringing various members of the family together and to express pent-up feelings toward their father in a safe way, and to support the mother.

Tom became slightly less difficult in the Unit but took the minimum initiative in any of the meetings. His words and phrases remained stereotyped and his deportment manneristic. His father moved to another site and said he wanted to take Tom home. His mother was opposed to this, but when we asked if she would try to stop it, said she would not. Since one parent no longer wished him to remain in the hospital, he was discharged.

Comment

A psychiatric label could have been put on Tom at admission and remained unchanged at discharge. If this had been the focus, there would have been professional anxiety about discharge with symptoms. He was discharged when the family was prepared to try again.

CONCLUSION—HOSPITAL ADMISSION, THERAPY, GROWTH, AND RESPONSIBILITY

One family, after a meeting with us and some staff from a psychiatric clinic, arranged to continue family therapy there. Some weeks later, the clinic psychiatrist telephoned to say that the parents now wanted to look around our Unit with a view to the admission of their daughter. We had few cases in at the time and it was an interesting family, so we warmed to this proposal and looked in the diary to fix a date. Then we remembered the family's decision the last time we met.

We asked if they had met at the clinic for the family therapy upon which they had then decided. The psychiatrist replied that they had not done so. We and the psychiatrist then thought that we both wished to support the family's earlier decision. The psychiatrist decided to share this thinking with the family and to offer an interview to see them at his office.

At times families do make decision for themselves. However, the family and professional systems together protect the homeostasis which maintains their traditional relationship. This casts the professional into the role of decision maker and the family gives him or her the power to reverse their decisions. It is always difficult for workers and clients not to have professionals (tinkerers) interfere, as if we had the knowledge of what was best. We rush to take responsibility. Often it is said the the "buck" stops with us. Perhaps the "buck" and the idea that we do know what is best are both illusions.

It looks as if hospitals are here to stay and we enjoy working in them. If we accept that we professionals do not always know best, then we may be able to promote a more positive direction for hospital development.

Hospitals are part of the therapeutic movement in our society, so we must look at what we mean by therapy. Although many of the same techniques may be used in both therapy and growth, we think that they are distinct. Therapy may be just a means to an end, but to what end?

We may be content with our lives, our work, and our relationships, but we may also have a view of ideals which includes the wish for ideal health. To approach this ideal and to grow, we involve ourselves in exercise classes, yoga, analysis, dental checkups, and so on. We create a pattern in which we must constantly achieve. Then something may happen which knocks us off this course, such as cancer, coronary thrombosis, divorce, bereavement. We may experience ourselves as being overcome by our own families, becoming depressed or hallucinate. The difference is between being and acting in a way which is acceptable to us and to others around us, or, being and acting in a way which is not. We usually call these coping and not coping. If we are coping, we do not need therapy; but we might want growth. If we are not coping, then we need therapy in order to help us cope. The way in which we are not coping may make it very difficult for us and others to live together. Someone starts to think about separation. We may then go into a different life style. One of these is called "being admitted to a hospital."

Our ideals may be based on any number of philosophical or religious beliefs but most of us accept that it is best to spend as little time as possible in the hospital. In physical medicine there is a strong move to this effect (early ambulation after surgery and early discharge after confinement).

When we enter a hospital, someone else's independently formed notion of our health may be used as a criterion for allowing us to leave. If this criterion is not met, we may not be allowed to leave, even though both we and the people we live with want to start living together again. If the professional's goal is treatment of the illness which he has diagnosed, then dialogue is difficult. If the goal is our reunion with our natural social networks, then dialogue can take place.

This, we maintain, is what therapy is about.

Therapy is different from growth. Therapy has to do with not coping and survival, while growth is coping and our continual search for our ideals. The main aim of therapy should be to help people spend as little time as possible in therapy or in a hospital; and to have them back living with other people as soon as possible. In our society, people usually live in families and therefore the focus of the work should be on family decisions to live together or not.

In an ideal world, Tom from the fairground (Case 7, above) would not have left his home and would have had all his problems instantly removed by some magic solution. We do not live in an ideal world and as practitioners in the mental health field, we are not magicians. We are mechanics. The problems which we mechanics are tackling are those concerning people who are bound together emotionally and who are trying to live together. Tom and his parents were not able to do that. They decided that he must come to us for a time and later decided that he should leave us and go back to live with one of them. It may be argued that the plan was risky. Our position was that that was not our business, but the business of the other state agencies who have responsibility for being society's watchdogs over children; a representative of one of them worked with us in the family therapy. Hospitals are one of the back-ups which those agencies and professional people can use.

Decisions about discharge and admission are often made on the basis of symptomatology and the likelihood of anticipated relief from those symptoms. Such a base is unclear if we define therapy as a means of enabling people to get back to living together. To achieve that aim we have to look at what is going on between the parties concerned—the stresses and strains of the relationships. Those caught up in these relationships should not be deflected from the responsibility of being decision makers. We can probably enjoy our work and do better at it if we release ourselves from the notion that we are responsible for making all the decisions.

REFERENCES

1. Balint, M. "The doctor's therapeutic function." *Lancet* i : 1177–80, 1965.
2. Bernstein, B. "Social class, speech systems and psychotherapy." *British Journal of Sociology* 15 : 54–64, 1964.
3. Bruggen, P.; Byng-Hall, J; and Pitt-Aikens, T. "The reason for admission as a focus of work in an adolescent unit." *British Journal of Psychiatry* 122 (568) March 1973.
4. Byng-Hall, J. and Bruggen, P. "Family admission decisions as a therapeutic tool." *Family Process* 13 (4), 1974.
5. Caplan, G. *Principles of Preventive Psychiatry.* London: Tavistock Publications, 1964.
6. Goffman, E. *Asylums.* New York: Doubleday-Anchor Books, 1961.
7. Jones, D. "Borders health board programme planning. Group-mental health services—interim assessment paper." Society of Clinical Psychiatrists Newsletter, 1977.
8. Jones, M. *Beyond the Therapeutic Community.* New Haven, CN: Yale University Press, 1968.
9. Langsley, D. and Kaplan, D. *The Treatment of Families in Crisis.* New York: Grune and Stratton, 1968.
10. Lear, T.E. and Pitt-Aikens, T. "A shift in emphasis in a psychiatric service." *Lancet* ii : 253–254, 1967.
11. Palazzoli, M.; Boscolo, L.; Ceechin, G.; and Prata, G. *Paradox and Counter Paradox.* New York: Jacob Aronson, 1978.
12. ——— "Hypothesizing—circularity—neutrality: three guidelines for the conductor of the session." *Family Process* 19 (1) March 1980.
13. Roemer, M. "How medical judgement affects hospital admissions." *Modern Hospital* 94, April 1960, p. 112.
14. Scott, R.D. and Ashworth, P.L. "Closure at the first schizophrenic breakdown: a family study." *British Journal of Medical Psychology* 40 : 109–145.
15. Trevelyan, G.M. *English Social History. A Survey of Six Centuries. Chaucer to Queen Victoria.* London: Longmans, 1944.

3

Strategic Family Therapy in the Prevention of Rehospitalization

CLOE MADANES

The current trend in psychiatry toward releasing patients from mental hospitals has exacerbated the problem of how to responsibly plan the disposition and social adjustment of patients after discharge. There is a need to ensure that whatever progress had been achieved in the hospital will be continued and rehospitalization will be prevented. If the discharge is not carefully planned, rapid rehospitalization is the consequence.

This chapter presents a method of therapy designed to prevent recurrent hospitalizations of adolescents and young adults with such diverse diagnoses as schizophrenia, manic-depressive psychosis, alcoholism, and drug addiction. This method of tertiary prevention is particularly indicated for severely disturbed young people who: (1) have been hospitalized one or several times, (2) remain in the hospital for continuous periods of less than one year and, (3) still maintain family ties.

When adolescents or young adults indulge in disturbing behavior —such as aggressive or self-destructive acts, abuse of drugs or alcohol, bizarre communication, extreme apathy or depression —family and community often respond by arranging that the youth be admitted into a psychiatric hospital. After the young person is pulled out of his social situation, family, community, and youth eventually calm down and the young person comes out of the hospital. If he begins to cause trouble again and is rehospitalized, the chances are that there will be more than one rehospitalization and that he has begun a career as a mental patient. The goal of the therapist in these cases is to prevent this cycle of hospitalization and rehospitalization.

Behaviors that precipitate hospitalizations can be seen as the expression of internal conflicts in the youth. However, if one asks what are the consequences of these behaviors not only for the youth but for his family, a different perspective emerges. The disruptive acts and the resulting hospitalizations keep a youth and his parents involved with each other in a special way. The young person is a constant source of concern for the parents, and the parents are the only significant relationship that the youth has, except for professional helpers. The disturbing acts, the repeated failures, and the trouble the young person causes become the main theme in the parents' lives. No matter what the personal problems of a parent (social, financial, health, or marital), they will be set aside as less important in contrast to the tragedy of the youth's life. Parents will neglect their own difficulties and overcome their own deficiencies, holding themselves together in order to help the youth. In this sense, the young person's disturbing behavior is helpful to the parents. This helpfulness, however, is unfortunate in that it merely distracts the parents from their problems and in this way prevents them from finding a solution. The disturbing behavior of the youth may take the form of passive threats of going crazy or of taking drugs, harming himself, or doing physical violence against the parents. Whatever the nature of the disturbing behavior, the parents become too incapacitated to help the youth because they are afraid of causing him harm or afraid that he will harm them. If the youth behaves normally he loses the power that the threats of extreme behavior give him over his parents. The youth is incompetent, defective, and dependent on the parents for protection, food, shelter, and money. The parents are in a superior position and provide and take care of him; yet simultaneously they are dominated by the youth because of his helplessness or threats of dangerous behavior. In this sense, two incongruous hierarchies are simultaneously defined in the family.

It is possible that the youth's disruptive behavior originally had a helpful function for the parents. However, the consequence of this helplessness is an increase in the youth's power over them. When the parents try to restore their position in the hierarchy by resorting to agents of social control (the police or the mental hospital), the youth is institutionalized and consequently, behaves more helplessly and with less control. Paradoxically, this gives him more power over the parents because they must focus more on him in their attempts to help him. Yet their helpfulness defines the youth as even more helpless (or out of control) and contributes to the power that can be derived from such helplessness. In this way, a system of interaction can be established that perpetuates itself over time, particularly if there is a certain stigma attached to the situation of the youth and if society (through social agencies) contributes to maintaining it. Whether the youth's behavior originally had a protective function, whether it was meant to prevent a separation between the parents, or whether it was only related to a bid for power is quite irrelevant. The issue is that to solve the problem, the hierarchy must be restored to one in which the youth does not dominate the parents through helplessness and abuse [3,4].

THE STAGES OF THERAPY

The therapist's problem is how to get the young person to give up the disturbed behavior that is the basis of his power. This cannot be done directly by the therapist. The youth's power is over his parents and it is the parents who must take it away from him.

The therapy of these difficult cases can be thought of in stages. In the first stage, the therapist lays down his agenda: to prevent further hospitalizations and to return the youth to a normal life involved in work or school. Parents are asked to make decisions about the youth and to take charge of his life. In the second stage, the parents react to the therapist's requests by attempting to avoid taking power over the youth and the therapist must respond with counteracting maneuvers to keep the parents in charge. In the third stage, there usually is a crisis in which the youth escalates his disturbing behavior. There may be suicide threats and hospitalization is considered. The therapist must offer alternatives to hospitalization and support the family through the crisis. In the fourth stage, the youth develops normal activities and gradually disengages from the therapist and the parents.

These four stages are discussed and a case illustrating the opening or first stage of therapy is presented below.

The First Stage of Therapy

Before the first interview the therapist must arrange to be in charge of the case so that he can state this fact clearly to the family. This includes responsibility for medication, discharge, and rehospitalization. If the therapist is not a physician, he must arrange for a physician to back him up in these decisions. If the therapy starts before release from the hospital, the discharge should be contingent upon the plans that the parents make for the youth. This gives power to both the therapist and the parents since the young person's release from the hospital is then dependent on them [1].

Parents must define their expectations for the youth when he comes out of the hospital in terms of where he will be living and what he will be doing. It is best if the youth comes home to his parents so that it is possible to reorganize the hierarchy in such a way that will enable the youth to ultimately be able to leave his parents successfully. The family should be told that at this time the young person needs the parents' guidance.

The parents must talk to each other and reach agreement on expectations and rules for the young person. These include issues of work or school, behavior in and out of the home, scheduling of activities, chores, the use of drugs or alcohol, and indulgence in violence. The rules must be as specific and practical as possible. Parents must also set consequences in case their rules are disobeyed. Depending upon the severity of the problem, the consequences can vary from mild to extreme. Coming home late may entail the loss of an allowance but use of drugs may necessitate house arrest. The young person should not be allowed to intervene while the parents are setting rules and consequences.

After the parents have agreed on rules and consequences, they must communicate them to the youth even though he has been present during the discussion. It is best if they can obtain some commitment from him that he will obey the rules. The young person will usually object and demand more independence. The therapist must then state that the youth's irresponsible or disturbing behavior has led to his hospitalization and that the parents must give him the guidance that he needs until he shows that he behaves like a responsible person.

If the youth's problem is apathy, the parents must set rules that will ensure activity and prescribe consequences if these rules are not followed. Often deadlines must be set for certain types of activities, such as finding a job, and there must be consequences if deadlines are not met. Only after the youth has begun to be active will he abandon his apathy.

If in the past the youth has indulged in violence, bizarre behavior, drugs, or alcohol, a recurrence must be anticipated and plans for future difficulties must be made. These acts must be defined as misbehavior and not mental illness or addiction, so that they are in the realm of expertise of parents, not professionals. Severe consequences should be planned ahead of time to discourage the youth from behaving in extreme ways. The parents must agree on a plan to handle the next episode of extreme behavior if it occurs. It is best to encourage the parents to use their own resources to control the youth even if this involves restraining him physically and requesting the help of relatives or neighbors. The therapist should make clear to the parents that hospitalization should not be part of their plan [3].

The young person should only be discharged from the hospital when the therapist is satisfied that there are clear rules about how he is to behave at home, consequences if he does not obey these rules, and a plan for what he is to do with regard to school or work [2].

The Second Stage of Therapy

Over the next several weeks, the therapist should review with the parents whether the rules have been followed, and if not, whether the consequences were applied. New rules and consequences must be set. The therapist must struggle to maintain the parents in a superior position as the young person puts them to the test. In this stage, not only the youth but also the parents respond negatively to the therapist's attempts to correct the hierarchy.

The parents typically avoid defining the family hierarchy as one in which they have power over their offspring. They do so for the following reasons: (1) the youth is more powerful than they, (2) society has intervened to take power away from them, (3) they are afraid to do the wrong thing and harm the youth, (4) they are afraid that they are to blame and wish to do no more harm, or (5) they are afraid to lose their child. Parents can decline to exert authority over the youth in various ways and the therapist must respond with counteracting maneuvers to keep the parents in charge.

Giving Authority to Experts

Parents might invoke the authority of experts by saying, for example, that the therapist or the chief of the ward should make the decisions concerning the disturbed young person. The therapist must transfer the power back to the parents by relabeling the young person's problem so that it is in the domain of the parents rather than medical or psychiatric experts. Even the most bizarre behavior can be redefined as discourteous communication, since others cannot understand it or find it upsetting. Then the youth can be asked to communicate more clearly and politely. Apathetic behavior can be reformulated as laziness so that the parents can be moved to demand regular activity. In drug addiction, the therapist can emphasize that it is not a physiological dependence that cannot be overcome:

If the youth is on medication, the therapist must state that he will reduce the medication and discontinue it altogether as soon as possible. As long as the young person is on medication, he is a mental patient under the care of a psychiatrist instead of a misbehaving son whose behavior must be changed by the parents. A similar issue often comes up with the question of whether the youth should be on disability benefits. If the therapist accepts this idea, he is defining the youth as a mental patient incapable of making a living like a normal person [3].

Parents often give authority to experts by expressing ignorance of what should be done. The therapist should persuade them that they must tackle the difficult task of giving clear guidance to their son so that his confusion about his life will be cleared. It would be a mistake to believe that the parents are actually ignorant; their expressions of ignorance serve the purpose of arranging for others to take charge.

The therapist should not set rules and consequences for the youth but should require instead that the parents do so.

Since the therapist wants a hierarchy with the parents in a superior position, he cannot put them down in front of the offspring by taking over a parental position. Only if the therapist feels strongly that the parents' decisions about the young person are seriously wrong should he undermine their authority by suggesting an alternative, and then this should be done with the parents alone, not in the presence of the youth [4].

Giving Authority to the Problem Youth

Sometimes the parents will offer the authority to the problem youth, turning to him for decisions and advice. The therapist must emphasize that it is necessary for the parents to provide the guidance, and that only when the youth is behaving properly will he be in charge of himself. In the meantime, the young person should live in a predictable world, with knowledge of his obligations and privileges.

At the beginning of therapy, chances are that every time the parents begin to talk to each other, the young person will call their attention to himself by behaving in bizarre or disruptive ways. This disturbing behavior will interrupt the possibility of an alliance between the parents that would give them power over their offspring. The therapist must quiet the youth or ask the parents to do so, so that they can proceed to talk to each other and reach agreements.

When a family with a severely disturbed youth comes to therapy there is a split between the parents. This split might be the result and not the cause of the pain, bickering, accusations, and guilt that inevitably surround this kind of problem. The disturbing behavior of the youth perpetuates the problem and, although it often prevents a separation and divorce since the parents must stay together to take care of their defective offspring, it also prevents the parents from coming together in joy and good feeling. It may be that the youth behaves disruptively both when the parents are too far apart (i.e., if they threaten to separate or divorce) or too close together (when there is agreement between them), because in both cases the young person loses power over the parents.

Sometimes parents will give authority to the problem youth by threatening to expel him from the family home as the only consequence for his misbehavior that is available to them. In this way the parents threaten to renounce their position in the hierarchy as parents who are responsible and in charge of their offspring. This threat must be blocked. The therapist must emphasize that separation from parents must happen when the youth is behaving competently and when they know and approve of where and how he is going to live. Expulsion is a threat that is rarely carried out and, in any case, the chances are that soon parents and youth will be involved with each other again and the cycle will be repeated.

Sometimes parents want to expel the youth from the house, put him in jail, hospitalize him, or enforce other extreme consequences. In these situations, it is important for the therapist to distinguish between firmness and rejection. Parents should be encouraged to be firm but kind. Rejection of the youth should be discouraged because it escalates the confrontation between parents and youth and increases a malevolent use of power rather than the benevolent guidance that the therapist seeks for the parents to establish.

Sometimes the young person makes a powerful bid for power by threatening suicide. In this case, there are two possibilities for the therapist: (1) to hospitalize the youth which means that the therapy will have to start all over again after discharge, or (2) to put the parents in charge of the youth and help them organize to prevent suicide. This is a difficult decision to make and should depend on: (1) the seriousness of the suicide threat, (2) whether there have been previous attempts, (3) an evaluation of the parents' investment in keeping their offspring alive, and (4) their ability to work together to prevent the suicide. If the therapist decides against hospitalization, he should carefully help the parents organize to prevent the suicide. They should institute a 24-hour watch so that the youth is never alone. This usually tests the limits of the parents' patience and helps them to take a more firm position in demanding normal behavior from the youth.

Defining Themselves as Inadequate

If a parent behaves in disruptive ways, for example, by crying, screaming, or threatening violence in a session, it is better for the therapist to deal with this behavior without the young person in the room. The therapist should emphasize all that the parent has done in the past, his kindness and dedication, and ask little of the parent—e.g., one more week of patience until there is a plan for what the young person will do with his life.

Disqualifying the Other Parent

Sometimes one parent will define the other as incompetent and disqualified for taking charge of the offspring. There are a series of tactics that the therapist can use to counteract this maneuver that prevents the parents from allying to guide the youth. He can say that this is a new situation where they will be working with the therapist who will help them to get together and jointly handle the situation. Whatever happened in the past is irrelevant. The therapist can reformulate the disqualified parent's behavior so that weakness becomes sensitivity, harshness or brutality becomes desperate attempts to provide guidance to a disoriented youth, depression and emotional instability become dedicated concern. Once the incompetence has been reformulated it can be discarded.

Disqualifying the Therapist

Putting down the therapist is another way that parents avoid being in charge, since they need not follow the directives of a therapist they do not respect. Parents may suggest that the therapist is incompetent and does not know what he is doing by quoting the opinion of other professionals whose position differs. The therapist can reply by suggesting the parents try his approach for a limited period of time, for example, three months. By this time they will understand the modality of therapy and can decide whether to continue. Also, after three months the young person might be on his feet and the therapy might no longer be necessary.

The Third Stage of Therapy

Changes in other relationships in the family can be expected to occur when there have been changes in the hierarchical relationship between parents and child:

Sometimes a sibling will make an alliance with the disturbed youth to support him against the parents and to reinstate an organization in which the parents are not in a superior position. Often a grandparent or other relative will ally with the youth, and there will be the danger that two incongruous hierarchies will again be defined in the family. In fact, the more disturbed the young person is at the beginning of therapy, the greater the possibility that as soon as the hierarchical organization of the nuclear family begins to become congruent, the therapist will discover involvements with extended kin that define a hierarchy that is incongruent with one in which the parents are in a superior position. The therapist must block these coalitions and shift the relative from allying with the disturbed youth to supporting the parents in their efforts to guide him. In order to do this, it is often necessary to have the relatives present at one or more sessions [3]

As the parents take charge, the young person may escalate his disturbing behavior to the point of becoming extremely bizarre or threatening and often there is a crisis situation. Parents then usually consider hospitalization. This would be an error since it goes against the efforts to put the parents in charge of the problem by giving authority to the hospital staff and going against the goal of the therapy which is to keep the young person out of the hospital. The therapist can suggest alternative consequences to the youth's extreme behavior, such as no money, no food, or confining him to his room. It can be suggested that the parents call the police if there are threats of violence. If hospitalization occurs, the therapy must start all over again, following the same steps that were carried out previously.

It is usually at this stage that important issues about money become explicit. If the family is poor, there is the issue of disability. If the young person begins to live normally, he and the family run the risk of losing these payments that sometimes help support several family members. In this instance, it is best for the therapist to insist that the youth can make an honest living like other people and refuse to collaborate in arranging for disability payments. If the family is in a good financial position, often there are quarrels about inheritances with implications that the mentally ill family member will have easier access to funds. Sometimes trusts have been explicitly established to pay out funds to the disturbed youth only if he is under psychiatric care. The therapist must discover and block these possibilities or the promise of a financially secure future may be more attractive to the youth and the family than the focus on work and school offered by the therapist.

The Fourth Stage of Therapy

As soon as the youth becomes regularly involved in a normal way of life centering on work or school, the therapist can begin to meet with him individually to plan tasks related to his activities and social relations. There should also be meetings with youth and parents to plan for possible eventualities and ultimate goals, such as the young person's social and financial independence from the parents. As various goals are met, the sessions are reduced in frequency until the therapy is discontinued.

SPECIAL CIRCUMSTANCES

The emphasis of this chapter has been on families consisting of two parents and a disturbed youth. However, a variety of family structures and circumstances are possible. For example, there may be a single parent or the young person may be married and the young spouse must then be considered in the therapy. Also, questions of organicity may complicate and confuse the goals of the therapy. These issues will be addressed here briefly.

In cases in which there is a single parent, it is best to try to include in the therapy a significant adult relative who is involved with the young person as a parental surrogate. This can be, for example, a grandmother, aunt, or parent's boyfriend. He or she should be the most significant parental person in the youth's life, apart from the parent. The therapy will proceed in the same way. If there is no relative to involve, the treatment plan will still be the same but the therapist will have to use himself more in the discussion with the single parent and will have to encourage and support the parent in making the decisions that are necessary during the course of therapy.

A word of caution is necessary about those cases in which the disturbed young person is married. It is a mistake to put the spouse in charge in the manner that has been described here for the parents. For parents to have extreme control of their children is appropriate in our culture during certain developmental stages. When things go wrong, it is proper to go back to those stages and put the parents in charge again until the youth accomplishes more mature behavior. It is not acceptable, however, in our culture, for one spouse to have extreme control of the other. To arrange this leads to an inappropriate hierarchy that may result in violent or suicidal behavior. Also, often the spouse who goes into a mental hospital is making a desperate attempt to escape an unfortunate marriage. To come out of the hospital under the control of the other spouse is not a helpful solution. It is better for the disturbed spouse to come home to his parents or to some other kind of living arrangement first, and then to slowly move back with the spouse or decide to separate. These steps should be carefully planned during the course of therapy.

Certain types of pathology that typically occur in young people (schizophrenia, manic-depression, etc.) may have an organic basis. The question, however, is irrelevant to therapy. Even if there is evidence for an organic or genetic base, the therapist must still organize a life as normal as possible for the young person, keeping him out of the mental hospital, and using medications only sparingly and with caution. In fact, this approach has been used in cases that were clearly organic, such as with the mentally retarded, the victims of tardive dyskinesia, epileptics, and young people with irreversible neurological damage from PCP use.

SUMMARY OF THE THERAPEUTIC STRATEGY

When a severely disturbed youth is coming out of a mental hospital, the therapist is typically presented with a situation in which there is an incongruity in the family hierarchy. The young person is a helpless patient who needs the parents to take care of him. At the same time, the youth maintains superior power over the parents by threatening them with his behavior and holding them together by providing them with crises that distract them from their problems but also prevent them from resolving their difficulties. If the youth abandons this behavior he loses his power over the parents. The therapist's goal is to get the young person to abandon the disturbed behavior that is the basis of his power, which means the parents must be able to gain control over the youth. They must set expectations and rules and establish consequences if these are not followed. The therapist must influence the parents to establish rules and consequences that are stringent enough to build up their power.

When the young person loses his power over the parents he will begin to behave normally. At this point, the therapist must help the parents to deal with their own difficulties without involving the youth. This task will be made easier because of the experience they acquired by expecting appropriate behavior and negotiating agreements with each other in the process of setting rules and enforcing consequences for the young person.

CASE ILLUSTRATION: A VIOLENT YOUTH

A transcript of a first interview will illustrate the approach to the opening stage of therapy.

Ralph is a 17-year old male who was hospitalized in a psychiatric ward because of outbursts of violent behavior. He also drank alcohol excessively. During the last year of high school he dropped out and stayed at home. His temper tantrums increased, as did his drinking. His violence consisted of breaking windows, punching holes in walls, and generally being destructive around the house. He had destroyed the door of his bedroom with his fists. He had also thrown heavy objects at his mother.

The young man had been adopted at six months of age and was aware and pleased about that. He is their only child. As a child he was considered hyperkinetic and had temper tantrums. Ritalin was tried without results. The father is a tall, thin man in his late fifties. The mother, a plump woman, had earned money on the side in illegal gambling. She earned more than the father who lost his job on the police force because of the mother's illegal gambling.

Just before this hospitalization the young man had had four interviews with a psychiatrist who gave him Dilantin; this was said to have had no effect. In the hospital he was also given Dilantin since his EEG showed a non-specific abnormality. He had one violent episode in a family session on the ward about the purchase of a coat. After three weeks in the hospital, which included family interviews on the ward, he was being considered for discharge. He was assigned to Dr. Hidalgo for outpatient therapy. She was part of a group of trainees being given "live" supervision at the Institute of Psychiatry and Human Behavior, University of Maryland Hospital. There was an extensive discussion between supervisor and therapist before the family was seen. It was important that they be in agreement on certain problems and that the supervisor suggest a plan for the interview. Their meeting resulted in the following plan.

1. The supervisor and therapist had to make a decision on how to approach the case when there was both a possible medical problem and a family problem. The supervisor recommended that the therapist approach the family with the view that the problem had to do with organization; the parents had to take charge and require that their son behave appropriately for his age. At the same time, there must be a discussion of the neurological and physiological aspect of the problem, as shown by the EEG findings. It was planned to tell the family simply that there was a possible neurological problem and that Dilantin would be given for that. However, the abnormality should be considered temporary and the medication would eventually be discontinued. They would be told that this medical problem often ends with adolescence so that they would not consider him a handicapped person. No connection would be made between the violent behavior and the possible neurological problem. If the parents suggested that there was a connection or questioned the therapist about this possibility, she would say that the son was responsible for his acts; the neurological problem could not be used as an excuse for his behavior.

2. It would be emphasized to the family that the therapist would be the only doctor to prescribe any medication and to decide on discharge from the hospital.

3. The therapist would emphasize that this was to be the last hospitalization. The young man's violence had to be controlled by the parents.

4. The young man was to stop drinking alcohol. The incompatibility between alcohol and Dilantin would be explained so that there would be a medical reason for him to stop.

5. The therapist would begin the interview by stating that discharge would be determined by what decisions were made in that session. The son wanted to get out of the hospital and the parents wanted him out, partly because their insurance did not cover the full cost. Arranging this emphasis gave the therapist power at the start.

6. The parents would discuss and agree on expectations and rules for the young man's behavior and there would be a special focus upon the period immediately after discharge. These rules would concern the issue of what was he going to do with his life and would require either return to school or work. Besides these goals, the therapist's agenda would include behavior outside and inside the home, and rules about drinking and violence. The rules set by the parents should be as specific and practical as possible. It was expected that the parents might bring up seemingly trivial matters, such as whether the son should take out the garbage—a typical issue in many families. The therapist would support the parents' authority and help them to agree on rules for the son. It is important to deal with these issues because, although apparently banal, they are often the context in which symptomatic behavior occurs; in this particular case, violence. However, the therapist would first make her agenda clear to the family. Other issues that the family might bring up would be dealt with only after the family had had some time to experience the therapy.

7. Agreement between the parents would be actively supported and any exploration of marital difficulties would be discouraged. It was assumed that the parents were in serious difficulty with each other, probably due in part to the fact that the father had lost his job because of the mother's illegal gambling. It was also assumed that the parents were quite distant from each other and had little conversation. The symptoms provided an issue that the parents had in common, something that they could talk about that brought some excitement into their lives, particularly now that the mother's illegal gambling, which had probably provided a great deal of excitement, had apparently ended. The therapist, however, would avoid any focus on their problems as a couple and would only deal with them as parents. It was hoped that if they could succeed at being parents to their son, their marital situation would improve. The hypothesis, therefore, was that the parents' usual subject of conversation at home was the son's misbehavior about which they disagreed and which they handled incompetently. In the therapy, they would still be talking about the son but they would reach agreement, take responsibility for him, and deal with his behavior competently.

8. While the parents discussed their expectations and rules, the son would listen and any interventions from him would be discouraged. The therapist would quiet him by saying that he would get a chance to speak later.

9. It was expected that the son would bring up his need for the independence that is appropriate for his age. The therapist would answer that the son's irresponsible behavior had landed him in the mental hospital and his parents had to give him the guidance he needed until he showed that he behaved like a responsible person.

10. The violence would be brought up and the parents would make plans for another possible episode of violence. They would agree on ways of restraining the son physically and on consequences for the son if such an episode occurred again. The possibility of another hospitalization for violent behavior would be blocked by the therapist who would state that the police route was more appropriate for this type of behavior than the hospital.

11. The parents would explain their expectations and rules to the son and would obtain a commitment from him to obey them.

12. The therapist would be optimistic and explain that if the parents cooperated the therapy would not take long.

Following is an edited transcript of the first interview.

Goals

Hidalgo: I called this meeting today because I was told by Dr. X that he has decided to discharge Ralph this Friday. (This interview is on Wednesday.) This meeting is very important because we have to be sure that this is the first and the last hospitalization. We have to plan his adjustment after his discharge in the community and in the family. I am in charge of the case right now, so it all depends on how we agree. If we don't achieve an agreement, Ralph will not be discharged this week. (To Ralph) I am also in charge of your medication from now on.

Ralph: Oh, you are?

Hidalgo: Yes.

Ralph: OK

In a brief opening statement the therapist has dealt with the basic issues of the interview: (1) the goal of the session is to determine whether to discharge Ralph that week; (2) the goal of the therapy is to prevent rehospitalization; (3) the therapist is in charge of medication and discharge. She has also stated that the interview is a planning session for his discharge into the community.

Expectations

Hidalgo: So I guess that we better start planning the first week at home. How is it going to be? What are your expectations for him?

Mother: Well, uh—you want to talk first, dear?

Father: Well, I've been on him for not cleaning up around his room enough. I know they've been training him at the hospital to pick up. He has to do it at home, too.

The father has gone at once to a too specific and rather banal issue, considering the magnitude of the young man's problems. Cleaning his room seems one of the least important among the issues at risk that weekend. The therapist must change what the father has offered but without disqualifying and putting him down, since she wishes to support his authority in the hierarchy. She takes what he says and accepts it by going even further, saying: "let's be a little more specific . . ." As they plan, the son behaves in a typical way by objecting to the hierarchy being established and by suggesting he do his own planning.

Hidalgo: Let's be a little bit more specific so Ralph won't have any doubts about it and doesn't start doing whatever he wants to do when he gets home. Let's start planning for Friday. What is he supposed to do Friday, Saturday, and Sunday?

Father: That's a lot of thinking.

Mother: Well, I—alright.

Ralph: You don't really do my thinking for me on the weekends.

Mother: Well, I expect him just to be a decent human being. Just to give us the courtesy, the same as we would give him the courtesy. Isn't that right?

Father: Right.

Mother: And—he's already planning a party Saturday night. This is in agreement with us because this is what he wanted to do

Ralph: This was decided three weeks ago. Matter of fact, it was supposed to be for my birthday, but then, all this hospitalization and stuff came up. And then I couldn't have it.

Mother: Yeah. It's sort of a belated thing because things were disrupted around his birthday.

Hidalgo: Well, it seems to me that after being in the hospital, it's nice to have some fun.

Mother: Uh huh.

Hidalgo: But—I know that you were going to school. And you were doing well in school. The two of you are expecting him to continue in school?

School

The therapist supports the idea of the party but then she immediately changes the subject to the serious issue of school. It is her style to say something pleasant about their discussion and then bring up a new, difficult problem.

Mother: Oh, absolutely. Absolutely.

Hidalgo: When are you expecting him to go back to school?

Mother: Monday.

Hidalgo: Monday?

Mother: That's right.

Hidalgo: O.K. How many credits are you expecting him to take?

Mother: Well, he started school in September, and he is just these three weeks out. So his schedule will continue when he goes back to school.

Hidalgo: What about if he doesn't? What would you do?

Mother: What will he do?

Hidalgo: The two of you will do?

Mother: Well, I would be very unhappy about it.

Father: He'd have to go to work. He wouldn't be able to sit around the house. We've already had that understanding.

Hidalgo: Who has that understanding?

Father: Him and I. That if he didn't go to school he's not going to lay in bed till 10 or 11 o'clock in the mornings. He's going to go to work.

Ralph: Like last year. (At a gesture from the therapist) Was I interrupting?

Hidalgo: Yes, a little bit.

Father: And I told him that work was hard to find. Men that actually have experience have a hard time finding work today. It would be better if he got through school, that would be better for him.

Hidalgo: Why don't you tell him that?

Father: Well, I could repeat myself, because I have told him that so many times.

Hidalgo: Maybe you have told him that many times, Yeah, one more time I'm sure would be useful.

Father: One more time — go to school. It's so hard for men to get jobs, that down at my job we actually have a college man who was a school teacher, from Loyola College, as a sales manager. That shows you how tight jobs are.

Ralph: You know, Dad, I have planned to go into the Navy and I cannot go in without high school, so that's why I want to go.

Father: Without high school and good grades.

Hidalgo: So you're saying if he doesn't go back to school and he decides to sit in the house and do nothing, he will have to work? You will send him to work?

Father: (Pause) Yes, I think I would.
Hidalgo: (To mother) Do you agree with that?

Here is the first time the therapist specifically asks for parental agreement; this is a major focus throughout the interview. She had already covered most of the major issues in the first ten minutes.

Mother: Absolutely, absolutely.
Hidalgo: And the two of you have talked about that already?
Mother: Absolutely. I will not tolerate him staying around the house and just doing nothing. We've discussed this before. As a matter of fact, last year when he decided to quit school/he quit school last year at one point. I told him I positively would not tolerate that. He either has to make a decision —either make a decision to go back to school, or he has to go to work.
Father: And he made a strong decision, because his best friend up the street quit around the same time, and he decided not to go back to school. And all he is doing is laying around. I know he's bored to death.
Mother: Well, Ralph even said that himself.
Hidalgo: Well, if not, you also have a chance to remind him about what happened.
Mother: Yeah.
Hidalgo: And you too.
Father: Yes.
Hidalgo: So school is a clear issue.
Mother: I'm pretty sure it is, yes. That's up to him.
Hidalgo: Even for Ralph, it's a clear issue?
Ralph: It is, definitely.

The Weekend

Hidalgo: OK. Let's go back to the first few days of discharge, Friday, Saturday, and Sunday. What are you expecting him to do? At what time are you expecting him to be in the house? For instance, for dinner. What kind of meals are you expecting him to participate in with the two of you? When is he allowed to go out? What is he supposed to do while he's out? That's very important to me. Let's talk about that.
Mother: I would like for him to be home Friday evenings for dinner. If he wants to go out for a couple of hours, but I don't expect him —

Hidalgo:	(Interrupting) You know, it seems to me that you have your own ideas. I'm wondering if you have had the chance to plan with your husband.
Mother:	No. No, I didn't.

The therapist can expect difficulty in getting the mother and father to talk to each other. She tries a direct request.

Hidalgo:	Why don't you go ahead and do it right here?
Mother:	Well —
Father:	(To son) Well, the room has to be —all your pictures have to come off the wall because the room is going to be painted. That's definite.
Ralph:	I'll do that during the day.
Father:	Yeah.
Ralph:	Friday, during the day.

The father has not addressed the issue or talked to his wife. The therapist wants the parents to talk together, and the son, who is sitting between the parents, to move out from between them. She asks him to move, using the excuse that they cannot see each other easily when they talk.

Hidalgo:	You know, I'm seeing the two of you a little bit like — trying to reach a — and how can you look at each other. Ralph, would you like to move? It seems your father and your mother want to discuss how they're going to plan what are their expectations.
Ralph:	For me?
Hidalgo:	Yeah.
Mother:	You move over there and let your Dad sit there.
Ralph:	(Moving out from between them, father takes the chair next to mother.) Plan for me? I usually plan for myself.
Hidalgo:	Did you say plan for yourself? But that's what got you in trouble, Ralph. That's what made you come to the hospital and you ended up in here —because you usually plan for yourself. Right now it's your parents chance to help you out.

It was expected that the son would question the hierarchy at some point in the interview and say he should decide for himself. Therefore the therapist was prepared in advance to make this intervention and so give authority to the parents.

Mother: (Turns to father) Well, Henry, I said I'd like for him to have dinner at home Friday. I'm going to plan a nice dinner. And for him to be around a couple of hours. If he wants to go out a decent hour, like 12:30, I think that should be a decent time to come in, because he's planning a party Saturday.

Father: Sounds good to me. It's alright with me.

There is a discussion of the time the son should come in and they decide on 12:30. Since the therapist does not want ambiguities in a rule, an exact time for the son to come home is important.

Hidalgo: Is that agreeable with you?

Father: Yes, it's agreeable to me.

Hidalgo: OK. What will happen if he doesn't show up by 12:30?

Mother: He won't have the car the next night. That's usually what happens.

Father: That's the usual punishment. Well, if he violates and he gets in late, much later, so then the next night he won't be able to have the car.

Mother: If he does violate this time, or any time he's out, he doesn't get the car the next night.

Father: (To son) I don't like that word "violations." You'd think you're on probation with us. Sorry, Ralph, I don't want you to think that way, OK?

Mother: Well, I do. I want him to think that way.

Drinking

Hidalgo: Let's see. Any ideas of what he is supposed to do and what he's not supposed to do while he's out of the house?

Mother: Well, not to get into trouble.

Hidalgo: What do you mean to not get into trouble? Be more specific.

Mother: Just getting into any fights, or any drinking, real heavy drinking, and things like that.

Hidalgo: Heavy drinking. We have to go into the subject of drinking.

Mother: That's right.

Hidalgo: In a few minutes. (Pause) What are you expecting him to do while he's out of the house. Let me put it this way: What is it that you don't want him to do at all when he's out of the house?

Father: I don't want him to overindulge in beer, or to get in fights, that's all. I don't have to worry about anything else, I mean he don't get into any other kind of trouble.

At this halfway point in the interview, the family is discussing violence and drinking, the primary issues. The discussion is in a context where the therapist has clarified her position in relation to the family and the hospital staff. She has made clear to the family what the therapy is about and has put the parents in charge. When the symptoms come up, it is with a clear idea of what the parents are expected to say about them. Often if symptoms are discussed at the beginning of a first interview, the family members go into their feelings about the symptoms or the origins of them, what happened in childhood, or what uncle had the same symptoms, and so on. They do this because the family is fishing to find out what the therapy approach is and what they should say. However, in this interview there is none of that fishing. The family knows perfectly well the approach of the therapist and what is expected of them. Therefore, they say "no drinking and fighting."

The therapist uses the issue of alcohol to give an explanation of the EEG, the illness, the medication, and to set her own rules about drinking.

Hidalgo: Alcohol is a problem for you, Ralph. You are taking Dilantin because there are some questions about your EEG. I know that people your age can have an EEG abnormality and that doesn't mean that they have a serious problem, or any problem at all. Maybe when they reach the age of 19 or 20, the EEG will turn normal and there is nothing. But there is a question about your EEG—that there are some abnormal dysrhythmia there and that is why you are on Dilantin. While you are on Dilantin you can't drink, absolutely.

Mother: Well, that's—

Hidalgo: There are people who can drink and nothing happens, but there are people that can't. And right now, you are one of those. And you can't drink and you have to accept the fact. So no alcohol.

Mother: (To son) This showed up Friday night, didn't it? Just what the doctor is saying—is exactly what happened Friday night.

Ralph: It wasn't my fault.

Mother: That's beside the point. The point is that you shouldn't have been drinking in the beginning. Isn't that right?

Ralph: I didn't drink that much.

Mother: Well, you were told by the doctor not to drink. That it would affect you, and it did, I think, to a point where you wound up getting into an argument. Don't you think that's what happened?

Ralph: I would have gotten into an argument if I was straight or not.

Father: Might have been provoked, but—

Ralph: (Interrupting) It was provoked. Someone hits me in the jaw, I'm not going to walk away.

Mother:	What I feel —
Father:	Your mother is saying that she thinks if you hadn't had any drinks at all, along with taking that medicine, you wouldn't have been provoked.
Ralph:	I'd have still beat him up.
Father:	Yeah?
Mother:	This is what I was saying, because Friday night when he went out he got into a fight with someone. He said it wasn't his fault, well, I'm inclined to believe him. But I'm saying that he shouldn't have been drinking in the beginning, because of the Dilantin. This is what I mean.
Hidalgo:	I also think that you should not drink. So this is something that also has to be in the expectations — not to drink.
Ralph:	I have no problem with that, I can go home and stop or whatever.
Mother:	(Simultaneously) Can you accept that, Ralph?
Hidalgo:	Good, very good.

It is important for the son to concede each time that he will follow the parents' and the therapist's rules. His wanting to get out of the hospital helps this.

Hidalgo:	I think that — let's go back to planning his coming home, his discharge.
Ralph:	I know what I have to do when I get home.
Mother:	What do you have to do?
Hidalgo:	Well, right now, you have to agree with what your parents decided.

When the son says that he knows what he has to do when he gets home the therapist might have encouraged him to say what that is, on the assumption that his initiative should be encouraged, or the therapist might be curious about what he would say. However, in this approach the primary focus at this stage of the therapy is the hierarchy in the family. The issue is not what is the son going to do, but how to organize the parents to decide what he is to do. Therefore the therapist emphasizes that the son is to do what the parents have agreed he should.

Ralph:	They're going to decide? Well, I'll tell you what I have to do. First when I get home I have to empty all the garbage cans, then I'll probably take all my posters down in my room and clean my room real good. Then, later on that night, I'll have to take the garbage out.
Father:	I've been handling the chores while you're gone.
Ralph:	All right. No drinking.
Mother:	You hear what you're saying right now. Hear what you're saying?

Ralph:	I hear you. I'll drink ginger ale.
Mother:	Now you're going to have a party Saturday night.
Ralph:	(Putting his finger to his head like a gun) Bang.
Father:	And it's going to be at your house. You're the host there, you know. You're not supposed to get out of hand when you're the host.
Ralph:	(Yawning and stretching) I have never gotten out of hand when I am the host, and I have never gotten out of hand otherwise.
Hidalgo:	I'm sure Ralph, that if you want, you really can control yourself.

The therapist accepts the son's assertion that he is never out of control by saying that he is capable of controlling himself and therefore that should be expected. This also supports her statements that the EEG findings should not excuse him from controlling himself.

Father:	He has a strong mind.
Hidalgo:	And you can control your anger, your irritability, and even your fights. You are telling us that, and I'm agreeing with you.
Father:	He can take his punishment, he can cut cigarettes out when he wants to, and he can cut out drinking. He's got a strong mind—a very strong mind.
Hidalgo:	So, we have to use that strong mind—
Father:	That's right.
Hidalgo:	(Continuing)—in the service of himself, for this is what we are here for, to help him out so this will never happen again. And, you know, Ralph, I don't think that because there was an irregularity in the EEG you have to think that you have mental illness; or because you have an abnormality in the EEG that that's something terrible. Many people have it and are functioning and this is what we look for with you. To function like a normal young man.

Chores

(Since the issue of drinking has been dealt with, the therapist begins a discussion of the chores.)

Hidalgo:	He has to take care of the room every day? Or how often?
Father:	Whenever it gets—looks a little too messed up, for him. Or in case some of his friends or anyone comes in, you know.
Hidalgo:	I wonder if it would be good to decide when he has to clean his room, maybe once a week, or twice a week, or whatever you decide—whatever you feel is appropriate.

Mother: Well, doctor, I didn't want to give him a set time to do his room.

Father: Yeah. He's a big boy, it's important for him to make up *his* mind.

Hidalgo: But you are still telling him when you think that the room is messed up. Maybe it's not too messed up for him.

Mother: Well, that's true too.

Hidalgo: You know you're expecting him to do that on his own. He should know, more or less, when he should clean it up, and take the garbage out, which is another issue.

Ralph: Nothing is dirty. Clothes are on the floor, the rest of the room is clean.

Mother: Well, he should pick up his clothes.

Father: Yeah, the rest of the room is clean.

Mother: In other words, then, that should be an everyday thing, that you should pick your clothes up.

Hidalgo: (To father) Do you agree with that? (As son interrupts she quiets him with a gesture.) Wait a minute, Ralph! (Turns to look at father.)

Father: Yes, I do.

Hidalgo: Every day? Tell him.

Mother: Every day.

Father: Just every day try to get the clothes off the floor and the towels off your bed, that's all.

Mother: We're not talking about general cleaning.

Hidalgo: OK.

Father: It's not a big thing, you're mother'll do the vacuuming of the floor and —

Hidalgo: What about the garbage?

Mother: He — twice a week, that is.

The Party

Hidalgo: Twice a week, that's been settled. And Saturday he's going to have the party, that is settled too.

Father: That's settled, yes.

Hidalgo: And that's an agreement between the two of you?

Mother: That's an agreement — but, now the party. He is going to . . . (Interrupted by father)

Father: Did you already pay for the party?

Mother: Yeah. Well, there's not really that much to pay for, because I'll probably fix some lunch meat, some platters for them. We agreed to pay for the quarter keg of beer. That's a small keg of beer and I told him we are not having any hard liquor at the party.

Hidalgo:	What could you do, Mr. Johnson, if one of his friends, for instance, this one that you're talking about, shows up at your house with the bottle of whiskey?
Father:	Just tell them they can't come in, that's all.
Hidalgo:	OK.
Ralph:	I wouldn't tell Sam that.
Mother:	I have told Sam that, and I have put Sam out of the house for that reason.
Hidalgo:	You know, I'm sure, Ralph, that you father would do it if he says that he will. I'm sure he would. What is going to happen on Sunday?
Mother:	Usually Ralph lies around on Sunday and watches TV.
Father:	We don't rush, you know, because I work all week.
Ralph:	Learn me how to drive that car.
Mother:	I imagine his father and him will go out Sunday.
Hidalgo:	(To mother, gesturing at father) Check it out.
Father:	I'm going to teach him how to drive my car. It's a four-shift car.
Hidalgo:	Did you have that in mind to do this Sunday?
Father:	Yes.

They talk about the possibility of going to a football game. After discussing these positive things, the therapist returns to the presenting problem which has not yet been discussed—the issue of violence.

Violence

Hidalgo:	Let's talk about the times that Ralph has become violent. And this is something that should not happen again.
Mother:	Absolutely.
Hidalgo:	So let's talk about the expectation in that area.
Mother:	Well, I think we encountered that the first weekend he was home, didn't we?
Father:	As to what?
Mother:	As far as him starting to become violent, and he settled himself down.
Father:	Yeah.
Mother:	We need more to talk things out instead of me getting as angry at Ralph. And that's usually what happens. Usually when Ralph is getting into this pitch, I'm getting as angry as—I get quite angry myself.
Father:	M-hmm.
Mother:	And I—I'm going to try to rationalize the situation and see if I can handle it better for him. I'm not saying he's right in what he's doing. What I'm saying is that I'm going to try to rationalize myself.

The mother seems to be implying that she provokes the violence. Possibly the idea was given to her in previous therapy. This therapist deals with it more matter of factly.

Hidalgo: What you're saying is that you're going to try not to lose your temper while he's losing his.

Mother: That's correct.

Hidalgo: But I really want you to tell him that that is not allowed any more in your house. Mr. Johnson, could you tell Ralph that?

Ralph: What is not allowed?

Hidalgo: To have a temper tantrum, to become violent, to put your fist against the window —the type of things that you would do prior to coming to the hospital. Could you tell him that?

Father: (To son) Do you think you've been here long enough to think you would know better than that?

Ralph: Yes.

Father: Not to do that.

Hidalgo: Suppose that he doesn't know that. I don't really know what he knows. But I want you to tell him that you are not going to tolerate any more of that kind of behavior. Tell him.

It is important that the therapist insist that the father tell the son he cannot be violent; then if the son becomes violent, he has disobeyed the father. It cannot be left implicit. It seems evident that the father is reluctant to draw a firm line against the violence, in contrast with the mother who wishes to. This is typical in families with violent young people: The parents are not in agreement about the seriousness of the violence and the need to see that it is stopped. Usually one parent is covertly siding with the child against the other parent in a cross-generation coalition which takes the appearance of one parent being nicer to the child with respect to these difficult issues.

Father: That's the way it is, Ralph, I'm not going to put up with it any more. I'm tired of putting in windows, and patching up holes in walls. I don't want it anymore, OK.?

Ralph: Right.

Father: One more hole to patch up.

Hidalgo: Let's see the alternative that we might have if he goes into one of his temper tantrums. What can be done? Hospitalization is not an option anymore. He will not come to the hospital for becoming violent. We have to look for other resources. I want you to understand that this is the chance for him to straighten out. OK.?

Father:	I understand what you mean. If he's still violent after being here three weeks we'll have to handle it in a different way.
Mother:	How we going to handle it?
Ralph:	You're going to lock me up like you did before?
Mother:	How are we going to handle it, Henry?
Father:	(Names an institution for juveniles) is all I know.
Mother:	Well, my thing is, if it happens again, I'm just not going to tolerate it—just like you told him you're not going to tolerate—I'm not going to tolerate.
Father:	It depends on what extent it is.
Hidalgo:	No, no, no—no extent. If he's angry, he can talk about being angry, he can say how he feels, but he doesn't have to destroy your property.
Mother:	That's right, that is our property.
Hidalgo:	It is your house. And he doesn't have to be disrespectful—you said it at the beginning.
Ralph:	I got three against one.
Father:	That's not three against one. She's just telling you facts. It's our house and we don't like you to bust it up. That's what she means, that's all.
Hidalgo:	I mean he can be angry, it's OK to be angry. He can express anger, but not by destroying the things in the house and making so much of a problem for the two of you.
Mother:	I fully agree with you in that. I will not tolerate it anymore and if it happens again, I will get on the phone and he will be arrested, and he will have to go wherever they put him.
Hidalgo:	This is important. By arrest you mean jail.
Mother:	That's—whatever—whatever they do.
Ralph:	I have never been there.
Hidalgo:	(To father) Do you agree with that?
Father:	I said it depends on the extent of it. Not if he justs gets a little tantrum . . .
Mother:	(Interrupting) Henry, you're giving him an out.
Hidalgo:	Let's try to see the alternatives. Would you be able to control him physically?
Father:	No.
Hidalgo:	Are there any friends, neighbors, somebody that you can call to come and help you control him physically, to restrain him.
Father:	We've done that already, we've done that before.
Ralph:	And I won.
Hidalgo:	You won? You're stronger than them?
Father:	Eddie? (Apparently a friend who helped restrain him.)
Ralph:	Yeah, I can beat Eddie up, it just takes me a while.
Father:	(Angry) Well, Ralph, what do you think you're doing?

Mother: You're still not accepting this, are you, Henry?

Father: Yes, I'm accepting it.

Hidalgo: What we can do right now is have the two of you decide the way you're going to handle him if he becomes violent again. You have to make the agreement, OK.?

Mother: Alright. If he does become violent again —we don't know if he's going to do it or not. You know that as well as I know it.

Father: Yeah, that's true.

Mother: What we're going to do, the only next step we have, is to call the police and have him arrested. You can't handle him physically, and neither can I. Isn't that correct?

Father: Yes.

Mother: Am I wrong?

Father: Yeah, well, if he don't do anything in their presence, they don't do anything about it —the police won't.

Mother: They certainly will do it. They did it before.

Ralph: That's because I ran out of the house.

Hidalgo: (To mother) I'm agreeing with you. If there is no other way to handle him, the police have to be called and he has to be arrested. (To father) But it sounds to me that you are not too agreeable with that. Then talk more with her.

Mother: Do you know why, really?

Father: I don't even like to think about it.

Mother: For the simple—well, we have to think about it. This is why this boy is here. This is exactly why this boy is here. More or less, this happens in my presence, more or less. Most of his violent tempers have happened in my presence. It has happened with his father at times, but it's happened more so with me. And I have threatened to, but I have never, ever called the police on him. His father has.

Ralph: Wait a minute, now come on.

Mother: (To son) Your father has —

Hidalgo: Leave him (the son) out of this.

Mother: His father has, at my agreement, but I have never. I have picked up the phone several times to do it and I haven't done it. I have left that decision up to him. The last time he had to do it, that was his decision, along with me. I haven't directly done it myself. But I see no other alternative. I'm hoping this discussion right now, what we're discussing is going to be just "if" because I hope it never happens again. We both hope that. Right?

Father: Well I certainly do.

Mother: But we have to face the facts if it does happen again.

Father: Right.

Mother:	That's what I'm saying.
Hidalgo:	So, what is the alternative? What is the decision then, for the two of you?
Father:	If he gets out of hand and starts busting up the house, we're going to call the police on him, that's all.
Hidalgo:	OK.
Mother:	But I—really, I've got full confidence in him. I've seen a difference in Ralph, a difference in his attitude, haven't you?
Father:	So have I.
Mother:	And I've got full confidence in him. I really do.
Hidalgo:	I'm also sure that, you know, he can make it.
Father:	He's strong.
Ralph:	And I'm moving out.

The son makes the threat of leaving them if they enforce rules upon him. This does not seem to have an effect on their willingness to continue to be firm.

Mother:	And everything in our power is at his disposal. We will do anything for him, to make him live more pleasantly and for us to live more pleasantly. I don't want to keep dominating the whole conversation, but I don't think Henry is really—he doesn't like to discuss things with other people. Just like with you and with the other doctor.
Hidalgo:	Sure. I understand that. And this is the first time that we've met.
Mother:	Yes, and that's why I'm sort of dominating the conversation.
Hidalgo:	(To Father) You see me as a stranger, I understand that.

As soon as the son threatens to leave the family, the mother turns against the father by disqualifying him in the eyes of the therapist, describing him as withdrawn and reluctant to participate. The threat of leaving the family is a strong bid for power. The mother's position is weakened; she turns against the father. The parental unity is threatened. The therapist helps the father to save face, excusing him for being shy with a stranger, rather than withdrawn with a therapist. At the same time she does not disagree with the mother.

Mother:	But I think things are going to work out, I really do. Believe me, at the point when he came into the hospital, I was growing quite afraid of Ralph. And this is my son, and I don't want to be afraid of my own child. And this is what was happening to me.
Hidalgo:	Uh huh.
Father:	(To son) Now don't she sound right? Don't you agree with her on that? Should she be afraid of you?

Mother: And I don't want to be afraid, I mean I just don't want to —I would rather not even see him ever again than to have to be afraid of him. And I mean what I'm saying.

Hidalgo: I'm sure that it's very painful for you to be afraid of him. It's a terrible thing.

Mother: That's right. It's a heart-breaking situation.

Hidalgo: Uh huh.

Mother: I'm sure he doesn't agree with us all the time. I'm sure Ralph doesn't agree with us. We're quite a bit older than him, you know, his generation and my generation are different. I understand that, but it's no way to solve things —busting things up.

Hidalgo: So you were able to explain the expectations for Ralph. Ralph agrees to follow your expectations. You also have already thought about resources, what to do in case he doesn't follow through.

Father: (To son) Do you think our expectations are too strong?

Ralph: No.

Mother: They shouldn't be, because you should make up your mind that you're not going to do it again.

Ralph: Naw, I ain't gonna do it again.

Hidalgo: Just one thing that I would like to say and make clear because I really believe it. If Ralph goes and does what he wants, he will end up in here again, in a state mental hospital, in jail —anywhere except in society, in the community, living a normal life.

The therapist outlines a bleak future if the problem is not solved. Sometimes it is helpful to project the parents into the future and have them discuss at greater length the misfortunes to come if they let their son down by not taking charge now.

Mother: That's right.

Hidalgo: So right now the two of you have to be in charge.

Ralph: I'm 17 years old. I'll be 18 next year.

Hidalgo: But they have to be in charge so you don't get into trouble.

Ralph: I don't get into trouble.

Hidalgo: I would call it being in trouble, Ralph, to be in a hospital at age 17. In a mental institution. Because this is where you ended up. And I don't want you to come back.

Ralph: Neither do I.

The therapist effectively points out the reality of the situation —the boy has not been able to stay out of trouble and therefore needs his parents. This is said in a matter-of-fact way, and it brings the youth over to her side.

Hidalgo: OK. And I'm sure that your parents don't want you to come back either. So it sounds pretty good to me.

Mother: I think so.

Ralph: So, they're going to start being stricter to me.

Mother: See, he's getting the wrong attitude —he's getting the wrong impression of this whole thing, I think. It's not the idea of being strict to you. The idea is that decisions have been made, period. You are not to get violent again. There's no question about that. How stricter are we getting? I'm not restricting your times of coming in or this and that.

Father: We're concerned.

Mother: We're making a decision here. You are not to get violent again in the house.

Ralph: OK.

Father: If you feel it coming on, the best thing to do is what I always tell you.

Ralph: I'll walk away from it. I'll get to the door and I'll walk away.

Father: Didn't I always tell you to do that?

Hidalgo: I'm really glad to see the two of you being able to agree and make the decisions that you have made, for Ralph's sake. We're going to end up now. He's coming out of the hospital this Friday.

CONCLUSION

The first interview brought out most of the issues that were dealt with as the therapy progressed. The therapist continued to meet with the family during the course of the next six months, anticipating difficulties, planning for the future, and helping them to solve problems. There was one more episode of violence but the son was not arrested since the parents handled it at home. He did not drink, but he had a couple of episodes of sniffing embalming fluid, a pastime among his friends. At the end of therapy the young man was in school and doing well, and he was not violent. The Dilantin was discontinued.

REFERENCES

1. Haley, J. *Leaving Home.* New York: Mc-Graw-Hill, 1980.
2. Harbin, H. "A family oriented psychiatric inpatient unit." *Family Process* 18 : 281–291, 1979.
3. Madanes, C. "The prevention of rehospitalization of adolescents and young adults." *Family Process* 19, June 1980.
4. Madanes, C. *Strategic Family Therapy,* San Francisco: Jossey-Bass, 1981.

4

Family Treatment of Patients with Chronic Schizophrenia: The Inpatient Phase

CAROL M. ANDERSON AND DOUGLAS J. REISS

Despite very real progress in our understanding of schizophrenic disorders, treatment outcome data continue to be grim. Undoubtedly, efforts at deinstitutionalization and the use of psychopharmacologic drugs have substantially reduced the length and frequency of hospitalizations. Nevertheless, the adjustment of patients discharged into the community is often marginal and plagued by frequent rehospitalizations. Schizophrenia remains the country's number one mental health problem.

It is estimated that of the approximately one million episodes of schizophrenia each year, two-thirds require inpatient care, 72 percent of whom have been hospitalized previously [43]. Without medication, approximately 80 percent of patients hospitalized with schizophrenia relapse within a year of discharge. Even with medication, it is estimated that as many as 40 percent relapse within a year [18,26,28,39].

The reasons for these high relapse rates are not entirely clear. Some patients apparently never stabilize; others fail to comply consistently with a treatment regimen. The failure to connect with after-care services appears to contribute strongly, as up to 50 percent discontinue treatment after just a few visits [43]. Whatever the reasons, many individuals with schizophrenia become the "chronic" patients who consume the majority of the time, effort, and resources of our mental health care systems. The National Institute of Mental Health estimates that this illness costs the country twenty billion dollars annually in mental health services and loss of human potential and resources [49], a toll which is magnified when the pain and hardship experienced by these patients and their families is taken into account.

We believe the problems that contribute to this "revolving door" phenomenon for patients with chronic schizophrenia can be decreased by the institution of the family-oriented program described here. This program begins with intensive support and education for the family during a patient's hospitalization which lays the foundation for ongoing outpatient interventions. These interventions aim to increase treatment compliance, sustain patients in the community, and prevent relapse. Although the inpatient phase is described in greater detail, the effective treatment of schizophrenia often requires many years, making it essential that inpatient and outpatient treatments be well integrated to insure continuity of care.

WHY A FAMILY-ORIENTED PROGRAM?

We do not yet know the cause of schizophrenia; the view generally held is that this crippling disorder is caused by an interaction of biochemical, genetic, and socio-environmental factors. Whatever the ultimate cause, schizophrenic patients do seem to have cognitive deficits which make it difficult for them to process and respond to complicated or excessive stimuli [13,44]. Stimulating environments in the home, workplace, or treatment setting have been shown to be correlated with high rates of relapse [10,19,27,34,35,46,48]. Of particular importance is the family environment. Although there is no evidence that family interaction causes schizophrenia, family interactions, even in normal families, involve intense emotion and complicated communications. Therefore, it is reasonable to assume that patients would have difficulty negotiating a family environment, particularly since families of schizophrenics tend to be different from normal families in ways that probably exacerbate the difficulties of patients who are sensitive to stimuli [20,29,30,31,40,41]. For instance, the families of schizophrenic patients have been found to exhibit more conflict and more ambiguous, fragmented, or vague communications. We do not know whether these family patterns predate and have a causal relationship to the illness, or whether they represent the residue of years of family attempts to cope with a very difficult situation. In either case, it would seem logical that the course and impact of schizophrenia can be mitigated or exacerbated by these family processes and relationships. This hypothesis appears to be supported by recent research. Conflict in the patient's home, for example, has been shown to be a predictor of relapse [27]. Patients who are members of families rated high in the expression of emotion, particularly criticism and overinvolvement, have a significantly greater chance of relapse than patients who are from more emotionally benign environments. When face-to-face contact between patients and relatives who have high rates of emotional expression exceeds 35 hours per week, the chance of relapse is even greater [10,47]. Thus emotionally charged family environments can lead to a pattern of repeated hospitalizations.

Clinically, it appears that the emotionality in these families is at least in part related to high levels of anxiety about the patient and the illness. During an acute episode most families of patients with schizophrenia are in crisis, and are crippled by fear, anxiety, and guilt about the illness. Family interventions which are client-centered, nondirective, or insight-oriented tend to increase anxiety and therefore are likely to aggravate rather than alleviate distress. For this reason, a family program which attempts to diminish the anxiety of families during the inpatient phase appears to be indicated. It is proposed that decreased patient vulnerability and improved cognitive functioning can often be achieved by pharmacotherapy, while the reduction of family anxiety can be achieved through support, structure, and education. Both of these changes produce a less intense home environment, and thus decrease the likelihood of repeated relapses for the patient. This program includes highly specific educative interventions that provide concrete, specific information and effective management techniques to accomplish attainable, realistic goals. While certain insights may result from changed behaviors, insight is neither a goal nor a prerequisite. The program strongly emphasizes that families probably are not the cause of schizophrenia, but nevertheless have the potential to positively or negatively influence the course of the illness.

The family program attempts to break the cycle of repeated admissions by putting the following principles into effect.

1. The creation of a hospital environment that promotes a supportive working relationship with the patient *and* the family while encouraging rapid return to the community.

2. The provision of information about the illness and its management to family members.

3. The creation of a low-key home/work environment that supports the patient staying in the community.

4. The creation of a sense of continuity of care and "institutional transference" for both patient and family.

THE HOSPITAL ENVIRONMENT

The type of environment created on an inpatient unit is crucial to the success of a program designed to prevent readmissions. There are several components to an effective program of this sort.

Cooperation Between Medical and Nonmedical Personnel

Whatever the etiology of this illness, both medication maintenance and psychotherapy clearly contribute to patient functioning and community tenure

[11,12,26,38]. A major reason for the failure of family therapy in an inpatient unit is the polarization that often occurs between family and medical approaches to treatment, suggesting that one type of intervention is less important than another. For this reason family therapists often have tended to avoid hospital settings, finding it difficult to cooperate with a medical model. Furthermore, many of those who do take on this challenge become entangled in fruitless power struggles with the medical power structure, wasting time seeking to prove their treatment as the treatment of choice. When this happens, staff can become more involved in their disagreements with one another rather than working together toward common goals. A family model usually loses in such power struggles; the treatment of the patient becomes the sole focus of the unit, and what work is done with the family is assigned to an inexperienced person without training, supervision, or support. Consequently the message family members get regarding their involvement is an ambivalent one at best, as they become unnecessarily confused by conflicting messages, and compliance suffers.

To circumvent this unnecessary polarization, an inpatient family program must have administrative backing to promote the integration of family issues into treatment planning. Time must be allocated to the discussion of family issues at rounds and team meetings, and, particularly, family needs must be considered when making treatment decisions. This is most likely to be implemented if a trained and skilled family therapist who knows what to do and how to do it is made a part of the treatment team.

A Team Approach

In the treatment of schizophrenia, effective therapy for patients and families begins with effective support for staff. A *group* of professionals, available to both the patient and the family, is central to an effective program with chronic patients. Patients with schizophrenia make progress slowly. Their families are often worn-out, frustrated, and, therefore, prone to what seems to be purposefully negative or irrational behavior. These cases take a great deal of time, energy, and patience. Months of therapeutic work can go down the drain because of an attempt to push the patient back to work before he is ready. Hard-won stability of functioning can be threatened by something as simple as a brief vacation for the therapist. For these reasons, staff treating patients with chronic disorders are unusually susceptible to therapist fatigue, hopelessness about change, and increased vulnerability to the acceptance of resistance. A team approach provides protection from these problems [7]. Team members can support one another and supply a dose of reality when one member becomes overinvolved or develops too high or too low expectations. Those members of a team who are less involved with day-to-day treatment can observe and identify subtle signs of change or progress, thus increasing objectivity and morale. Team members can cover for one another's absences, thus providing ongoing availability to patients and families. Furthermore, rather than encouraging an intensive relationship between the patient/family and one professional (an intensity which in itself can be stressful to these patients), patients and their families are encouraged to use the entire treatment team as a resource. An "institutional transference" is stressed, one in which all members of the unit are regarded as "the therapist."

A Philosophy of Rapid Discharge

The major goals of inpatient care are to provide the patient with a beginning sense of control and the family with a brief respite from having to cope with the illness. No focus is placed on behavior, insight, or feelings that do not directly aid the patient's return to the community. In this way the goals of inpatient treatment are kept specific and attainable, and the focus is on concrete issues and practical management techniques. When the hospital staff is no longer involved, most families will once again be the primary caretakers of the patient. Therefore, the need for ongoing compliance with aftercare services is encouraged. It is repeatedly stressed that the greater part of the treatment program will take place on an outpatient basis after the crisis has passed. With this philosophy, the pace of the inpatient program can be fast without being intense, since the emphasis is on a rapid return to the community rather than on a total cure.

A Working Relationship: Partners in Treatment

The fourth component of the hospital program is the establishment of a working relationship with the patient *and* the family. The staff of most hospital systems find it easy to establish a relationship with the patient, since his pain and disorganization are obvious. As the staff come to know the patient and to identify with his problems, it is natural that they tend to view the patient as victim, and by implication, the family as villain. However, since they have not had to spend 24-hours a day with a decompensated patient in an uncontrolled environment, staff are more likely to be judgmental about the family's attempts to cope. Such attitudes may lead to the alienation of the family, making it impossible to establish a treatment alliance [1,3,24,33]. For this reason, special attention must be given to the formation of a supportive relationship with the family.

Support

The establishment of a working relationship with a family begins by providing the family with support and an orientation to the hospital program. The issue of early support for the family is a crucial one. When a patient is admitted to the hospital the search for historical information and precipitating events often unwittingly suggests to the family that staff are attempting to discover what the family did wrong. This is not surprising, since history taking usually focuses entirely on what was abnormal or atypical about the patient's development; the family's interaction; or their social, genetic, or biological history. Even family-oriented professionals who espouse belief in the systems concept of circular causality behave in ways that imply linear thinking about family problems. They look for family communications that make patients crazy. In ongoing family work, they often allow sessions to focus primarily on parental shortcomings or become a forum solely for the airing of the patient's complaints, real or not. Such therapists can too easily give an implicit or explicit message that the family must continuously alter their lifestyle to accommodate the patient's needs. This process perpetuates family guilt and increases family anxiety. Family members who already feel bad about themselves can begin to feel helpless and as though they cannot possibly cope with the patient or be good parents.

Familial Concerns

The initial assessment of the family on admission, therefore, must attend to the needs of family members as well as those of the patient. For instance, an attempt must be made to discover current stresses experienced by each family member. In so doing, attention is paid to stresses and resources in the workplace, the extended family, and in the family's social network. Particular attention, however, is paid to potential stresses brought on by the patient's illness and hospitalization. The assessment explores the family's reaction to the illness, and the effect of the illness on the instrumental and psychological roles the patient has played in the family. Families experience a great deal of pain, frustration, and anger before turning to hospitalization of a disturbed member. A discussion of these issues provides the family with a chance to decompress the impact of these events and see the therapist as understanding of their difficulties. For this reason common emotional responses experienced by all families are explored. The most universal emotional reaction is that of guilt. Most families ask "What did we do wrong?" or "Where did we miss the boat?" Most families also experience stigma, since many behaviors related to this illness are socially embarrassing. For instance, some patients accuse neighbors or employers of attempting to poison them; others remove their clothes in public. Other patients lack social skills, rudely ignoring other people's needs. Many patients have imposed strange rules or unreasonable rituals upon the family. Since some families have tolerated humiliating behaviors for years before resorting to hospitalization, it is not surprising that they have come to feel hopeless or angry.

In fact, it is more often surprising that they have coped so well for so long. Those families who are not angry are often overwhelmed by sadness, feeling that their loved one never will be the same again. They are painfully aware that the patient's capabilities have diminished and the hopes and dreams they had for the future may be lost.

Most families try their best to help, and attempt to adapt to the patient's strange behaviors. Contrary to reports which suggest that families wish to rid themselves of the burden of the patient, most families attempt to maintain the patient in the community if it is at all possible. To avoid hospitalization, they try to normalize what is going on as much as possible by attempting to coax the patient to behave according to society's rules and to reason with him about his unusual ideas. Many families try to ignore bizarre behaviors, make sense out of nonsensical communications, or take on extra chores in order to compensate for what the patient no longer appears able or willing to do.

They watch the patient to make sure he does not kill himself or hurt someone else. In order to protect the patient, they usually curtail their own activities, both social and professional. Sometimes the patient is maintained in the home only because the entire family has learned to ignore their own needs. By definition, these methods have not worked for families with a chronic patient.

After serious and prolonged pain and anguish they have had to turn to an institution for help. Whatever temporary relief the hospital provides, most families wish to avoid hospitalization. Furthermore, the patient often resents the hospital *and* his family for admitting him, particularly if the admission was a forced one. Most families of patients with chronic schizophrenia have had past negative experiences with hospitals. Thus, they expect to pay again the emotional price exacted by both the patient's reaction and the staff's intolerance.

During this assessment process, the clinician carefully adheres to the principle of "joining the family" before attempting change-producing interventions [37]. If the clinician takes the time to become a part of the system, the family's tendencies toward resistance, rejection, and discontinuance are diminished. For this reason, the clinician begins each session with appropriate social conversation and makes attempts to increase the family's level of comfort and feelings of being accepted and understood. Whenever possible, the clinician also attempts to use the family's style of relating and the family's terms for behaviors.

In early sessions with the family, support is emphasized by designating the team member they see as the family's consultant and ombudsman. This helps to avoid the common tendency to ignore or neglect family members during a hospitalization [1,3,14,24,32]. Since families of chronic patients may have had negative experiences with other mental health professionals, the family's reactions to past treatment attempts are discussed and every attempt is made to stress that this treatment approach is different from past treatment efforts. Reassurance is given that the clinician will protect the family's interests and that the treatment team is made up of competent professionals who expect and can facilitate change.

The need for the family's participation in treatment is made explicit by the creation of a treatment contract. Such a contract involves a mutual agreement about the goals, content, length, and methods of therapy. The family's main complaints and concerns are translated by the therapist into clear, specific, and attainable goals. If a complaint is unreasonable or a goal is unattainable, the clinician negotiates with the family toward "the possible." If there are crucial goals the family has not mentioned spontaneously, the clinician suggests they be placed on the treatment agenda.

The mutuality of the contract is emphasized. The family agrees to attend sessions and to work on the goals that have been established. The clinician agrees to include the family in all decision making about the patient and his treatment; to keep the family informed of ward decisions regarding the patient and the treatment plan; and to provide advice, support, and information about the hospital, its staff, and its procedures.

Furthermore, not only the patient's problems, but also the needs of the family (established in the assessment phase) are considered as necessary data in making these decisions. The family's current emotional, financial, and social state are part of the data used to make decisions regarding the patient's continuing care.

PROVIDING INFORMATION

Considering the nature of schizophrenia, the normal responses of both patients and families to the crisis of illness and hospitalization may not always be the most helpful ones. Most families attempt to support the patient by becoming intensely involved, attempting to make sense out of the nonsensical, and by avoiding setting limits on someone they view as sick. For a patient who has trouble responding to stimulation, these seemingly helpful responses can make things worse, since they tend to create more stimulation rather than establish more distance and control. Therefore, information is given which provides families and patients with an understanding of the illness, as well as with specific behaviors which will help to create a more controlled, predictable, low-key environiment.

This information can be provided in a number of ways. It can be imparted gradually during regular sessions, in a series of teaching sessions during the patient's hospitalization, or in a day-long workshop format as we have described elsewhere [2]. The last two methods are particularly advantageous since a multiple-family format can be used. This format is not only less threatening to family members who otherwise may be reluctant to ask questions, but it also can help to begin a process of de-isolation and peer group support. Regardless of the format, the following topics should be covered.

Information About Etiology and Treatment

It is important that this information be given early in the treatment phase since it provides not only basic knowledge about schizophrenia, but sets the tone and establishes the themes for the family treatment program. Facts and major theories about schizophrenia are summarized in understandable language, including theories about the potential biological, genetic, and familial contributions to the illness. It is emphasized that there is no conclusive evidence for any theory of causation.

Information about major behavioral symptomatology, including the likelihood of the patient's sensitivity to stimuli and his potential cognitive deficits, are explained, along with examples of how these phenomena manifest themselves in family life. In order that the family truly understand what the patient is experiencing, material written by expatients is distributed [5,36].

This information usually results in an increased understanding by both the family and patient of what is known about the etiology, course, prognosis, symptomatology, and effective management of the illness. By stressing nonfamilial etiologies, this understanding serves to decrease guilt and increase the amount of sense they can make of their experiences with the patient. This in turn helps the family to modulate their level of emotional involvement.

In this process, the patient is labeled as someone with a serious illness. This is a controversial step, since it has been suggested in the literature that labeling causes or at least perpetuates illness, and may fixate patient-type behaviors [16,17]. It is possible, however, that labeling has advantages that outweigh its disadvantages [21]. When a patient is behaving in a deeply disturbed way, viewing him as ill makes it far more likely that the family will be able to continue to support the patient during those times when he is unable to function at full capacity. Furthermore, labeling the patient as having an illness decreases the tendency to assign negative and emotional meanings to symptoms. If the family can believe that the patient is neither malingering nor attempting to communicate a malicious message, there is decreased anger at the patient and the treatment team.

The educational session(s) should connect information with the goals of ongoing treatment. The legitimacy of these goals is supported by data which indicate that if patients can be maintained in reasonably good health and with reasonably good social skills, some of the perils of the illness diminish in time.

All points made in this process of education will relate to the goals of decreasing patient vulnerability and creating a home/work environment that will contribute to keeping the patient in the community. Specific information related to these two goals can be gone over in some detail.

Decreasing Patient Vulnerability Through Medication

Because families can facilitate or impede the implementation of a medication program, information is shared which increases the likelihood of the family's support. Medication is stressed as one way to decrease the patient's vulnerability to stimulation and families are given information about its potential importance and its negative side effects. The risks of taking medication versus not taking it are discussed as well as the differences among various medications. The family is told that most patients are ambivalent about taking medication. Some are made uncomfortable by some of the side effects, while others wish to stop it as soon as they begin to feel better. Fortunately or unfortunately, the positive effects of medication often linger for several weeks after it has been discontinued, while the negative side effects diminish more rapidly. It is very hard, therefore, for patients to appreciate the connection between medication and well-being. Thus noncompliance with a medication regime is common. When the patient is resistant, many family members find it difficult to support a medication program, even with information. This is particularly true if the patient appears lethargic, withdrawn, or overly sedated. Therefore, a great deal of time must be given to weighing the costs and benefits of a medication regime. Statistics demonstrating the relationship between medication compliance and community tenure are useful.

Creating a Low-Key Home/Work Environment

Families are helped to see that they can influence the course of schizophrenia by an explanation of the negative role stress plays in the disorder [9,10,19,45,47]. The need to decrease stimulation and stress is explained as central to an eventual decrease in patient vulnerability. The family is told that, for the patient, the illness produces diminished stress tolerance, including a diminished tolerance for the interpersonal stresses common to family life. As stated previously, studies of the post-hospital adjustment of schizophrenic patients have demonstrated that relapse is related to the amount of stimulation in the patient's environment, and particularly, the amount of expressed emotion of the family. To decrease emotionality it is necessary to create a more benign low-key family environment. Conflict, simultaneous multiple interactions, unclear power structures, and diffuse generational or interpersonal boundaries will be difficult for the schizophrenic patient to tolerate.

The family is helped to see that certain instinctive behaviors of families in crisis are less helpful than other behaviors. Generally, these less helpful behaviors can be put into three categories: (1) increased conflict and criticism between one another and toward the patient; (2) extreme involvement with the patient, be that involvement positive or negative; (3) decreased involvement with the family member's own social support network or other potential gratifications beyond the nuclear family.

Although these behaviors can be described as normal responses to a serious illness of any sort, the family can be helped to see that they are not useful given the special symptoms of schizophrenia. In order to avoid the paralysis caused by fear, guilt, anger, and lack of knowledge about what is the "right way" to intervene, the family is given specific coping strategies to substitute for these highly stimulating responses. The mobilization of a family's positive abilities and powers to help, reinvolves them in the patient's life in a potentially constructive way and may help to diminish guilt, anger, and criticism.

An attempt is also made to help the family to allow the patient psychological space in order to diminish the intensity of his personal environment. This psychological space is created by stressing decreased expectations, setting reasonable limits, and encouraging involvement for both patient and family with extrafamilial contacts.

Temporarily modified or decreased familial expectations of the patient make the family less likely to be surprised, or "let down" by the patient's behaviors. To facilitate these more realistic expectations, the course, symptoms, and duration of schizophrenia are discussed with the entire family. Such information may also help the patient to have more appropriate expectations for his own behavior and thus cause him to be less likely to become discouraged and thereby stressed by comparing himself to healthy peers.

A series of suggestions are given to the family relating to the creation of barriers which prevent overstimulation. Much like the Muzak heard in department stores and dentist offices, the family is asked to diminish the highs and the lows in their family interaction, to create a family attitude of "benign indifference." They are encouraged to minimize nagging, rejection, fights, and conflicts, as well as extreme concern, overly positive encouragement, and excessive enthusiasm. They are asked to create distance without rejecting the patient. They are taught to allow the patient to withdraw when he seems to need to do so, and to recognize signals that the patient needs time out from interaction or activity. To avoid regression, the family is encouraged to offer the patient activities, such as going to a movie or going bowling, but to accept the patient's refusal if he seems to need to be by himself. Another method of discouraging overstimulation is the creation of reasonable rules and their reinforcement through limit setting. The family is instructed not to confuse the need for low stimulation with permissiveness. Because the patient is sick does not mean that the family must do whatever he asks. The family is helped to understand that limits are reassuring to the patient. Rituals and strange irritating behaviors that upset the family are not helpful to the family or the patient. The family is asked to set limits clearly and without too much detailed discussion. The importance of setting limits before the tension builds and blow ups occur is stressed.

The only exception to setting limits on these kinds of behaviors has to do with paranoid delusions. It has been our experience that if a family member sets a limit on a paranoid idea directly, the patient often at best becomes more agitated and at worst begins to believe the family member is a part of the plot against him. In these cases, we suggest that the family respond to the patient by saying, "That doesn't make sense to me, but I can appreciate your anxiety if you believe it."

Finally, specific training regarding a limited number of communication skills may be conducted. This training suggests that the content of interaction matters less than clarity, simplicity, structure, and control of intensity. The family is asked to keep their communication simple with an appropriate amount of details and a moderate level of specificity. Some families have an obsessive style and become very involved in details. Such a style would not cause trouble in other circumstances, but schizophrenic patients may find such interaction too stimulating or confusing. Family members often contribute to nonsensical conversations by searching for a core element of rationality in the patient's delusional statement. They should be encouraged not to try to discern the meanings of nonsensical communication. Rigorous training in communication effectiveness is avoided since such a task is thought to be too ambitious, frustrating, and anxiety-provoking for both family and therapist. Thus, only four points are emphasized:

1. The ability to differentiate description from evaluation. (The ability to say what happened as opposed to how they feel about it.)
2. The ability to acknowledge the statements of others and to accept responsibility for one's own communications.
3. The ability to keep things at a moderate level of specificity (avoiding excessive detail or excessive abstraction.)
4. The ability to express and emphasize positive messages and supportive comments.

The family is helped to see the patient as ill, but as having continuing assets. As time goes on, an increasing attempt is made to diminish unidimensional views of the patient, particularly those that regard him as totally incompetent because he is ill. If families believe that the patient's behavior is beyond his control, they tend to react with overinvolvement, excessive concern, and exaggerated attempts to support, close ranks, and fill in for his deficits. While some amount of protection is necessary, overprotection can lead the family to be too tolerant of patient-type behaviors and too easy with limits, thereby discouraging the growth and development of which the patient is capable. While overprotective families are less likely to impose unrealistic expectations on the patient, they are also unable to provide the structure and increasing separateness necessary to simplify the environment and diminish chaos.

Unidimensional views of the patient as having some sort of "character deficit" are also discouraged. If families believe the patient can control his behavior, but chooses not to do so because he is lazy or evil, the family usually responds with criticism, anger, hostility, and suggestions that he eliminate problem behaviors by sheer "will."

Family responses to the patient may in part be dependent on the meaning the family attaches to the patient's aberrant behavior and whether they are the "target" of his delusions, fears, or upsets. However, families may attribute different meanings to behaviors at different stages of the illness. Thus the family's view of the patient is a repeated focus of the education process, particularly when things are not progressing or tensions seem to be building. At all times an attempt is made to decrease conflict among family members about the meaning of the illness, the patient's capabilities, and the most helpful way of responding to him. Family conflict is more likely if the meaning of the patient's behavior is viewed differently by different family members. This conflict is likely to decrease the ability of family members to provide support for one another in a time of crisis and may adversely affect the course of treatment.

Family Support Networks

Most families with a schizophrenic member become increasingly isolated over time. Those families with fewer or less available social supports outside the immediate family probably have a lower tolerance for stress and deviance within the family [10, 47]. For this reason, these family members may also tend to be more overinvolved and critical since they have fewer people to substitute for needs which are less likely to be met by an increasingly dysfunctional patient, and fewer confidants with whom to discuss the pain they are experiencing about the patient's illness.

Families are taught the importance of maintaining a support system beyond that of nuclear family. Family members are encouraged to talk of their difficulties to friends and extended family and to engage such people in psychological and instrumental support services. Three types of extrafamilial contacts are stressed:

(1) Interpersonal supports: the use of others to serve as outlets for discussion of concerns, tensions, needs, and to give support and reassurance.

(2) Social and/or recreational outlets: the use of others to serve to distract, amuse, and stimulate areas of interest that would decrease the totality of the family's investment in the patient and his illness.

(3) Work and/or service: emphasis on alternative areas of personal competence, altruism, and ability to contribute to others.

This directive is one of the most difficult for family members to accept. Many families consider their own needs as unimportant when a family member is in crisis. Therefore, the emphasis must be on helping the family to consider their own needs for survival as essential, *in order to be able to help the patient* on an ongoing basis. The message is given that if they deplete themselves, in the long run they are less able to help one another or the patient. While ongoing social and work activities are often impossible during the acute phase of the illness, the family is encouraged to see the need for different management techniques for the "long haul." Long-term management techniques must include a life style that does not entirely center on the patient and his needs. Stressing the needs for support of other family members helps to reduce the emotional intensity of the family's relationship with the patient.

It is also common, especially in chronic conditions, for patients to become socially isolated and devoid of external activities or support systems. Family members at times complain that the lack of friends forces the patient to spend an inordinate amount of time at home, thus enhancing the chances for conflict. It certainly is likely that patients with fewer or less available social supports outside the immediate family are more vulnerable to family intensity and family stress, since they are more involved in and dependent on the family. Gradually, an attempt is made to decrease the intensity of family relationships by distributing this intensity throughout a larger network.

CONTINUITY OF CARE: AFTERCARE

The inpatient phase must be used to educate the patient and the family about the necessity of follow-up care and the importance of the tasks that must be addressed once the patient is discharged. This message is extremely important since it is estimated that 50 percent of schizophrenic patients never engage in aftercare services and that those who do tend to drop out prematurely [43]. In regard to continuity of care it would be most desirable if the same therapeutic team could do both inpatient and outpatient treatment. Since this is not always feasible, preparation for discharge should include at least one meeting with the outpatient team. The establishment of at least a verbal agreement to ongoing treatment aids in transfer to the aftercare team. The team asks the family for a commitment to attend sessions for at least a year, although these sessions need not occur weekly.

Such a long period often seems overwhelming or unnecessary to the patient and the family, but is essential since the length of the recuperative process tends to be very slow.

Preparation for Discharge

In preparation for discharge, we attempt to give families very practical help in dealing with problems of daily living. The family is asked to do a number of things as the patient is reintegrated into the family. First, the need for revised expectations of the patient is stressed again. It is emphasized that the fact that the hospitalization was short-term does not mean that the patient's illness is not a very serious one. It is suggested that the family regard the patient as though he has a very serious illness which will require a long process of recuperation. The need for increased rest, sleep, and limited activity for a period of time is predicted. It can be suggested that this is the body's response to a debilitating stress, and therefore may be adaptive. However, whether it is adaptive or not, it is in fact inevitable. This is a crucial component of any preparation for discharge since after the initial stabilization, a period of inactivity, decreased motivation, and excessive sleep usually follows, creating the impression that the patient is healthy, but lazy. If the family can believe that this apparent laziness merely represents another stage of the illness, it will help them to tolerate behavior that is otherwise extremely irritating. The therapist is established as someone who will help them to make decisions regarding sickness versus malingering. Furthermore, the therapist helps the family to use what one of our patients called "an internal yardstick," that is, helping the patient and family to compare their progress to where they were a month ago rather than to where someone else is today. This monitoring process helps in sensitizing the patient and the family to small steps of progress, thus avoiding discouragement.

The family also is asked to normalize the family routine as much as possible in preparation for aftercare and living together again. We ask that they not center their life on the patient. In an acute illness, it is necessary for a family to focus their attentions and their energies on the patient when he is ill, but in any long-term illness (like diabetes, heart disease, or schizophrenia), life must go on for others. If not, the illness will be more debilitating to the family, and family members may experience so much stress that they will be unable to offer support and may even cause additional problems for the patient. If family members begin to be debilitated by the patient's illness, patients often feel responsible, thereby experiencing the family as a burden not a support.

The need to attend to other children in the family is also emphasized. A chronic illness, such as schizophrenia, often leads to disproportionate amounts of attention to the patient, often at the expense of the needs of his or her siblings. Siblings frequently complain that their parents side with the patient while they always are expected to understand and avoid conflict. Our goal is to give the siblings and patient problem-solving tools to help diffuse potential conflicts as they erupt. Further attempts are made to help parents to attend to the needs of their other children. Finally, all family members are encouraged to engage in activities and to establish supports outside the family.

Signals for Help

The family is asked to become aware of and discuss those behaviors that tend to signal increased stress or difficulty for this particular patient. Together, the family and the patient identify which behaviors require the family's help or support, and which signal the need for psychological space. To decrease family anxiety, emphasis is placed on the fact that withdrawal is not always a negative symptom, but at times an adaptive one. A review of signals helps to avoid the tendency of families to over-respond to every patient symptom as if it means he is getting sick again, or the tendency to under-respond by ignoring all messages in order to avoid confrontations. Both the patient and the family are helped to become aware of early indications of decompensation. They are taught about what can be done to initiate fast and appropriate interventions that may avert a psychotic episode [25].

The inpatient phase is a time when families can be prepared to use professional help productively on an ongoing basis. Some families require education regarding the appropriate use of therapeutic resources. Since many families are reluctant to intrude or impose on the clinician, his availability for crisis intervention on an emergency basis is stressed. The family clinician is available for emergency phone and in-person contacts, and continues his role as an ombudsman for the family regarding other therapeutic and rehabilitation systems, services, and mental health personnel.

Families are helped to differentiate between the kinds of questions that can be saved for therapeutic sessions and the kinds they should regard as emergencies. This includes the anticipation of problems that can occur so that they can be avoided, connecting with those people who will be responsible for aftercare treatment, and essentially the selling of the idea of ongoing family involvement as an effective mechanism of help.

The use of professional help is also encouraged by verbally rewarding family members for bringing issues to family sessions and for simply attending. The importance of every member's input is stressed repeatedly. It is predicted that some stages of therapy will seem slow and painful, causing families occasionally to wish to discontinue treatment. The need to persevere is stressed.

The aftercare treatment team helps the patient and family walk a fine line between the exacerbation of the positive symptoms of schizophrenia (delusions, hallucinations, loose associations, etc.) and the solidification of negative symptoms (lethargy, amotivation, excessive sleep, loss of work or social skills, etc.). To avoid relapse, the patient is allowed to withdraw from stimulation. However, to prevent a habitual dysfunctional state, the patient is urged to re-engage. This creates a seeming double-bind situation for clinician, patient, and family. The proper resolution of this dilemma requires clinical skill and careful intervention.

The answer rests in the timing of the push for patients to make an effort at reactivation. Based on research and our clinical experience, it seems that most patients can tolerate only minimal stressors during the first 12 to 18 *months* following an acute break [26]. Thus our most active therapeutic thrust takes place after these time constraints. The actual time parameters are monitored continually by watching the patient's responses to a series of assigned structural tasks that increase in required responsibility in a slow step-by-step fashion.

Avoiding Too Rapid Emancipation

The subject with the most potential for causing excessive stimulation and relapse is too early, too fast emancipation from the family, and/or too rapid return to work. The patient's response to his family and the family's response to the patient is generally characterized by ambivalence in the area of differentiation/ emancipation. Most patients and their families will demonstrate some difficulty achieving a satisfactory balance of togetherness versus separation. If the onset of the illness is in adolescence, which appears most common, the emancipation process is often impaired. The tasks of adolescence are stressful ones for normal teenagers, and patients with schizophrenia have extra difficulty establishing themselves as separate, independent adults. If the family's style is overly protective or intrusive, as is common when an illness has occurred, the patient and the family probably will have more than the usual difficulty maintaining strong interpersonal boundaries.

Although it is likely that increased differentiation and decreased contact between the patient and his family will decrease stress and thus decrease the potential for relapse, a sudden push toward emancipation produces stress in and of itself. For these reasons, it is best to avoid dealing with the goal of emancipation during the inpatient phase or during the early stages of aftercare. However strongly these families or patients claim to desire emancipation, increased differentiation and/or independence is to them a controversial and difficult task. The introduction of such an issue during or immediately following hospitalization for psychosis creates stresses rather than diminishing them. Furthermore, a focus on emancipation early in treatment often causes the "emmeshed" family to feel overwhelmed or criticized, pushing them to resist or even discontinue therapy. Discharge planning that pushes "emancipation" through a transitional living placement is often sabotaged by the patient, the family, or both. Even after months of gradual preparation, many of these families react to the introduction of the issue of separation catastrophically, attempting to totally reject or totally engulf the patient. This polarization is to be avoided for patient survival and survival of the treatment relationship.

Therefore, simple tasks which provide structure are strongly suggested as first steps toward more complete responsibility and reintegration into the world beyond the family. The level of difficulty of these tasks is based on an ongoing assessment of the maximum amount of stimulation the patient can tolerate without relapse.

For instance, after hospitalization, the patient frequently does not take responsibility for chores around the house, often sleeping for inordinate amounts of time. Small, time-limited, structured chores can be assigned, with a slow movement toward larger, more independent activities. Often joint chores (done with another family member) are assigned to promote positive familial interaction as well as give the patient a support and guide. After the accomplishment of initial household tasks, social activities involving the patient and a nonconflictual immediate family member can be prescribed, followed by time-limited social outings with members of the extended family or close friends. Later in treatment, the patient can be urged to engage in more structured social outings such as those conducted by neighborhood organizations. In this way, the patient gradually is moved toward greater independence.

Of particular importance in this entire treatment process is the idea of making one change at a time. For example, if the patient has obtained a new job, it is not the time to discontinue his medication. If he has moved into a new apartment, it is not the time to change jobs. This point must be stressed repeatedly for two reasons. One, patients often become impatient because they are so far behind their peers in accomplishing developmental tasks. When they feel good, therefore, they often try to do everything simultaneously. Two, therapists, particularly young ones, so highly value emancipation that they tend to push for its attainment unrealistically. This is often reinforced by the idea that the family is disturbed and destructive, and therefore the patient should be helped to "escape" immediately. Most families are not destructive, just anxious. However, even if the family is destructive, the patient must take one step at a time and only when he is ready to do so.

Ongoing Treatment

Aftercare sessions begin just before the patient is discharged from the hospital and continue after the patient returns home, at a gradually decreasing frequency. Since the primary goal is a gradual re-engagement of the patient, weekly meetings appear to be counterproductive, implying that we anticipate rapid progress. A less frequent schedule sets a more appropriate therapeutic pace and is more comfortable for the patient, the family, and the therapist. Since this is the time of highest risk for relapse, the emphasis during these sessions is on dealing with ideas, conflicts, or problems that interfere with the effective functioning of the patient and the family. The therapist and the family choose issues from the established treatment contract which must be resolved in order for the family to begin to live together with a minimum of chaos. Individual or family issues not related to patient survival are introduced only after an extended period of stable functioning and only when discussion of such issues is desired by all concerned.

Ongoing Support

To begin a process of de-isolation and desensitization of the families, we suggest exposing family members to other families struggling with similar issues and problems. This can best be accomplished through the use of inpatient and outpatient multiple-family groups or self-help organizations [4,6,8,15,22,42]. Within these groups common themes and emotional reactions can be shared and coping mechanisms can be passed from one family to another. In our groups, family members who have not yet been able to follow through on the clinician's suggestions have passed the same suggestion on to a member of another family struggling with a similar issue. As families mutually reinforce one another and their attempts to cope, the clinician's job is made easier.

DISCUSSION

The method of intervention described in this chapter is different from traditional family therapy in a variety of ways. It is suggested as an alternative to traditional family therapy for the following reasons.

Most professionals who have attempted family therapy with chronic schizophrenic patients have found that traditional family therapy is often unsuccessful and at times even stimulates noncompliance, crises, or relapse. There are probably several reasons for this failure. Perhaps the most significant is the number of potentially negative metacommunications given by family therapy itself. These metacommunications needlessly erect obstacles and resistances to family interventions, and exact a price from the family in terms of pain, guilt, anxiety, and diminished self-respect.

For instance, many family therapists communicate that change is best obtained through family sessions alone. For schizophrenic families, this communications implicitly suggests that we know what schizophrenia is (a family disease), what causes it (families), and what cures it (family therapy). To suggest that change can occur by family therapy alone suggests that it is not necessary to cooperate with the rest of the multidisciplinary team. Noncompliance with medication is subtly encouraged, a process that is not only potentially problematic to the patients and their families, but also creates problems with colleagues. Furthermore, to suggest cavalierly that family therapy is *the* method of treating this serious problem is evidence of unwarranted arrogance. There is little data to support *any* current explanation of the origins of schizophrenia, much less evidence that we can effectively influence the course of this illness. For this reason, it would seem best to keep all options open and all resources available.

Furthermore, the institution of family therapy often contains the unwitting metacommunication that the family is to blame. While claiming to have a systems focus, many family therapists begin their assessment by attempting to determine how a family keeps a poor struggling young person sick. They search historically or in the here and now for familial causes of this illness. Rarely is a thought given to the potential impact on family members of years of bizarre behavior on the part of the patient. Unusual family behavior is rarely viewed as responsive rather than causal.

Also, family therapy too often includes the implicit or explicit message that the patient is not "ill" but is a symptom of a "family problem." This message requires that families, in order to be helped, deny their version of reality. With little respect for the family's perspective, families are asked to accept the professional's view that the patient's inappropriate, paranoid, or bizarre behavior is a response to family tensions or communications. The communication that schizophrenia is a family problem leaves families confused, helpless, and angry at both the patient and the therapist. This request is reminiscent of what Laing called "mind bending," a process viewed as destructive when it involves parents and their children. Furthermore, defining the family as the problem too often decreases parental authority by putting them in a "one-down" position, confused and anxious about their abilities. This is counter-productive to the very goals we seek to attain, namely—the reinforcement of healthy generational boundaries, clear power structures, and effective communication within families.

Another metacommunication of many family therapy approaches is that increased understanding or better communication will enable the patient to function better. If an illness severe enough to require hospitalization has occurred, the patient is usually behaving in a bizarre manner and the family is in crisis. When things have gone this far, increased understanding or better communication may or may not help the patient to function. However, sessions which attempt to increase family understanding and communication without clearly tying this focus to the patient's ability to function tend to alienate families from professionals who are attempting to help them.

This is not to say that traditional family therapy will never work with chronic patients. Some patients and some families will respond, whether through the sheer force of the therapist's personality and persistence or because they manage to take the good and ignore the bad. We believe our family approach is more humane *and* more effective.

The family approach proposed here specifically avoids the pitfall of unwittingly increasing family anxiety by implicitly blaming them for the patients' problems. Messages are given to families that specifically undercut the attribution of family causality and blame for the illness. Information is given which mobilizes family anxiety and concern into productive coping mechanisms. This family approach is based on ongoing cooperation and communication between professionals of various disciplines. In this way it helps to provide continuity of care, while avoiding pointless power struggles and therapist burn-out. In this approach clinicians are able to support patients, families, and one another when fatigue and hopelessness set in.

SUMMARY

We have described a method of intervention for families of patients with schizophrenia which begins with the admission to the hospital and continues after the patient's discharge. Our program stresses a structured step-by-step approach toward decreased family criticism and involvement and increased patient independence. The key elements are the provision of support and information to family members to decrease anxiety and maximize the family's use of internal and external resources. The goals are to educate and inform family members to help restructure family interactional styles; to increase familial support systems; and help the patient and his family move at a slow, nonthreatening pace toward individuation and emancipation. What we believe is unique about this program is the interaction and cooperation between the medical treatments (hospitalization and medication), family therapy interventions, and the introduction of educative sessions for family members. Although it is described as a program for chronic schizophrenics and their families, we believe the principles are sound and applicable to family work with any long-term serious physical or mental illness.

REFERENCES

1. Anderson, C.M. "Family intervention with severely disturbed inpatients." *Archives of General Psychiatry* 34 : 697–702, 1977.
2. Anderson, C.M.; Hogarty, G.E.; and Reiss, D.J. "Family treatment of adult schizophrenic patients: a psycho-educational approach." *Schizophrenia Bulletin* 6 : 490–505, 1980.
3. Appleton, W.S. "Mistreatment of patients' families by psychiatrists." *American Journal of Psychiatry* 131 : 6, 655–657, 1974.
4. Atwood, N. and Williams, M. "Group support for the families of the mentally ill." *Schizophrenia Bulletin* 4(3) : 415–426, 1978.

5. Bachman, B.J. "Re-entering the community: A former patient's view." *Hospital and Community Psychiatry* 22 : 119–122, 1971.
6. Barcai, A. "An adventure in multiple family therapy," *Family Process* 6 : 185–192, 1967.
7. Beels, C.C. "Family and social management of schizophrenia." *Schizophrenia Bulletin* 1(13) : 97–118, 1975.
8. Berman, K. "Multiple family therapy: its possibilities in preventing readmission." In: G.D. Erickson and T.P. Hogan (eds). *Family Therapy: An Introduction to Theory and Technique.* Monterey, CA: Brooks/Cole Publishing Company, 1972, pp. 279–284.
9. Brown, G.W. and Birley, J.L.T. "Crises and life change and the onset of schizophrenia. *Journal of Health and Social Behavior* 9 : 203–214, 1968.
10. Brown, G.W.; Birley, J.L.T.; and Wing, J.H. "The influence of family life on the course of schizophrenic disorders. A replication." *British Journal of Psychology* 121 : 241–258, 1972.
11. Cole, J.O.; Goldberg, S.C.; and Davis, J.M. "Drugs in the treatment of psychosis: Controlled studies." In: P. Solomon (ed.) *Psychiatric Drugs.* New York: Grune & Stratton, Inc., 1966, pp. 153–180.
12. Cole, J.O.; Goldberg, S.C.; and Klerman, G.L. "Phenothiazine treatment in acute schizophrenia." *Archives of General Psychiatry* 10 : 246–261, 1964.
13. Corbett, L. "Perceptual dyscontrol: a possible organizing principle for schizophrenia research." *Schizophrenia Bulletin* 2 : 249–265, 1976.
14. Deasy, L.C. and Quinn, O.W. "The wife of the mental patient and the hospital psychiatrist." *Journal of Social Issues* 11 : 49–60, 1955.
15. Detre, T.P.; Sayers, J.; Norton, N.M.; and Lewis, H.C. "An experimental approach to the treatment of the acutely ill psychiatric patient in the general hospital." *Connecticut Medicine* 25 : 613–619, 1961.
16. Doherty, E.G. "Labeling effects in psychiatric hospitalization." *Archives of General Psychiatry* 32 : 562–568, 1975.
17. Erikson, K.T. "Notes on the sociology of deviance." *Social Problems* 9 : 307–314, 1962.
18. Falloon, I.R.H.; Liberman, R.P.; Simpson, G.M.; and Talbot, R.E. Family therapy with relapsing schizophrenics: a research proposal. Unpublished manuscript, 1978.
19. Goldberg, S.C.; Schooler, N.R.; Hogarty, G.E.; and Roper, M. "Prediction of relapse in schizophrenic outpatients treated by drug and social therapy." *Archives of General Psychiatry* 34 : 171–184, 1977.
20. Goldstein, M. and Rodnick, E. "The family's contribution to the etiology of schizophrenia: current status." *Schizophrenia Bulletin* 1(14) : 48–63, 1975.
21. Greenley, J.R. "Familial expectations, post-hospital adjustment and the societal reaction perspective on mental illness." *Journal of Health and Social Behavior* 20 : 217–227, 1979.
22. Harrow, M.; Astrachan, B.M.; Becker, R.E.; Detre, T.P.; and Schwartz, A.H. "An investigation into the nature of the patient-family therapy group." *American Journal of Orthopsychiatry* 37 : 888–899, 1967.
23. Hatfield, A.B. "The family as partners in the treatment of mental illness." *Hospital and Community Psychiatry* 30(5) : 338–340, 1979.
24. Hatfield, A.B. "Psychological cost of schizophrenia." *Social Work* 23(5) : 355–359, 1978.
25. Herz, M.I. and Melville, C. "Relapse in schizophrenics." *American Journal of Psychiatry* 137 : 801–805, 1980.
26. Hogarty, G.E.; Goldberg, S.C.; and Schooler, N.R. "Drug and sociotherapy in the aftercare of schizophrenic patients." *Archives of General Psychiatry* 31 : 609–618, 1974.
27. Hogarty, G.E.; Schooler, N.R.; Ulrich, R.; Mussare, F.; Ferro, P.; and Herron, E. Fluphenazine and social therapy in the aftercare of schizophrenic patients." *Archives of General Psychiatry* 36 : 1283–1294, 1979.
28. Hogarty, G.E. and Ulrich, R.F. "Temporal effects of drug and placebo in delaying relapse in schizophrenic outpatients." *Archives of General Psychiatry* 34 : 297–301, 1977.

29. Jacob, T. "Family interaction in disturbed and normal families: a methodological and substantive review." *Psychological Bulletin* 82 : 33–65, 1975.

30. Jones, J.E. "Patterns of transactional style deviance in the TAT's of parents of schizophrenics." *Family Process* 16 : 327–337, 1977.

31. Jones, J.E.; Rodnick, E.; Goldstein, M.; McPherson, S.; and West, K. "Parental transactional style deviance as a possible indicator of risk for schizophrenia." *Archives of General Psychiatry* 34 : 71–74, 1977.

32. Kreisman, D.E. and Joy, V.D. "Family response to the mental illness of a relative: a review of the literature." *Schizophrenia Bulletin*, 1(10) : 34–54, 1974.

33. Lamb, H.R. and Oliphaint, E. "Schizophrenia through the eyes of families." *Hospital and Community Psychiatry* 29(12) : 805–806, 1978.

34. Linn, N.W.; Caffey, E.M.; Lett, C.J.; Hogarty, G.E.; and Lamb, H.R. "Day treatment and psychotropic drugs in the aftercare of schizophrenic patients." *Archives of General Psychiatry* 36 : 1055–1066, 1979.

35. Linn, M.W.; Klett, C.J.; and Caffey, E.M. "Foster home characteristics and psychiatric patient outcome." *Archives of General Psychiatry* 37 : 129–132, 1980.

36. McDonald, N. "The other side: living with schizophrenia." *Canadian Medical Association Journal* 82 : 218–221, 1960.

37. Minuchin, S. "Structural family therapy." In: S. Arieti (ed.) *American Handbook of Psychiatry*, Vol. II. New York: Basic Books, Inc., 1974, pp. 178–192.

38. Mosher, L.R. and Keith, S.J. "Psychosocial Treatment: individual, group, family, and community support approaches." *Schizophrenia Bulletin* 6 : 10–41, 1980.

39. Schooler, N.R.; Levine, J.; Severe, J.B.; Brauzer, B.; DiMascio, A.; Klerman, G.L.J.; and Tuason, V.B. "Prevention of relapse in schizophrenia: an evaluation of fluphenazine decanoate." *Archives of General Psychiatry* 37 : 16–24, 1980.

40. Singer, M.T., and Wynne, L.C. "Thought disorder and family relations of schizophrenics." *Archives of General Psychiatry* 12 : 187–212, 1965.

41. Singer, M.T., and Wynne, L.C. "Communication styles in parents of normals, neurotics, and schizophrenics." *Psychiatric Research Reports* 20 : 25–38, 1966.

42. Strelnick, A.H. Multiple family group therapy: A review of the literature." *Family Process* 16 : 307–326, 1977.

43. Taube, C. "Readmissions to inpatient services of state and county mental hospitals 1972. Statistical Note 110. Biometry Branch, NIMH, 1974.

44. Tecce, J.J. and Cole, J.O. "The distraction-arousal hypothesis, CNV, and schizophrenia. In: D.I. Mostofsky (ed.) *Behavior Control and Modification of Physiological Activity*. Englewood Cliffs, N.J.: Prentice-Hall, Inc., 1976.

45. Torrey, E.F. "Is schizophrenia universal? An open question." *Schizophrenia Bulletin* 7 : 53–59, 1973.

46. Van Putten, T. and May, P.R.A. "Milieu therapy of the schizophrenias. In: L.J. West and P.E. Flinn (eds.) *Treatment of Schizophrenia*. New York: Grune & Stratton, Inc., 1976, pp. 217–243.

47. Vaughn, C.E. and Leff, J.P. "The influence of family and social factors on the course of psychiatric illness." *British Journal of Psychiatry* 129 : 125–137, 1976.

48. Wing, J.K., and Brown, G.W. *Institutionalism and Schizophrenia*. Cambridge: Cambridge University Press, 1970.

49. Wyatt, R. Frontiers of research: an overview of NIMH research, research around the world, medication effects and patient therapies. Presented at the Annual Conference of the National Alliance for the Mentally Ill, 1980.

5

Multiple-Family Therapy in the Psychiatric Hospital

WILLIAM R. McFARLANE

Multiple-family therapy is, simply, the treatment of several families simultaneously through the vehicle of a group meeting led by therapists. This approach has been, and continues to be, closely identified with psychiatric hospitals and the patients most often treated there. Many applications of multiple-family therapy (MFT, hereafter) have developed over the course of the past 20 years, centering on outpatient clinics and nonpsychotic patients. But the most striking results and the most experimentation are occurring within the context of services oriented to the more severely disturbed patient population. The reasons for this phenomenon are complex and are examined in detail below, but part of the explanation is contained within the story of the origins of one of the first multiple-family groups, (MFG, hereafter).

During the late 1950s, Laqueur was in charge of a research unit at Creedmoor State Hospital, Queens, New York [26]. Initially, treatment emphasis was on insulin coma therapy and later, chemotherapy. In addition, Laquer and the staff organized the ward as a therapeutic community in order to maximize therapeutic efforts. Having elected to hold one of the principle community meetings during visiting hours, the staff was faced with a situation in which many of the patients, most of whom were young adult schizophrenics, would drift out of the meeting to spend time with their families, especially their parents. When the staff attempted to intercede, the parents began protesting the lack of consideration for their needs. Hoping to salvage their ward meeting, some of the staff were assigned to meet weekly with the parents as a group, to explain ward policy, their therapeutic intents, the progress of the patients, and so forth. This meeting was held simultaneously with the patients' meeting, but in another location. While one segment of the staff was struggling to create a cohesive group of patients, many of whom were psychotic, another was attempting to create a parents' committee. The latter turned out to be somewhat dull and fragmented, although many of the relatives expressed appreciation for the information they received from this new service.

After a few weeks, some of the patients again drifted out of the community meeting, this time insisting on joining the parents' group. Laqueur noted that a few of the patients who preferred the parents' committee behaved significantly better there than in the therapeutic community meeting. They were more attuned to their surroundings, behaved in a less bizarre manner, and were capable of surprisingly appropriate interactions. He decided to combine the two groups into a joint session; the results were astonishing to everyone concerned. This new group was remarkably cohesive, almost immediately. The activity level of patients and relatives was increased, with only a few minor episodes of agitation and family quarrels. Although the staff initially maintained a committee format, they also began to see family interaction directly and to sense that the parents and other relatives felt reasonably supported by the staff and each other, and thus relatively safe. This combination presented an irresistible opportunity to make therapeutic interventions. Gradually, the "committee" became an MFT group which began to have gratifyingly positive effects on both patients and relatives. Probably of equal importance, the staff was fascinated and energized by the meetings and — paradoxically — found them easier to lead than either of the previous formats. The families found the group valuable; most relatives and patients became highly invested in it. Attendance and punctuality improved. Within a short time, this new modality had become the central focus of the ward's activities. The rest of the development of this group is described elsewhere [27].

It is unclear how much of this tale is myth, but it does tell a great deal about some of the distinctive features of MFT. MFGs often develop into highly cohesive and nearly self-directed "small societies" [37] that generate strong feelings of loyalty and enthusiasm and a surprising amount of openness to change among the members [6,16,25,32,39]. In retrospect, it appears that Laqueur's group had a centripetal, cohesive quality before it was actually formed; the families created the group for the staff. Furthermore, the sense of support and reassurance that families appeared to gain from the group was evident within a few meetings. Also, the process unique to MFT — the often uncanny accuracy of group members' observations about other families' dysfunctional interactions and the willingness of members to accept and utilize these comments — appeared very early in that group and with minimal initiative on the part of the staff. In addition, the improvement in patients' symptomatology consequent to the MFGs formation resulted from the group's capacity to diffuse intrafamily intensity while simultaneously validating and encouraging the family's identity as a family [8,28,29,32,33]. Finally, the enthusiastic response of the therapists to the original MFG has been replicated regularly in the subsequent experience of most practitioners. This virtue may seem less relevant, but from the perspective of the mass of unmet service needs still facing the mental health professions, any modality that is effective and economical and also tends to build staff morale will be more useful than those that are simply effective. This will be especially true when the modality is built on previous skills—group and family therapy.

SOLVING PROBLEMS OF HOSPITALIZATION

As a means of better understanding the role that MFT can play in a psychiatric hospital setting, it is useful to outline some of the problems that are inherent in the institutionalization of the psychotic patient and review how MFT can ameliorate or solve them.

Family Alienation

Hospitalization inevitably creates a focus on the individual patient and his psychosis as the principle priorities of treatment. The needs of family members tend thereby to become secondary. At the same time, it is a dramatic event, full of implications of failure and defect. One effect of these phenomena is to promote the family's preexisting sense of powerlessness and guilt. Add to that the effects of the widespread belief that families do something to cause mental illness, and the result is a set of relatives—especially parents—who feel helpless, blamed, and estranged [1,2]. Some unsophisticated family therapy has tended to worsen the situation by implying that family disturbance alone has caused the psychosis.

Multiple-family therapy addresses this problem in several ways. When the leaders work to foster cohesion, group support, and problem-solving efforts, the effects include: (1) a ready sharing of profound feelings of guilt and shame, with the consequent development of an equally profound sense of relief, in the parents, particularly; (2) an implicit and explicit empowering of the relatives and patients to find means of diminishing family conflict and of fostering the best possible atmosphere for the prevention of exacerbations of the illness; (3) a marked and often surprising degree of openness about the severe family problems that do exist. In short, once the family members feel validated by the group and the staff, they become remarkably available to therapeutic intervention. Further, MFT reduces and usually reverses the family's sense of estrangement by giving the members a structured role and set of expectations within the total treatment plan, without necessarily impugning them with having caused the patient's decompensation.

Family Fragmentation

Hospitalization, with the important exception of partial hospitalization, fragments the family. Although hospitalization tends to interrupt positive-feedback cycles within the family, this advantage is usually short-lived [23]. The catch, of course, is that most families with a psychotic member are more or less fragmented even in equilibrium. So, as happens so often, what is at one time a solution — the physical removal of the patient from the family — tends to then become a problem in itself. The family has usually attempted to overcome fragmentation by visiting. The results of family visits to the patient on the ward are well known to most clinicians; too often, visits are followed by relapse. Another traditional solution, having the family seen by a therapist other than the one treating the patient, results in more fragmentation of family and staff. Single-family therapy is capable of building family integration and diffusing the members' anxiety, confusion, and triangulation processes but requires great skill and a tremendous investment of the therapist's energy. A significant contribution to the fragmentation on many busy wards is the difficulty the family has in obtaining information that is consistent and understandable about both the specifics of the illness and the more general aspects of treatment, prognosis, availability of ancillary services, and so on.

Multiple-family therapy has many positive effects on these fragmenting processes. The family is able to meet together, but under a controlled situation in which the more blatant forms of family dysfunction can be interrupted by therapists or group members. Family members are able to see how their relative is doing, and can obtain direct information from staff. Since the latter are outnumbered by patients and relatives, they tend to give more straightforward answers. Many MFG leaders have reported that they have come to see this as a major advantage to the modality. All concerned seem to be able to give and receive information in a more efficient, relevant and less defensive manner [12,22,32]. Additionally, the presence of other families that are undergoing similar disasters and are engaged in the group as a way to deal with them promotes a sense of family cohesion and more positive family identity. The reduction in guilt commonly noted in MFGs also contributes to the development of family integration. In a larger sense, the staff and the families become better integrated, since they have an explicit common goal and are meeting conjointly. Since most MFG leaders attempt to remain neutral in their treatment of patients and relatives, the fragmenting effect of the staff's tendency to take the patients' side will be reduced. Usually when leaders do unwittingly take sides, other group members will make compensatory maneuvers.

Exacerbation of Enmeshment

Most families with a psychotic member are enmeshed and hospitalization tends to exacerbate the situation [9,30,35]. When the ill member is physically absent from the home, most families become even more emotionally involved with the patient than previously. Traditional efforts to isolate the patient from the parents or spouse usually have the same effect. This process is comprehensible from a family systems viewpoint — as an example of triangulation — but most therapeutic efforts aimed at detriangulation simply are inadequate to stop the process in a psychotic-level family. Increasingly, clinicians and researchers are recognizing that much of the enmeshment and tenacity of these families derives from the more obvious sources of guilt and family loyalty [1,2,3,17]. That is, when faced with the catastrophe that is mental illness in a loved one (frequently the family's "special child"), the *least* likely response is that the family would disengage from the ill member. Thus, when the patient is separated, the stage is set for a series of overloaded interactions at visiting hours — even during family therapy sessions — that are likely to overwhelm the fragile emotional and perceptual capacities of the patient. This also occurs at discharge time, or even during discharge planning, provoking decompensation and requiring readmission [44].

This tendency toward enmeshment has been widely recognized as a key factor in, at the very least, the aggravation of psychotic illnesses; it has not as yet been demonstrated to be either universal or etiological. The reasons that most conventional forms of family therapy are usually unsuccessful in decreasing enmeshment in these families are complex and still not well understood. What is clear is that the therapist working with such families is presented with an extraordinarily delicate task. He must be able to simultaneously support every member of the crucial triad, while also making the necessary structural shifts in the family's relationship patterns. This is frequently beyond the capacities of most mortal therapists. In fact, one could argue that in the most severely disturbed families, it is theoretically impossible.

The MFG, particularly when made available to the patient's family well beyond the period of hospitalization, can accomplish significant degrees of disenmeshment. The process involved is quite complex, but the major aspects can be isolated. First, MFGs promote a remarkable degree of freedom of expression and openness of communication. Second, this openness leads to direct comments between group members about concrete examples of enmeshment, overinvolvement and overprotectiveness, many of which are enacted in the session itself. Third, though such interventions provoke considerable anxiety in the recipient, there is such a large pool of actual and potential supportive alliances available in the group that it is rare that the recipient finds the observation and its implications intolerable. That is, someone, usually a fellow-sufferer, is able to soften whatever blow is delivered, while other members tend to keep the process sufficiently on track so that the issue is not lost, or the effect neutralized. Fourth, over longer periods of time a group culture develops that tends to hold each family responsible for following through on instituting suggested alternatives and maintaining them. Finally, when groups are run indefinitely, parents especially begin to develop real social relationships within the group that in a structural sense replace the overinvested bonds with the patient.

Family Isolation

Family socialization through MFT solves another problem that hospitalization — as well as the illness itself — tends to worsen: the social isolation of the family of the psychotic person. Throughout the past 20 years there have appeared sporadic reports that families of schizophrenic and manic-depressive patients have remarkably restricted social networks [5,9,13,18,20,36,40,44]. From a systems point of view, social isolation and enmeshment at the family level are complementary aspects of the same problem: a relatively impermeable social boundary around the family. Wynne has referred to this as the familiar "rubber-fence" phenomenon. In practical terms, this implies that it is equally as hard for family members to make social and even instrumental connections outside the family boundary as it is for nonfamily (specifically non-kin [39] to penetrate the boundary and establish reciprocal and satisfying connections with family members. These same reports present a glimmering of evidence that this phenomenon precedes the onset of the psychotic process *per se*. The functional relationship between enmeshment and isolation is rather straightforward: the degree of isolation is in direct proportion to the likelihood that enmeshment and positive feedback processes go uninterrupted. This in turn increases the likelihood of a return of symptoms in the vulnerable individual.

What does hospitalization have to do with this process? For most families and patients the process of commitment represents a crystallization of the powerful stigma that is still carried by mental illness. As such, it almost inevitably exacerbates demoralization, a sense of defeat, and the guilt-anxiety-overinvolvement cycle. These factors alone tend to lead to a further withdrawal from social life. Additionally, the family's *sense* of isolation is increased by their perception that others may be withdrawing from them consequent to learning of the family's misfortune. In essence, the family frequently is left with no one to relate to but the patient, and that is often in a pathological manner.

A well-led MFG within a hospital setting reverses many of these pathology-amplifying tendencies toward isolation. One author has described the

MFG and network therapy as social rituals for the family in a situation in which there are none, at least none that provide social and cognitive assistance [4]. Multiple-family therapy offers a structured social milieu with fairly well-defined tasks and roles for the participants. The members' isolation is usually converted to a sense of belonging, of being known, acknowledged, and validated. Stigma becomes the ticket of admission to an exclusive social organization. The sense of relief and enhanced self-esteem resulting from this process is almost always verbalized by many members of the group and is probably the precondition for any substantive structural change within these families. As noted above, MFT goes beyond relieving the members' feelings of isolation by offering actual social connections and supports that are acceptable and appreciated, and yet not so intense or obligatory that the family members feel compelled to flee. By being given a specific role in the treatment without having to accept blame for having caused their relative's illness, family members are often mobilized to attempt alternative ways of relating to the patient and each other. At a cognitive level, they develop a shared meaning and significance to one another in relation to the illness. It might be remembered that outside Western culture, large groups involving whole families are the normative mechanism for most healing and preventive efforts. Thus MFT can be seen as a modern form of tribal social organization created specifically for the healing and health-maintenance of afflicted members. In short, an MFG can correct for the essential isolation of many families with a psychotic member and compensates for some of the factors in hospitalization that tend to increase that isolation.

Family Non-Compliance

At the risk of sounding trivial and simplistic, it should be stated that most of the treatment modalities offered to psychotic patients and their relatives are experienced by them as unpleasant, stressful, and rarely of obvious help. In the author's experience, patients simply do not like individual therapy, pharmacotherapy, milieu therapy, group therapy, and family therapy. Patients' family members often have negative reactions to these modalities, except perhaps to medication, as long as it is not for them. The reactions of both parties to hospitalization itself needs no comment. The reason that these considerations are not trivial lies in the fact that most of the psychoses are not discrete illness episodes, but exacerbations of severe and fundamental dysfunction at several levels. For the time being, schizophrenia and manic-depressive illness are generally life-long processes. Therefore, it becomes essential to provide an effective treatment over long periods of time that is *experienced* as helpful, as well as being so, to maximize the chance that the patient and family will continue to participate in treatment. That is, most people will not continue to involve themselves in an unpleasant activity for most of their adult lives if it appears that there is any chance that avoiding it will not have disastrous consequences.

Most patients and their family members seem to enjoy multiple family groups. This observation was stressed in the earliest reports on MFT, has been consistent over the ensuing years, and has been noted by the author consistently in his experience [16,21,39]. It is not at all uncommon for most of the members of a time-limited MFG to insist that it continue. Attendance remains high with frequent spontaneous requests that other involved family members be admitted.

Continuity of Care

One problem, while perhaps not inherent in hospital treatment but so common that it appears to be so, is the great difficulty most services have in providing a continuous format for therapy that bridges inpatient and outpatient phases. The evidence that such continuity aids, or is possibly essential to, prevention of early relapse is beyond the scope of this chapter. However, the reader is most likely aware of the issues involved. He is probably aware also of the tendency of patients to discontinue most after-care programs prematurely and then to require readmission. One key factor in this drop-out problem is the lack of involvement of family members in the after-care process. Having been somewhat excluded from the inpatient phase, many family members assume that it is the hospital's responsibility to handle issues of continuity. They tend not to press the patient to persist in treatment and often decide that the therapist is aware of the reappearance of minor signs and symptoms, sometimes when the patient is not attending clinic at all. Added to this is the all-too-forgivable hope that somehow the illness is over and will just go away on its own, like most other episodic medical diseases. Too often this denial is abetted by simple lack of information as to what to expect. Some workers have been taking this problem quite seriously in recent experimental programs [1,2,17,30]. Most have elected to use the multiple-family format, though in some instances without the presence of the patient for some or all of the process.

The impact that an MFG can have on problems of continuity is often significant. By involving family members in treatment before discharge, the way is paved for an easier transition to community life. Multiple-family therapy creates a social milieu that is organized around desire to keep the gains made in the hospital and to expedite whatever further improvement is possible after discharge. Since the MFG frequently becomes the principle focus of attention for staff, patients, and family during hospitalization, there is a tendency to see the major part of the treatment as continuous; the actual discharge becomes a much less significant event. If the group has achieved a moderate cohesion, it will tolerate a change of therapists with minimal regression. This makes simpler many of the administrative problems that make continuity so difficult to achieve in many settings. Since MFT promotes a more rapid social adjustment, the patient makes a smoother transition to community living [38]. Finally, if providing more complete information about the psychoses to patients and their families is demonstrated to reduce relapse rates and enhance compliance of patients and their families, the MFG is the logical format for undertaking this difficult task.

PROCESS AND TECHNIQUE IN MULTIPLE-FAMILY GROUPS

For heuristic purposes, a discussion of techniques can be divided into two approaches: one for younger, nonpsychotic hospitalized patients and the other for the chronically or periodically psychotic population. While these are typical MFT applications, they also represent the extremes of a continuum with many intermediate forms. (Not discussed are couples' groups and MFGs for family subunits, but the principles are essentially similar.) Certain aspects, however, apply for both patient types and are reviewed briefly.

The administrative and clinical context of the group must be supportive and enthusiastic; MFT is greatly facilitated when it is the central psychosocial modality in the unit or after-care program. This is necessary for several reasons. An MFG is very demanding of staff energy and time in the opening phase. If the MFG is competing with other modalities for staff and family attention, it will rarely get started at all. Also, many families will avoid an MFG — even though they will usually prefer it once participating — if offered other alternatives. The ideal treatment program on an inpatient service is to combine a therapeutic milieu with MFT and abundant occupational therapy programs, plus good psychiatric coverage for medication. For after-care, an MFG with access to a crisis team and regular medication review is adequate and effective.

All MFGs share with most other group modalities a good deal of difficulty in getting started [41]. Anxiety runs fairly high all around. A number of technical interventions can greatly facilitate moving beyond this opening phase. Family preparation, sometimes running to four or five sessions, is usually necessary before joining the group in order to evaluate family dynamics, reduce anxiety, orient the family to the process, and build a trusting alliance with the therapists. Leadership style during the first few group meetings must be active, directive, confident, educative, warm, even humorous, and inviting of therapist-family interaction. The author uses elaborate introduction rituals, asking the family members to tell their story with emphasis on the positive aspects of life together and allowing each member to make a brief speech about himself and his perceptions and feelings about the family. Also, a paradoxical injunction against seriously discussing any family problems in the first two sessions will greatly allay anxiety, especially if framed as necessary to "get to know one another as normal people." The leaders should describe the goals, methods, and ground rules in detail. Emphasis is needed on regular participation, punctuality, and, when likely, violence should be explicitly proscribed. The desired types of interaction should be overtly encouraged and modeled by the therapists. Some groups require a one-person-at-a-time rule to control private conversations and simultaneous contributions by several members. Physically, the room should be large, comfortable, and supplied with enough chairs oriented so that everyone can see the other participants.

The therapists should ideally be quite familiar with each other's work and have an explicit contract to candidly discuss their individual interventions. Once the group gets underway, affect runs very high in an MFG and intense family dramas unfold regularly. The opportunities for countertransference reactions are thereby made most numerous and can quickly lead to splitting and/or replication of a family's dysfunctional relationships by the therapists. The most effective antidote to these tendencies is consistent and honest communication between therapists in post-session meetings. The number of therapists needed depends on many factors, but two is probably the minimum for all but the most seasoned clinicians. Having both sexes represented is almost a necessity and the racial composition of the group should be reflected in the therapist team. Many centers use trainees as observers or video operators to great advantage. However, it is inadvisable to have MFGs in a hospital setting led entirely by inexperienced staff unless live supervision is provided for each meeting. The leaders should ideally be experienced in group methods and also with family therapy. To be maximally effective, the therapists should have roughly comparable views on family systems, since they need a consistent and coherent model of family functioning, normal and pathological, against which to measure family process as seen in the group and to assess group-derived strategies for family change. The author has found that a combination of structural and strategic models is the most useful theoretical and pragmatic base to deal with the severely disturbed families seen in a hospital practice [19;35].

The Nonpsychotic MFG

Further description of therapeutic technique requires differentiation between psychotic and nonpsychotic populations. In a largely nonpsychotic group, the goal is to restructure family relationship patterns so that the family no longer requires the patient's symptomatic behavior for its stability. The MFG is most useful with more isolated and fragile families, regardless of diagnosis.* Thus, the group can include borderline, depressed, severely obsessive, and psychosomatic patients, as well as a few young people with behavior disorders. Substance abuse, when it is the chief complaint, usually is an indication for a homogeneous group. The MFG should be composed of like family types, such as parents with patients at home, married couples, and so forth. If the unit is treating a large number of adolescents with behavior disorders, it is advisable to put them together in an MFG specifically for this type of problem. If combined with neurotic patients, the latter's issues are submerged in concern with management and control.

Since most hospital units treating such patients have length-of-stay restrictions, these MFGs are usually open and rotating in membership. For best results, groups should be kept small—four or five families—and several run concurrently so that new families can be distributed more diffusely. The goal is to maximize group cohesion under administrative conditions that make cohesion rather difficult to achieve. For the same reason, arrangements should be made to allow families to continue in the same group after discharge. It is preferable to start groups and keep them closed through termination. In the rotating MFG, each new family will have to be introduced and the group can be expected to withdraw from active therapeutic work for a session or two while the newcomers are woven into the group's fabric. The therapists can expedite the process by sanctioning it, making ample allowances for the new family's anxieties and the group's frustration, and allowing the new family to sit on the sidelines until they are fully ready to present their problems in detail to the group.

Once the group has achieved a minimal level of cohesion, the therapists can begin to promote in-depth discussion of family issues. Initially there is much accusation, especially of parents by offspring, and the therapists may have to directly support the former, while beginning to promote role-specific interaction to ensure that parents do not feel overly blamed. Usually one family spontaneously volunteers itself as the subject for discussion. Early in the group's development, the therapists provide the major portion of therapeutic intervention themselves, almost as if the other families were not there. However, they should shift as rapidly as possible toward diffusing interaction to the other families. This is done through familiar group techniques, such as inviting comparisons and asking for others' observations, suggestions or similar experiences. After a few sessions, the therapists should begin to insist on the

---

* As a general rule, neurotic-level families in which hospitalization is unnecessary are better treated in single-family therapy. Multiple-family therapy is effective with this type of family, but progress is not as rapid. It can be justified when issues of economy are significant, since the difference in effectiveness is small. Adolescents may constitute an exception, in that many outpatient MFGs for this population have been remarkably effective.

group's accepting the major responsibility for handling each family's presentation, while increasingly monitoring the adequacy of the group's performance and filling in when needed. The group leaders should keep discussion on track and summarize the members' comments and suggestions.

Usually by the time this shift becomes possible, blaming has subsided, family boundaries have been dissolved in the group, and a variety of *ad hoc* subgroups come into play—fathers, families with common interests, cross-parenting alliances, etc. Also, most of the intrinsic mechanisms will have been in evidence (see section "Therapeutic Mechanisms in Multiple-Family groups, below). During this intermediate stage, the therapists must ensure that each family is brought into focus at least once, and that each is undergoing structural shifts. Usually a follow-up session will be necessary. In "good" groups, the members take on some of the monitoring function, bringing in the recalcitrant and eliciting the necessary interaction. The therapists can promote this development if the membership stays stable for a long enough period. By this time, not only will a rapid improvement be seen in the identified patient, but a remarkable equality will be developed between generations in the group. Many formerly split families will be seen to be experiencing a new cohesion, harmony, and role structure. If the group remains together long enough, the parents will gradually begin using it to explore solutions to marital and personal problems relating to their offspring's original symptoms. However, therapists must guard against trying to promote this phase prematurely: it is only possible when the identified patient is well on the way to recovery.

In most settings, the nonpsychotic patient group tends to be composed of adolescents and young adults. With them, issues of autonomy, parental control, personal responsibility, and generational alienation usually emerge as the dominant themes. The therapists should make these themes quite explicit and use them to keep discussion focused. When the group is dominated by borderline and depressed patients, there is often concern with rejection, criticism, and emotional deprivation, in addition to the themes noted above.

The Psychotic-Level MFG

By contrast, an MFG composed of families with a chronically or periodically psychotic member has a different orientation, style, and basic purpose. For this population the major therapeutic benefit derives from continued participation and, to a lesser extent, to direct intervention by the therapists or group members. The therapists' main task is to create a viable social network, composed of families afflicted with a psychosis. If therapeutic gains can be accomplished, their potential benefit has to be carefully weighed against the risk of the family's leaving the group. It is implicit in this type of group that most of the families are quite disturbed, with major structural and communication problems and a strong tendency toward being overwhelmed by anxiety. Thus the therapists will rely heavily on the intrinsic mechanisms, especially resocialization, disenmeshment, and stigmatic reversal (see section "Therapeutic Mechanisms in Multiple-Family Groups, below). Also, they will strive to magnify these processes by promoting a wide variety of interactions among group members.

Patient selection should be guided by a few simple rules. Isolation at the family level is the principle indication for MFT, given a diagnosis of psychosis that requires hospitalization. Therefore, very isolated families should be grouped together. Second, the group should be relatively homogeneous as to diagnosis. Manic patients do not do well with schizophrenics and should be put in a separate MFG, if possible. If the situation permits, psychotically depressive patients and their families should meet together. The rule for inclusion of families is straightforward: insist on the attendance of those who significantly affect the patient, especially if living at home. These groups can be larger than the nonpsychotic versions — up to eight families and 30 to 35 people are manageable. Larger size is preferable in that each family will feel less exposed while having a greater variety of people with whom to establish contact. For best results, the group should start with all families joining simultaneously and then be closed, except to replace dropouts. The group should be completely open-ended; the longer it persists, the better. In many settings such groups have a more frequent turnover of participants than is desirable. This is tolerable, but tends to reduce the perceived safety of the group. Obviously, continuation after discharge should be the rule and with the same therapists, if possible.

The phases of a chronic MFG are similar to those described above, but evolve more slowly. Thus, the therapists in the beginning phase have to remain active and invite interaction to occur through them for many sessions, sometimes for months. Affect, especially related to guilt and blaming, has to be kept at a much lower level, basically until it subsides or can be addressed by the parents at an intellectual level. Moving affective issues to the cognitive level proves to be a useful device for controlling anxiety without simply ignoring these vital concerns. From time to time, the therapists should allow more intense interaction to run its course as a means of assessing the capacity of the group to contain and utilize it effectively. Groups vary tremendously in the speed with which they develop, and only trial and error and clinical judgment can accurately evaluate the state of any given MFG. During the early phase, general discussions of what appear to be everyday problems should not be interrupted. The goal is to develop a solid small society; the therapists should remind themselves that they rarely use discussion of severe family difficulties as the medium of conversation when they are making new connections in a strange social environment. The author consciously models interventions in this phase after what would be appropriate host behavior at the initial meetings of a new task-oriented community organization, rather than a psychoanalytically oriented therapy group. Also, the therapists should go to great lengths to emphasize family strengths, positive interactions, and small indications of progress, rather than pathology and dysfunction.

With time, and if the therapists work diligently to create an atmosphere of support, empathy, and social unity, families can be encouraged to discuss their individual difficulties. At the same time the group can be increasingly brought into the discussion, not only as co-sufferers, but as resources for providing feedback and problem solving. Themes that usually arise are overinvolvement of parents, conflict and confusion over reasonable expectations for the identified patient, using psychosis as a means of maintaining an unnecessary degree of dependency, and the needs of parents outside their concern for their psychotic offspring. The therapists should be supportive of increasing the social and occupational role performance of the patients, while gradually but persistently using their own and the group's influence to build more appropriate boundaries between parents and children.

It helps at this stage if movements toward outside socialization by the families with each other is encouraged by the group leaders. This gives the parents a concrete demonstration that there is a tolerable life for them outside of caring for their patient-children. Likewise, some of the patients may make moves to live away from home, and the group can be used to assess the reasonableness of the idea and help the family through the inevitable reactions to separation. The same applies to moves by patients to get involved in jobs, occupational training programs, social organizations, and friendships. Gradually throughout this stage of the group, the therapists will be moving away from their earlier position of being voluntarily triangulated toward being the facilitators, monitors, referees, summarizers, and sources of clinical information for the group.

In some groups, if they persist for two to three years with roughly the same membership, a third stage is reached in which the therapists are almost irrelevant, except as links to the hospital, sources of medication, and occasionally, crisis interveners. By this time relapse rates will have sunk to almost zero, some significant gains will have been made by some patients, and the group will perceive itself as capable, legitimate, and largely self-sufficient. Unfortunately, many hospital settings are too unstable to be able to allow groups to develop to this point, but it is the ultimate goal of an MFG for psychotic-level families. A group at this stage is an excellent vehicle for the training of mental health professionals. Family members often take great pride in teaching trainees a thing or two about the management of psychotic patients and what they have learned through the group. To be sure, the psychosis as a disease will not have been cured, but major parts of the morbidity will have been neutralized.

THERAPEUTIC MECHANISMS IN MULTIPLE-FAMILY GROUPS

There are nine processes or mechanisms that occur within an MFG, some of which are inherent and some of which depend on the skill of the therapist. Assumed here but not discussed are the many well-studied group effects that are not specific to, but usually active in, most MFGs. These include group empathy, belongingness, universalization, tolerance of deviance, ventilation and catharsis, the "helper effect," as well as therapist-induced clarification, interpretation, confrontation, guidance, and so forth [31]. Similarly, the family therapist using MFT will have opportunities to induce de-triangulation, create boundaries, reframe problems and processes, and improve communication, as in single-family work.

Several key phenomena in MFT are essentially intrinsic, so that the therapist makes them available to the members by starting the group and avoiding interference in their evolution. They derive more from group membership — its structure and its social role — than from the activity or skill of the therapist. In the author's experience, with families containing a psychotic member, they are the more powerful effects.

1. *Modulated disenmeshment.* Given that the MFG is a controlled social environment, it uniquely allows gradual, regulable reduction in family enmeshment simultaneously and interdependently with the creation of new interactional and relational bonds with members of other families. At the same time, family bonds are preserved and validated [42]. This process is modulated by the group to proceed at a rate that is tolerable to the family. Thus the all-too-frequent development of overwhelming anxiety that accompanies attempts at intervening in overinvolvement in single-family therapy is avoided. One example is cross-parenting, in which parents develop much more helpful and appropriate relationships with the patient offspring of other families. Also, members first try new forms of interaction with members of other families before proceeding to try them with their own.

2. *Rapid resocialization.* MFT by its very nature puts whole families in contact with one another. Since most families of psychotic patients and many severely disturbed nonpsychotics are socially isolated, a format that increases their social interaction without requiring the skill and integration needed for less

structured and more competitive social situations corrects one major deficit in these families. This major change in function is accomplished simply by the family's attendance. Each family then has available a surrogate neighborhood or social network. Given the evidence that psychopathology is almost linearly associated with isolation of the family and individual, much of the effectiveness of MFT may derive from this mechanism [15,43].

Elements of this process that are therapeutic include: the provision of a rich variety of available supports, periodic scrutiny of family interaction by relatively empathetic others, social pressure toward societal norms of family structure and communication, and a greatly increased quantity of potential ideas and information regarding instrumental aspects of the families' lives (especially the problematic areas). Because enmeshment and isolation are system correlates, disenmeshment and resocialization go hand in hand. It is very difficult to promote the former without the latter.

3. *Stigmatic reversal.* The irony of an MFG is that families are admitted by virtue of a major stigma: mental illness. From a position of marked shame and guilt, most families in MFT experience group acceptance and often develop pride and group identity that are based in sharing concerns and dealing more effectively with psychosis. Since rejection and avoidance are common responses to mental illness, family isolation is also family alienation. Thus an MFG is experienced as a relief because it is a reversal of the rejecting tendencies of most other social groups. It is the author's impression that the high level of group interest and loyalty observed by most MFG leaders follows partly from the conversion of stigma to membership in a special society.

4. *Indirect restructuring.* Family members in MFGs appear to see very clearly the structural and interactional dysfunctions in other families. They also appear to apply these observations to their own families without necessarily making them explicit to themselves. Often, seemingly uninvolved families undergo shifts in relationship patterns after similar shifts are explicitly discussed with respect to another family. It is unfortunate that this phenomenon is so poorly understood; it is conceivable that family members discuss their own similarities to other families outside the group, but this has not been documented. Laqueur's concept of "identification constellation" is one of the elements of this process [29]. The most common example of this mechanism occurs is discussion of subsystem issues — mother and son overinvolvement, inter-sibling inequality, marital problems, in-law interference, and so forth. In some instances, especially with more highly functional families, the similarities are made explicit by another family in the group and an implicit request is made of the group to help the family clarify and modify its own version of the issue under discussion.

5. *Inter-family competition.* In a cohesive MFG, it is quite common for families to become competitive with respect to group participation and clinical

improvement. This is not so surprising from a sociological viewpoint, in that similar processes occur whenever small societies have subgroups, especially families. It may be surprising, however, to the group therapist of psychotic patients, who often seem to compete for the role of the most disabled, and to the family therapist of the same population, who is often faced with similar tendencies toward "one-downmanship" within individual families. The exposure of whole families to one another appears to provoke normative responses in these very disturbed families. Gradually, this competition creates in the group a set of expectations of higher levels of functioning; this in turn has highly beneficial effects on the rate of clinical progress of individual families.

Some mechanisms in MFT depend heavily on the orientation and skill of the therapist. That is, although they may be characteristic of this modality, they are not inherent and will not necessarily operate without the specific intervention of the group leaders.

6. *Inter-family support and confrontation.* An MFG provides a unique opportunity for a rich variety of therapeutic interactions among members of different families. Interactions can range from profound empathy or enthusiastic side taking in a conflict to candid and very accurate confrontation regarding another member's contribution to dysfunctional relationships. In many instances the same words coming from a therapist would lead to denial or panic but, when offered by a group member, they are usually accepted. This can occur between role peers — mother to mother, patient to patient — between families and across roles — child in family A to parent in family B. This process depends on the therapists having modelled these interactions in the early phases of the group and actively and continually promoting interaction among families. From a theoretical standpoint, the different effects of therapist and group member interventions is predictable from communication theory: therapist comments are inherently complementary and occur in a vertical social structure while most member comments are symmetrical and socially horizontal. Thus, the two types of interventions, even if identical in content, are members of different classes of communication.

7. *Positive feedback stabilization.* Much of the morbidity in the chronic psychoses can be attributed to "runaway" processes in the family that lead to relapse in the identified patient. MFT, by diffusing family intensity and providing diversionary avenues for interaction and relationship, can do much to prevent circular processes from reaching pathological levels. In addition, the group leaders can enhance this effect by focusing attention on the specific types of interaction in each family that produce these runaways, and help the group work toward alternative ways of handling affectively loaded situations. Most often this involves interceding in over-close relationships in the family, leading to transfer of involvement from the patient to other members of the group and/or other family members. Frequently, it is also necessary to promote new

relationships within the group for the patient. It may be that simple observation of other families' behavior is a diversion sufficiently powerful to act as a break in circular intrafamily processes.

8. *Tertiary prevention.* Although actually a specific example of stabilization, the capacity of an MFG to arrest incipient relapse and handle small and moderate family crises warrants attention separately. Both group leaders and members will be able to note early signs of psychotic decompensation and/or family crisis and make restitutive moves. Since many decompensations follow life events that affect other family members more directly than the patient, the leaders can anticipate and counteract relapse by helping the group deal with losses and other traumatic events that affect either family members or patients. Once the precedent is established, most MFGs will perform this function almost automatically. The leaders should help families learn to anticipate the consequences of life events and how they tend to affect different family members.

9. *Medication maintenance.* A long-term MFG enhances the use of medication in several ways. Families can be informed of the uses, side effects, and limitations of psychotropic medication, as a group affair. In many cases the therapeutic effects of the group will permit lowering maintenance dosages and will carry patients through drug holidays, when they are indicated. Family resistance and sabotage of necessary drug regimens can be dealt with by the group culture, if handled properly. As Beels has pointed out, the general clinical state of the patient can be assessed inconspicuously, without undue questioning [3]. Since attendance at MFT is usually better than for individual or group therapy, clinicians are more likely to detect emerging signs of tardive dyskinesia and other major side effects. For the same reason, drug dosages can be made more flexible—low during periods of stable functioning and higher during incipient crises. Patient tendencies to stop taking medication precisely when it is needed most can be confronted and overcome by other group members.

THE VARIETIES OF HOSPITAL-BASED MFT: A REVIEW

Multiple-family therapy is most often used with inpatient and psychotic-level populations. It might be useful to review briefly what has been attempted and evaluate, to the extent possible without controlled studies, what these groups have been able to accomplish. The lack of direct comparisons with other modalities has become a serious issue within the small field of MFT, because the impression of nearly every practitioner, published and unpublished, is that with the severely disturbed patient, MFT seems the most effective psychosocial modality. When combined with medication and milieu therapy, one could argue that it is without parallel. However, no one has attempted to demonstrate such a claim with the use of controls, cross-over procedures, or even self-controlled methods. The one exception is a study using a multiple-couples group in the treatment of chronic alcoholism [10]. In this work, 40 couples were distributed between group and individual treatment. The group was a weekly, 90-minute meeting of five couples. At the conclusion of the study, 7 of 20 of the MFG patients were drinking to excess, while essentially all the controls had relapsed. Half of the experimental group were abstaining altogether. Aside from this, what has been reported has been enthusiastic and is probably reflective of a significant trend toward improved clinical effectiveness, but it is singularly difficult to demonstrate such a claim conclusively.

Publication of MFG applications began with three reports appearing in the early 1960s, one from Laqueur and two from the Grace-New Haven (now Yale-New Haven) Hospital [16,22,27]. All three used the modality as part of a larger treatment plan; in one case [16], quite an involved and seemingly thoughtful one. All described characteristic processes: the rapid development of cohesion, spontaneous moves toward openness by relatives, a sense that the MFG had quickly become the focus of the major portion of therapeutic attention, and a sense of the staff having been surprised by it all. At Grace-New Haven, since the group was being conducted twice weekly on an acute inpatient service of a general hospital, the families only participated for the duration of the inpatient stay [16]. Goals included the reduction of family isolation and staff fragmentation, and the maximization of positive aspects of family interaction. At Creedmore, Laqueur's group was relatively closed and ran for long periods with the same membership. This was a function of the research orientation of the service. Laqueur was explicit as to goals: improvement in intrafamily communication and improved insight into disturbed interaction. In spite of what might be described as a difference of orientation reminiscent of the supportive versus insight dialectic, the groups in all three reports were described as affectively intense, rich were psychotherapeutic group confrontation *and* support, and seemingly leading to substantive change. As to technique, Laqueur went to some lengths to recommend a high level of therapist activity, use of the therapists as role models for communication and management of affect, directing the process to "basic values," and bringing to light hidden messages and communication patterns within the family. The Yale report restricted discussion of technique to the promotion of reciprocal support between relatives. Both groups seem to have been roughly equivalent in their effectiveness. Laqueur noted that 67 percent of the families in his project reported improved communication and family "understanding"; the Detre group reported rehospitalization rates of 12 to 18 percent two to three years after the index admission [16].

The other report from Grace-New Haven emphasized the use of MFT within an integrated group-oriented treatment program [22]. The service was an inpatient ward, open to patients with acute psychoses, with a moderate length of stay and referral to other agencies for follow up on discharge. Family involvement was a condition of admission. The therapeutic protocol included three groups: a patient group, a relatives group and an MFG, all weekly and all led by the same clinicians. The MFG quickly became the most intense of the groups, sometimes approaching the limits of manageability. At the same time it became the arena for change in the members' behavior and attitudes. The other two groups became "auxiliary to the mixed sessions [MFG]." The patient group allowed the participants a chance to gain some support in dealing with the strong reactions elicited by the MFG, while also providing an opportunity for patients to confront one another about relating to others using habitual family patterns. The relatives group allowed parents to share their guilt and hostility toward the hospitalized family member without having to worry about untoward effects. The therapists got a chance to see some of the personal strengths of the relatives, something that was not usually possible in the MFG where relatives often presented pictures of severe personality disturbance. Thus, although MFT was the central element in this approach, its interdigitation with the other groups enhanced its effectiveness.

In subsequent reports, MFT has been used within two broad categories: as a primary or ancillary treatment during hospitalization and as the primary after-care therapy. Although some reports describe using the group for both functions, the great majority of the reported applications fall discretely into one or the other category. In addition, it is possible to distinguish groups on the basis of the stated intentions of the therapists. Some have seen the group as a means of fostering more efficient and effective contact and communication between staff and family members, especially during the inpatient phase of treatment. Others have used MFGs as means of alleviating some of the acute situational disturbances within the family, especially feelings of guilt, demoralization, isolation, and hostility toward the identified patient. The third group includes clinicians who have used the MFG format to achieve substantive change in the ongoing structural and communicational dysfunction in the family. As is seen below, these distinctions are far from clear cut, since many authors have described goals that have changed during the course of the group. In all such instances the evolution was toward more change-directed therapeutic processes.

Two reports from the Langley-Porter Institute illustrate the process of change in the orientation of the group. Levin described a group that grew out of the residents' frustrations with the inadequate amount of time they had to spend with their patients' families [32]. The service was an active acute inpatient ward with an emphasis on milieu therapy. The group was presented to family members as a means of answering questions and discussing feelings about hospitalization. In addition, most families were seen in single-family therapy. Some continuation after discharge was allowed, usually at the family's request.

After several sessions, the group developed more affective intensity and suppressed conflict was exposed and resolved. Of interest was the positive effect the group had on staff morale and effectiveness, since it provided a means for many channels of communication while allowing the staff to obtain a more comprehensive and useful picture of the patient's situation. Curry, writing about the same service, described a more therapeutic orientation [11]. Seeing the role of the therapists as promoting guidance and counseling, he framed the goals as "limited." His descriptions of these groups, which were open-ended and quite heterogeneous in composition, included themes of ventilation, clarification of intrafamily communication, cross-family comparison and problem-solving, while dealing with denial, guilt, blame, and questions about the etiology of psychosis.

Daniels described an MFG that grew directly out of a relatives-only meeting on a therapeutic community inpatient service in a general hospital [12]. There were many advantages in the MFG format as opposed to the relatives-only meetings, and the MFG persisted as the preferable alternative. He reported a reduction in family suspiciousness and staff-patient-family triangulation. There was improved comprehension of, and cooperation in, the treatment plan by the family. This report, as well as others, includes vignettes that clearly describe major structural and communicational shifts within families. In this report, as in Levin's and Curry's, the MFG was a central but not exclusive treatment modality used while some patients were at least semi-acutely psychotic, was quite heterogeneous as to diagnosis and other parameters and was led by multiple therapists (often the patient's primary therapist). Participation by any given family was confined to the duration of the admission.

Other practitioners have seen the MFG as the means by which acute disruptions within the family are compensated, thus promoting more directly remission of the identified patient's psychosis. They appeared to operate within a psychoanalytic framework and thus saw such therapeutic effects as relatively superficial, although useful. One example is the first report coming from the Langley-Porter group; their groups were conducted within the setting described above [7]. Their efforts were more intense, however, in that both MFG and single-family meetings occurred twice weekly. Their descriptions reiterate most of the features included above. In addition they emphasized the therapeutic power of simple exposure and scrutiny of family processes and the inevitably ensuing social pressure toward nondeviant structure and communication. They were surprised by the facility and directness with which group members confronted the deviant communication and linguistic style of other families. They also consciously encouraged the development of the group as a semiautonomous social entity through "the creation of family-focused recreational and occupational therapies, with a group of families having dinners and parties which they plan and implement as part of the hospital program."

They encouraged patients without available families to remain in the group, which then functioned as a surrogate family/social network with surprisingly positive effects.

Another paper has described similar processes in an MFG that was part of a partial hospitalization program within a general hospital/community mental health center [14]. This MFG ran as an open-ended, rotating membership meeting. The leaders quickly learned that homogeneity of diagnosis and level of ego function markedly enhanced the cohesion and effectiveness of the group. Another report on a partial hospital application illustrates the entire range of possible goals and approaches in MFT [33]. Within a strongly family-oriented state hospital program serving chronic schizophrenics and some borderline patients, the group grew out of separate patient and relative groups which had proved unsatisfactory because the sick/well dichotomy of patient and family was seemingly being exacerbated. The MFG was initially undertaken to reverse this trend, as well as to prevent patient isolation and family fragmentation. Within the first session, families spontaneously began discussing family relationships with remarkable intensity — with frequent expressions of anger punctuating increasingly direct exploration of family conflict — followed by significant improvement in family communication, conflict resolution, and cohesiveness. The patients' improvement paralleled that of their families.

A third group of MFT clinicians has set out ambitious therapeutic goals for their work, seeing the meetings as a unique opportunity to accomplish substantive change in families with a psychotic member. Julian and her co-workers at McLean Hospital described a group of young schizophrenic patients and their mothers [24]. Here, the MFG — part of an intensive therapeutic milieu — was continued after discharge, closed to new members after the initial phase, and conducted by the patients' individual therapists. Their goals included provision of support for patients and mothers, staff economy, creation of mutual identification, clarification of family interaction patterns, and rehabilitation through improved and more open communication. Perhaps as a result of the closed-group format, the process described was quite intense and included the expression of profound hostility between patients and mothers, the discussion of rejection, suicide, and murder and the exposure of serious intrafamily splits. With time and the development of cross-family bonds, the aggressive interchanges diminished and were followed by depression, then improved family integration and more cross-family support and problem solving. Subsequently, mostly after patient discharge, the mothers increasingly utilized the group to explore their own problems. Laqueur's experience probably equalled that of all other authors combined, since he led and supervised MFGs at Creedmoor and Vermont State Hospital continuously for 20 years. By choice, he worked entirely within state hospital contexts and thereby with a largely chronically psychotic population. He was one of the few MFT enthusiasts whose theoretical frame of reference lay within that of family systems and communication theory. Thus he saw the goal of MFT to be the disruption and normalization of habitual, dysfunctional, and probably pathogenic family interaction and communication patterns. At the same time he had become aware of the great difficulty that single-family therapists had in making any major changes in communication dysfunction [29]. He saw MFT as the means by which families learned new patterns, largely indirectly, through "analogy, indirect interpretation, mimicking and identification" [28]. This avoided the nearly inevitable and counter-therapeutic anxiety, denial, and resistance that occur with more direct interpretation, clarification, or confrontation by therapists. Thus, one very apt description is that an MFG is "A sheltered workshop in family communication" [27].

In later writings, Laqueur noted the capacity of an MFG to both provoke family crisis by disrupting negative feedback (homeostatic) mechanisms, and to promote new ones that include the possibility of growth without decompensation. It is important to observe, however, that the success of Laqueur's groups in achieving his stated goals owed much to their long-term, relatively stable and homogeneous nature. He brought families into the group as soon as the identified patient was able to tolerate it, but attempted to keep the groups' membership stable, or "semi-closed." The later groups functioned autonomously of the patient's ward, and each family's participation was encouraged after the patient's discharge.

Two other reports are worthy of note, primarily because of their use of MFT with a diagnostically specific set of patients. Marx and Ludwig describe a moderately successful attempt to reinvolve the family of markedly chronic schizophrenics who had seemingly been abandoned by their relatives [34]. This turned out to be a difficult task that had serious negative side effects involving staff, patients, and family members. Nevertheless, major gains were achieved by helping patients and family members to abandon pseudoharmony and infantilizing. In the end, chronically debilitated patients were provoked to clinical improvement.

Davenport and her research group at the NIMH have developed a couples-group approach to manic-depressive patients that appears to be the psychosocial treatment of choice for this very difficult group [13]. Their groups are very long-term, closed, and intense. The central themes are fear of loss; marital, child-rearing, and extended family conflict; and tendencies toward inter-spouse provocativeness. The groups promoted conflict expression and resolution and the creation of a larger social network. They generate considerable empathy and understanding both about the biological dimension of their illness and the relational difficulties that tend to trigger relapse. Practical advantages include easy medication monitoring and peer-group pressure toward medication compliance. The group has had a profound effect on relapse rates.

Although these long-term, reconstructively oriented MFGs have often extended into the post-discharge phase, two reports deal with the use of this modality primarily as an after-care treatment. Beels, as part of an ambitious family-oriented treatment service at Bronx State Hospital, used MFGs and crisis intervention as the principle psychosocial modalities in the aftercare of a population of exclusively chronic patients [3]. Although the MFT aspect of his program is as yet unpublished, the MFGs reduced recidivism among those patients who continued in the groups to remarkably low levels —often leading to significant gains in the patient's social and occupational functioning, and improvement in family functioning. Of particular importance was the service's policy of keeping some MFGs as closed and as long-lived as possible, although other groups were kept open to newly discharged patients and their families. His intent was to create a new social network for the families. The effect of this approach was to gradually shift the burden of clinical and social maintenance and even crisis intervention onto the group. This took place over very long periods of time, however, and could only have occurred under such conditions. (One group was still meeting when the service was administratively dismantled, after five years.)

Lansky and his co-workers used a similar model in their application in a Veterans Administration Hospital [25]. These essentially closed groups were very homogeneous as to diagnosis; they were the only psychosocial therapy and means for medication maintenance after discharge. If a patient was rehospitalized, he and his family continued in the group. Their explicit goal was to intercede in the families' contribution to the residua of the acute illness, but they found that they initially had to take "scapegoating" and practical issues of living with a psychotic and a psychosis at their face value. Once this was done, the group members tended to move beyond triangulation on their own. Again, relapse rates dropped precipitously. They conducted separate groups for married and unmarried schizophrenic patients, finding that the issues in the two groups were quite different. Unfortunately, the married couples did not achieve nearly the same success as the parents-offspring group.

Brief mention should be made of recent efforts to work with the parents of schizophrenic patients in groups that specifically exclude the identified patients. The question of whether these are MFGs is academic, since many features and goals are essentially similar to those of the groups previously reviewed. Leff and his colleagues in England have been using the parents groups format to teach "high emotional expression" relatives to be less so [30]. The teachers are the "low EE" parents who in some ways compensate for the patient's deficits rather than exacerbating them. In a small sample they have shown promising results in reducing relapse rates of schizophrenics from the high EE families. Atwood and Williams used the parents' group format to develop support for families, then helped the group in its efforts to promote more autonomy in the patients and more emotional distance on the part of key relatives.

Finally, Anderson is using MFT to accomplish several goals [1]. Essentially, this complex and multifaceted approach to schizophrenia is "psycho-educational" in its orientation. In what are called "survival skills workshops," a group of four or five families meet for an entire day and, by popular request, at bi-monthly intervals, to hear explicit information about schizophrenia, discuss information about management issues, work indirectly on family communication, encourage concern for self in the relatives, and promote a free exchange of experience among the different families. These groups are preceded by single-family sessions, some with and some without the patient, and are followed by family therapy sessions that aim at individualizing the lessons gained in the MFG. Their ultimate goal is to deintensify the social environment of the patient. It is too early to assess outcome, but this program addresses many problematic aspects in a direct way.

A CONCLUDING UNSCIENTIFIC POSTSCRIPT

Presented here is an overview of the rationale, experience, process, and technique of multiple-family therapy. The field is still, after 20 years of existence on the margins of the larger mental health movement, in a preliminary state of development. It is hoped that readers will be moved to add the modality to their repertoire and that they will be willing to experiment with new forms of MFT. There is no definitive use or technique for MFT and there is a great need both for more clinical experience in, and rigorous study of, the modality. Its potential in severe syndromes seems well-established, but the best means for applying MFT is not at all clear and not demonstrable scientifically. Although this is a great deficit, it is also a great opportunity for the contribution of new data and therapeutic techniques.

REFERENCES

1. Anderson, C.M.; Hogarty, Gerard; Reiss, D.J. "Family treatment of adult schizophrenic patients: a research-based psycho-educational approach." *Schizophrenia Bulletin* 6 : 490–505,1980.
2. Atwood, N. and Williams, M.E.D. "Group support for the families of the mentally ill." *Schizophrenia Bulletin* 4 : 415–425, 1978.
3. Beels, C.C. "Family and social management of schizophrenia." *Schizophrenia Bulletin* 13 : 97–118, 1975.
4. Beels, C.C. "Social networks, the family, and the psychiatric patient." *Schizophrenia Bulletin* 4 : 512–521, 1978.
5. Beels, C.C. "Social networks, and schizophrenia," *Psychiatric Quarterly*, 51 : 209–215, 1979.
6. Berman, K.K. "Multiple family therapy: its possibilities in preventing readmission." *Mental Hygiene* 50 : 367–70, 1966.

7. Blinder, M.C.; Colman, A.; Curray, A.; and Kessler, D. "MFGT: simultaneous treatment of several families." *American Journal of Psychotherapy* 19 : 559–69, 1965.

8. Bowen, M. "Principles and techniques of multiple family therapy." In J.O. Bradt and C.J. Moyniham (eds.) *Systems Therapy.* Washington, D.C., private publisher, 1972.

9. Brown, G.W.; Birley, J.L.T.; and Wing, J.K. The influence of family life on schizophrenic disorders: A replication." *British Journal of Psychiatry* 121 : 241–258, 1972.

10. Cadogan, D.A. "Marital group therapy in the treatment of alcoholism." *Quarterly Journal of Studies on Alcohol* 34 : 1187–94, 1973.

11. Curry, A.E., "Therapeutic management of multiple family groups." *International Journal of Group Psychotherapy* 15 : 90–5, 1965.

12. Daniels, N. "Participation of relatives in a group-centered program." *International Journal of Group Psychotherapy* 17 : 336–42, 1967.

13. Davenport, Y.B.; Adland, M.L.; Gold, P.W.; and Goodwin, F.K. "Manic-depressive illness: Psychodynamic features of multi-generational families." *American Journal of Orthopsychiatry* 49 : 24–35, 1979.

14. Davies, I.J.; Ellison, G.; and Young, R. "Therapy with a group of families in a psychiatric day center." *American Journal of Orthopsychiatry* 36 : 134–46, 1966.

15. Dean, A. and Lin, N., "The stress-buffering role of social support." *Journal of Nervous and Mental Disease* 165 : 403–16, 1977.

16. Detre, T.; Sayers, J.; Norton, N.; and Lewis, H. "An experimental approach to the treatment of the acutely ill psychiatric patient in the general hospital." *Connecticut Medicine* 25 : 613–9, 1961.

17. Dincin, J.; Selleck, V.; and Streicker, S. "Restructuring parental attitudes—Working with parents of the adult mentally ill." *Schizophrenia Bulletin* 4 : 597–608, 1978.

18. Garrison, V. "Support systems of schizophrenic and non-schizophrenic Puerto Rican migrant women in New York City." *Schizophrenia Bulletin* 4 : 561–96, 1978.

19. Haley, J. *Problem-Solving Therapy.* San Francisco: Jossey-Bass, 1977.

20. Hammer, M.; Makiesky-Barrow, S.; and Gutwirth, L. "Social networks and schizophrenia." *Schizophrenia Bulletin* 4 : 522–545, 1978.

21. Harrow, M.; Astrachan, B.; Becker, R.; Detre, T.; and Schwartz, A. "An investigation into the nature of the patient-family therapy group." *American Journal of Orthopsychiatry* 37 : 888–99, 1967.

22. Hes, J. and Handler, S. "Multidimensional group psychotherapy." *Archives of General Psychiatry* 5 : 92–7, 1961.

23. Hoffman, L. "Deviation-amplifying processes in natural groups." In Haley, J., ed. *Changing Families.* New York: Grune and Stratton, 1971.

24. Julian B.; Ventrola, L.; and Christ, J. Multiple family therapy: The interaction of young hospitalized patients with their mothers." *International Journal of Group Psychotherapy* 19 : 501–9, 1969.

25. Lansky, M.R.; Bley, C.R.; McVey, G.G.; and Brotman, B. "Multiple family groups as aftercare." *International Journal of Group Psychotherapy* 28 : 211–24, 1978.

26. Laqueur, H.P., Personal communication.

27. Laqueur, H.P.; LaBurt, H.A.; and Morong, E. "Multiple family therapy: Further developments. " *International Journal of Social Psychiatry,* Congress Issue, 1964.

28. Laqueur, H.P. "Multiple family therapy and general systems theory." *International Psychiatry Clinics* 7 : 99–124, 1970.

29. Laqueur, H.P. "Mechanisms of change in multiple family therapy." In: C.J. Sager and H.S. Kaplan, eds. *Progress in Group and Family Therapy.* New York: Brunner/Mazel, 1972.

30. Leff, J.P. "Developments in family treatment of schizophrenia." *Psychiatric Quarterly,* 51 : 216–232, 1979.

31. Leichter, E. "Interplay of group and family treatment techniques in multi-family group therapy." *International Journal of Group Psychotherapy*, 22 : 167–76, 1972.
32. Levin, E.C. "Therapeutic multiple family groups." *International Journal of Group Psychotherapy*, 19 : 203–8, 1966.
33. Lewis, J.C. and Glasser, N. "Evolution of a treatment approach to families: Group family therapy." *International Journal of Group Psychotherapy* 15 : 505–15, 1965.
34. Marx, A. and Ludwig, A. "Resurrection of the family of the chronic schizophrenic." *American Journal of Psychotherapy* 23 : 37–52, 1969.
35. Minuchin, S. *Families and Family Therapy*. Cambridge: Harvard University Press, 1974.
36. Pattison, E.M. Forest hospital conference on family therapy, Chicago, IL, October 1976.
37. Reiss, D. and Costell, R. "The multiple family group as a small society: Family regulation of interaction with nonmembers." *American Journal of Psychiatry*, 134 : 21–4, 1977.
38. Schaeffer, D.S. "Effects of frequent hospitalizations on behavior of psychotic patients in multiple family therapy." *Journal of Clinical Psychology* 25 : 104–5, 1969.
39. Sculthorpe, W. and Blumenthal, I.J. "Combined patient-relative group psychotherapy in schizophrenia." *Mental Hygiene* 49 : 569–73, 1965.
40. Sokolovsky, J.; Cohen, I.C.; Berger, D.; and Geiger, J. "Personal networks of ex-mental patients in a Manhattan SRO hotel." *Human Organization* 37 : 5–15, 1978.
41. Strelnick, A.H. "Multiple family therapy: a review of the literature." *Family Process* 16 : 307–25, 1977.
42. Strelnick, A.H. "Multiple family therapy and family change: an exploratory clinical study." Unpublished report.
43. Tolsdorf, C.C. "Social networks, support and coping: an exploratory study." *Family Process* 15 : 407–17, 1976.
44. Vaughn, C.E. and Leff, J.P. "The influence of family and social factors on the course of psychiatric illness." *British Journal of Psychiatry* 129 : 125–37, 1976.

6

Pediatric Hospitalization in the Treatment of Anorexia Nervosa

Gordon Hodas, Ronald Liebman, and MarJeanne Collins

INTRODUCTION

Anorexia nervosa is a potentially life-threatening disorder which is difficult to treat, and has a mortality rate, according to some authors, of 2 to 15 percent. [3,8,2]. Its incidence is increasing dramatically [1]. In defining anorexia nervosa we adhere to Minuchin et al.'s physical and psychological criteria:

The physical symptoms include a loss of over 25% of the body weight [in the absence of a primary medical disorder] as well as one or more of the following conditions: amenorrhea, hyperactivity, and hypothermia. The psychological symptoms include a pursuit of thinness, fear of gaining weight, denial of hunger, distorted body image, sense of ineffectiveness, and struggle for control [3].

In this chapter, we describe the indications and methods of hospitalizing anorectic patients on a medical unit while working with the family.

In treating patients, we are guided by four general principles:

1. The treatment must be collaborative, involving both psychotherapist and pediatrician, whether or not the patient is hospitalized.
2. The treatment involves the active participation of the family, whether or not the patient is hospitalized.
3. Whenever possible, we treat anorectics on an outpatient rather than inpatient basis.
4. When hospitalization is required, we utilize a pediatric rather than psychiatric inpatient unit.

The treatment of anorexia nervosa requires a collaborative psychiatric-pediatric approach because neither discipline alone can adequately treat the disorder. The pediatrician rules out possible organic causes of weight loss and monitors the patient's nutritional status. The therapist, working with the anorectic and her family, confronts the non-eating behavior and those factors that have maintained the symptom.

Currently, less than 25 percent of anorectic patients treated in family therapy at the Philadelphia Child Guidance Clinic first require hospitalization at the Children's Hospital of Philadelphia. This figure is lower than the 57 percent described in Minuchin et al.'s original study [3]. As can be seen in Table 6-1, the indications for pediatric hospitalization are primarily medical.

Table 6.1   **Indications for Pediatric Hospitalization**

1. Severe acute or unremitting weight loss
2. Intercurrent infection in a severely cachectic anorectic
3. Alterations in vital signs (postural hypotension, bradycardia, hypothermia) and absence of urinary ketone bodies
4. Electrolyte abnormalities (often resulting from laxative abuse and/or recurrent vomiting)
5. Cases accepted on transfer with medical complications
6. Marked family disturbance (massive denial or inability to engage in outpatient therapy)

We prefer to treat anorectics on an outpatient rather than inpatient basis with their families because this enables the therapist to work with the anorectic in her natural context—the family—rather than separating her from those with whom she interacts on a daily basis. The family's symptom-maintaining behaviors can be more easily understood and the family's assets can be mobilized to help the anorectic's recovery, with the patient at home. Outpatient treatment also allows the patient to continue attending school and to maintain peer contacts and age-appropriate activities.

A pediatric rather than psychiatric hospital is utilized since a medical setting is best equipped to treat serious medical problems and to rule out possible organic causes for the weight loss. Pediatric hospitalization avoids the stigma of "a mental hospital" that psychiatric confinement may entail, and is less threatening to patient and family. In addition, emphasis on the severity of the medical symptoms helps mobilize parents to action. Parents confronted by a child on a medical unit with a life-threatening refusal to eat can more easily identify the patient as rebellious and controlling rather than pitiful and weak. With teen-age anorectics, we utilize a medical adolescent unit within the pediatric hospital.

THREE PHASES OF TREATMENT FOR
HOSPITALIZED ANORECTICS

For the anorectic requiring hospitalization, pediatric hospitalization initiates the treatment process, which consists of three phases: (1) The inpatient phase, (2) a transitional phase, and (3) the outpatient phase. It is only by keeping the goals of each phase in perspective that the total treatment of anorexia can be integrated and effective.

The Inpatient Phase

The inpatient phase is intended to be brief, usually a period of three weeks. There are several important goals for this phase: (1) ruling out organic causes of the weight loss, (2) treating any medical complications of the anorexia, (3) engaging the family in the treatment process, (4) beginning informal contact between psychotherapist and patient, and (5) having the anorectic regain about half of her lost weight. The pediatrician determines the ideal weight for the anorectic (based on standard HEW height-weight charts). A gain of one half of the amount of lost weight prior to admission is necessary for discharge from the hospital into outpatient therapy. During the early inpatient phase the pediatrician is in charge of the case, with therapist serving as a consultant.

The Transitional Phase

During the transitional phase, the primary responsibility for treatment begins to shift from the pediatrician to the therapist. A formal family meeting run by pediatrician and therapist usually occurs about seven to ten days after hospitalization. The diagnosis of anorexia nervosa is confirmed for patient and family, and the medical evaluation is reviewed. The pediatrician introduces the therapist to the family, and the needs for family therapy are outlined and discussed. Frequently, the family meeting is immediately followed by a family lunch session in which the patient, family, and therapist all eat lunch together in the office so that the non-eating behavior can be directly observed and confronted [3]. Following the family meeting and family lunch session, the therapist assumes increased responsibility in the case until the time of discharge, holding additional family meetings and lunch sessions as needed.

The Outpatient Phase

By the time of medical discharge, the anorectic has reached the required discharge weight and the family is committed to the treatment process. Discharge is planned so that the first outpatient family meeting occurs on the day of or shortly after the patient's return home. During the outpatient phase, which typically involves 6 to 12 months of weekly outpatient family meetings, the therapist has primary responsibility for the case and the pediatrician is available in a consultative capacity. The goals of outpatient treatment are to help the anorectic reach and maintain her ideal weight; to change the structure and functioning of the family, rendering anorectic behavior unnecessary; and to encourage the patient to deal more effectively with such age-appropriate tasks as increasing autonomy and peer relationships.

CREATING A UNIFIED NETWORK
DURING THE INPATIENT PHASE

A successful inpatient phase requires that all persons involved in the treatment process communicate frequently, thereby creating a single united treatment network. Each person must understand and confine himself to his particular role in the overall treatment, so that inadvertent undermining is avoided.

The Weight Gain Program

The weight gain program is implemented only for those inpatient anorectics with no serious medical complications which first require attention. As can be seen in Table 6-2, progress is measured in daily weight gain, and the results of each weighing-in determine the extent of the patient's activities for that day.

Table 6-2.   Weight Gain Program for Inpatient Anorectics

1. The patient, after discussion with the dietitian, is given a 2500-3000 calorie diet each day, and orders most of the items herself. The patient determines how much food she consumes; the staff makes no attempt to force or cajole the patient to eat.
2. The patient is weighed each morning at the same time dressed in nightgown only. A weight gain of 0.25 kg entitles the patient to full privileges on the unit. Weight gain of less than 0.25 kg or weight loss results in loss of privileges for that day.
3. If the patient fails to gain 0.25 kg on a given day, her activity is restricted in the following ways:
    —no visitors or phone calls, including parents
    —confinement to bed with curtain drawn without access to television or reading material
    —no bathroom privileges for that day
4. When bedrest is enforced, the patient is told that this is medically necessary in order that she conserve her limited calories and concentrate more effectively on gaining weight. The purpose of the bedrest is medical, not punitive.
5. Once the patient has reached her previously set discharge weight, she is discharged into outpatient family therapy.

In general, it is important that the weight gain program be enforced with consistency and that modifications be avoided. At the same time, the program is tailored to each individual patient and occasionally unexpected developments require flexibility, as with the patient who water loads and needs additional random weighings, or the patient who becomes psychotic necessitating increased social contact and the use of psychotropic medication.

Simple reassurance supplements the behavioral program. The patient is reassured that the goal of the hospitalization is to help her, not punish her. She will be helped to regain positive control of her body by following the prescribed weight gain program. If the anorectic fails to gain the necessary weight on a particular day, she is reminded that she will have another chance to succeed the next day. The anorectic is also reassured that she will not be permitted to "get fat," thereby addressing a frequently voiced concern.

Collaboration Between Pediatrician and Psychotherapist

Collaboration between pediatrician and therapist is essential throughout the entire treatment process. Following the initial call of inquiry by the family, the pediatrician and a psychiatric consultant meet to review the data, discuss therapist assignment, and decide whether hospitalization is required. Strategies for engaging the family are discussed. Once the anorectic is hospitalized, the pediatrician and consultant meet to discuss the specialized needs of patient and family, the responses of other staff members to the patient, and the progress made in the hospital. Particular emphasis is placed on anticipating potential problems involving the patient, family, and staff. Formal interdisciplinary meetings with pediatrician, house staff, nurses, social worker, and therapist are held to discuss the case and implement the treatment plan. Important decisions are written in the patient's chart after the multidisciplinary discussions.

It is essential that the patient and family experience the pediatrician and therapist as working together. By meeting together with the patient and family, the pediatrician and therapist demonstrate that the treatment program is integrated. For this reason, it is mandatory that the pediatrician and therapist are physically present together with the family during the inpatient and transitional phases of treatment.

The Role of the Family

During the inpatient phase, the locus of responsibility for the anorectic's weight gain shifts from the parents to the patient in the hospital. In this way, the hospitalization offers a temporary "time-out" period for the family in which conflicts over food are suspended, and the patient is given an opportunity to exert control in a positive direction and begin reclaiming her own body. At times the anorectic, after an initial testing period, begins to eat normally and gain weight. At other times, weight gain is minimal until the time of the family lunch session led by the therapist. The goal of the lunch session is to bring the non-eating behavior into the room, where it can be confronted directly by the family with the help of the therapist and pediatrician [4]. The possible outcomes are:

1. The anorectic eats uneventfully, which enables the therapist to reframe the problem as not an eating problem but a problem of growing up, communication, or other interpersonal issues.

2. The anorectic refuses to eat and the parents are given the responsibility of getting their daughter to eat. If the parents do not succeed initially, they are told to continue working together until the patient begins to cooperate.

3. The anorectic refuses to eat and the parents fail in their attempts to get her to eat. With this outcome, the therapist points out the power that the patient has over the parents and how she has defeated them. The parents are told that they will continue to fail unless they are able to work more effectively together and stimulate greater cooperation from the patient.

Regardless of the specific outcome, the family lunch session is frequently a turning point in the treatment and hospital course of the patient, even if prior weight gain has occurred in the hospital. Often, rapid weight gain follows the lunch session, permitting discharge of the patient into ongoing outpatient therapy. In more resistant cases, additional family lunch sessions may be necessary during the inpatient phase. Thus, while initially the parents are relieved of responsibility for their daughter's weight, at the time of the lunch session they are again involved in the daughter's non-eating behavior, but this time, with the help of the therapist and pediatrician, a more positive outcome results [3].

The parents also play an important role during the hospitalization in ways not directly related to eating. They are expected to inform their daughter of their explicit support for the treatment program and to remain united with the pediatric staff, resisting their daughter's appeals to undermine or terminate treatment. The parents tell their daughter that they will visit or talk to her only if she gains the required weight for that day; since the anorectic has strong ties to her family, the desire to see her parents becomes a further motivation for her to eat.

There are many reasons why the parents cooperate with the treatment program. From the outset the pediatrician explains thoroughly the goals and expectations of the program to the parents, and agreement with these goals is a precondition of entry into treatment. At the time of admission, the pediatrician meets with the parents and patient to review the goals, and contact is maintained throughout the hospitalization by meetings and telephone. The parents fear that their anorectic daughter may die and find adherence to the treatment program preferable to that alternative. The pediatrician and therapist convey hopefulness to the family, sharing with them their prior experience in treating anorexia. The pediatrician serves as a role model for the parents, in such areas as limit-setting, flexibility, and communication. The parents are encouraged to call the pediatrician if any questions or concerns arise. Whenever possible, potential problems are anticipated, as when the pediatrician calls the parents to let them know the first time that their daughter is upset about being confined to bed after losing weight. The parents can respond to their daughter's distress by encouraging her to gain weight so that she can return home.

It is crucial that the parents understand that the successful treatment of anorexia involves more than the patient's gaining weight in the hospital. The parents are told from the beginning that the treatment typically requires a 6-to-12 month commitment by the entire family, with most of the treatment on an outpatient basis. This message is repeated at the time of hospitalization and reinforced by the entry of the therapist and subsequent family meetings. Unless pediatrician and therapist can adequately engage the family, treatment will not succeed.

The Role of the Nursing Staff

The nurses have the greatest frequency of contact with the patient. They relate to her respectfully and objectively, avoiding overidentification with her plight or the parents' dilemma. They resist the divisive tactics of the anorectic and make no attempt to "do therapy" with her. The nurses carefully record the eating of the patient but make no attempt to force or cajole her into eating. Given the many management problems that an anorectic may create, it is important that staff experienced in the treatment of anorexia be employed on the unit.

The Role of the House Officer

The house staff are in a different position with anorectic patients since they rotate every four weeks and usually have little or no prior experience with anorectics. In contrast to other medical patients for whom they bear primary responsibility, the house officer of an anorectic has a limited role, with major decisions made by the staff pediatrician. Efforts are made by the staff pediatrician and therapist to include the house officer in the treatment process and to educate him about anorexia and its total treatment. The house officer is invited to observe family lunch sessions and family meetings, and to offer his opinions. His relationships with patient and family is discussed so that his efforts mesh with those of the staff pediatrician and the therapist.

The Role of the Dietician

Upon admission the patient meets with the dietician, who reviews basic nutritional principles with the patient, explains the 2500-to-3500 calorie diet, and elicits the patient's eating preferences. Great flexibility in diet is provided, as long as the patient eats balanced meals and takes in sufficient calories. If she does, she will gain weight; otherwise, she will stay the same or lose weight.

The Role of the Patient

The anorectic is treated with respectful objectivity by the inpatient staff, thereby avoiding the traps of overprotectiveness and proximity that usually characterize the parents' unsuccessful approach to their daughter. The patient is told that the staff is available to help her, but that she must take responsibility for herself. Expectations for weight gain and necessary nutritional information are clearly stated, enabling the patient's response and behavior to determine her hospital course. Nurses, pediatricians, and therapists are all alert to attempts on the part of the anorectic to "divide and conquer" by misrepresenting staff members or playing one person against another. The consistent message given is that the staff is united in wanting to help the patient begin behaving in more age-appropriate ways.

DISCUSSION

The treatment program described here differs from other treatments of anorexia nervosa along three parameters: (1) the conceptualization of the problem, (2) the purpose of the hospitalization, and (3) the systems approach to hospitalization with family involvement during and after the inpatient phase.

The Conceptualization of the Problem

The work of Minuchin et al. supports the view of anorexia nervosa as primarily the outcome of a dysfunctional family system [3]. The anorexia emerges in the context of a family that is overprotective toward the anorectic and unable to deal effectively with conflict. The family, despite its good intentions, does not promote the autonomy of the anorectic because unresolved marital and family issues may require the anorectic's presence as a conflict-avoidance mechanism. In addition, family loyalties may be so strong that growing up and moving away may be seen as acts of family betrayal. In such families, where food has been a symbol of the closeness from which the anorectic is seeking distance and separation, the symptom of anorexia develops.

   Hospitalizing the anorectic patient becomes necessary when her symptoms endanger life and require immediate intensive interventions. It is obligatory to involve the family in treatment because the factors reinforcing the anorexia extend beyond the patient herself.

The Purpose of the Hospitalization

Hospitalization may be used in various ways in the treatment of anorexia nervosa. Even with the use of pediatric hospitalization, significant differences in goals may exist. For example, Silverman customarily initiates treatment with a three-month pediatric hospitalization, during which time intensive individual psychodynamic psychotherapy (four sessions per week) is begun. There are strict limitations of ongoing contact between parents and patient in conjoint family therapy. To foster a "realistic regression," the patient receives "total care" and is relieved of all decision making on a temporary basis [6,7].

In our program, hospitalization of the anorectic is employed only when absolutely necessary; the major indications for hospitalization are medical, and less than 25 percent of referred patients are hospitalized. During the hospitalization, the family is involved in ongoing family therapy while the patient on the unit is encouraged to accept age-appropriate responsibility in all areas of functioning. Because the most significant changes occur at home after the patient's discharge, hospitalization is made brief (an average of three weeks).

The Systems Approach and the Involvement
of the Family

Just as the anorectic is part of a larger system—the family system—and must be viewed within that context, the hospital setting also constitutes a social system which must be understood as a unit and seen in terms of the mutual interaction of its various parts. The pediatrician, house staff, nursing staff, dietician, and therapist all comprise parts of the hospital treatment context requiring coordination and unity. The impact of the anorectic on other medical patients, who in turn impact on the anorectic, should be taken into account. The role of the parents, as potential allies or potential adversaries, must be appreciated. The goal is to create a united medical network, and a therapeutic partnership between that medical network, the patient, and the family.

As described, the family plays a significant role during the hospitalization of the anorectic. The family lunch session, in addition to signaling the beginning of formal family therapy, serves another therapeutic function: it enables therapist and family to begin to move from the symptom of non-eating to the interpersonal issues and transactions that sustain the non-eating behavior. Successful therapy requires that nonconstructive discussions about food be replaced as quickly as possible by focusing on family relationships, with the emergence of improved family transactional patterns as therapeutic goals.

OUTCOME

Minuchin et al. described the treatment of 53 anorectics seen over a seven-year period by 16 different therapists. The median age for the group, of which 89 percent were females, was 14½ years, with 60 percent between the ages of 13 and 16. The medical weight loss was 30 percent, with a range of 20 to 50 percent. Other characteristics of the patient population are described.

The authors measured treatment outcome along two dimensions: weight gain and psychological adjustment. They found, with follow-up periods of from 1½ to 7 years (80 percent followed for at least 2 years), that 86 percent of the treated anorectics (all but three families completed treatment) showed recovery in terms of both weight gain and psychosocial adjustment [3, 5].

Of the 23 anorectics that we have subsequently hospitalized on the inpatient unit from 1975–79, 17 of the patients ranged in age from 12 to 15 and 6 were from 16 to 19. The average weight gain for the entire group was 12½ pounds, and the average and mean length of stay was 21 days. The effectiveness of the inpatient phase can be measured along two parameters: (1) achievement of discharge weight, and (2) successful engagement of the family into outpatient therapy following discharge. Of the 23 patients, 18 attained their weight goal for discharge and all continued in subsequent outpatient therapy. One patient, accepted on transfer from another hospital having already lost 50 percent of her body weight, died from a cardiac arrhythmia despite treatment with central hyperalimentation. Another patient left the hospital against medical advice. Three patients who failed to gain to their optimal discharge weights had their initial discharge weights reduced by the attending physician in order to effect an earlier discharge and avoid further power struggles.

While data on the outcome of the outpatient therapy of the latter hospital-treated anorectics is not yet available, the trend appears to be one of improvement in psychosocial and interpersonal parameters in addition to maintenance of a normal weight.

CONCLUSIONS

The successful treatment of anorexia nervosa requires a collaborative pediatric-psychiatric approach. The role of the family is essential whether or not hospitalization is employed. More than 75 percent of referred anorectics receive outpatient treatment alone; pediatric hospitalization is reserved for those patients whose medical condition makes hospitalization mandatory. On occasion, pediatric hospitalization is also strategically used to engage a particularly resistant or disturbed family as a part of the treatment program.

The goal during the hospitalization of the anorectic is to create a unified medical network simultaneously with the development of a therapeutic partnership between the hospital staff and the family.

Three factors which, in combination, tend to differentiate our treatment approach from those used at other centers are:

1. The view of anorexia as a disorder of a dysfunctional family system necessitating family involvement throughout the treatment process.

2. The use of brief medical hospitalization which encourages the patient to accept responsibility for herself while simultaneously engaging the family in treatment.

3. The use of a systems perspective in working with the anorectic family and in organizing a therapeutic hospital treatment context.

Data indicates that this approach has been effective for both the inpatient management of anorexia and its long-term outpatient treatment. It is essential that the family commit itself to ongoing treatment for 6-to-12 months in order to stabilize weight gain and to develop new family transactional patterns which promote the growth and development of family members.

REFERENCES

1. Crisp, A.H.; Palmer, R.L.; Kalucy, R.S. "How common is anorexia nervosa? a prevalence study. *British Journal of Psychiatry* 128 : 549–544, 1976.
2. Hsu L.K.G.; Harding B.; Crisp, A.H. "Outcome of Anorexia Nervosa." *Lancet* 61–65, January 1979.
3. Minuchen, S.; Rosman, B.; and Baker, L. *Psychosomatic Families: Anorexia Nervosa in Context.* Cambridge, MA: Harvard University Press, 1978, pp. 2–130.
4. Rosman, B.; Minuchin, S.; and Liebman, R. "Family lunch session: an introduction to family therapy in anorexia nervosa. *American Journal of Orthopsychiatry*, 45 : 846–853, 1975.
5. Rosman, B.; Minuchin, S.; Baker, L.; and Liebman, R. In: R.A. Vigersky (ed.) *A Family Approach to Anorexia Nervosa: Study, Treatment and Outcome.* New York: Raven Press, 1977.
6. Silverman, J. Anorexia nervosa: clinical observations in a successful treatment plan. Journal of Pediatrics 84 : 68–73, 1974.
7. Silverman, J. "Anorexia nervosa: clinical and metabolic observations in a successful treatment plan. In: R.A. Vigersky (Ed.) *Anorexia Nervosa.* New York, Raven Press, 1977, pp. 331–339.
8. Van der Wiele, R.I. "Anorexia nervosa and the hypothalmus." *Hospital Practice* 45–51, December 1977.

7

The Family Changes the Hospital?

THOMAS KRAJEWSKI AND HENRY T. HARBIN

Families of psychiatrically ill persons usually look to the hospital for relief and support. They hope that the staff will take custody of the patient, work with him, and ultimately cure his illness. Usually the family members view themselves as outsiders vis-à-vis the hospital in this treatment process. They may want to visit and/or provide emotional and financial support for the patient/family member. Families rarely think that the hospital treatment program will have a significant impact upon them directly. They usually do not expect that the way they deal with each other will be altered during the hospitalization process. Yet the manner in which the staff perceives and communicates with the patient and family does significantly influence the family. Families receive a variety of messages from the hospital staff—sometimes direct but more often indirect—as to how they should interact with each other and the patient. Frequently, the patient himself is the bearer of the hospital's messages to the family. The patient may directly quote staff members who have made suggestions about how he should be handled by the family or should have been treated in the past. Often, staff demands for the family to change are implicit and covert, such as when the hospital staff assess the patient as ready for discharge even though the behavior for which the family brought the patient to the hospital persists. This is an interesting message to the family that could be understood by them in multiple ways, perhaps the family: (1) should have handled the patient in a different manner, (2) should reassess their views of the behavior as abnormal, or (3) must change their expectations of the hospital. In the traditional psychiatric hospital, staff attempts to influence the family are usually random, unplanned, nonsystematic, uncoordinated, and generally lacking in a purposeful goal. Yet there are significant hospital effects upon the family even if unintended; some of these are perceived as positive, some not so. When psychiatric hospitals set out to involve and change the family directly as part of an inpatient family-oriented treatment program, then naturally the impact upon the family is intensified [1,2,3].

Whether family change is planned by the hospital or not, families will have a wide variety of reactions to the hospital's influence upon them. Many perceive the hospital staff's expectation for change as creating excessive pressure and will make attempts to reduce the level of this new stress. This may be particularly upsetting for a family if they have just reached a new internal equilibrium dependent upon the hospital's total care of the patient/family member. When an inpatient unit utilizes conjoint family therapy, the family's new steady state may be disrupted by the therapist's giving directives or making uncomfortable interpretations. Essentially, the family will be asked to gradually work through a conflictive process in order to resolve the identified problem. It is hoped that the experienced hospital therapist will manage the pressures on the family so that they may participate constructively. Yet there will be occasions in which the stress of change will be too much for some families.

In this chapter the authors attempt to provide a simple classification of some common types of family reactions to the patient and the hospital clinical staff. We focus upon how some families attempt to change the activities of the clinical staff, the hospital administration, or the suprasystem of the hospital, e.g., outside budgetary control agencies. The kind of intervention the family makes and their motives grow out of the type of relationship that the family has developed, first with the patient and then with the ward treatment staff, particularly the primary therapist. The major precipitating event that provokes a family to try to change the hospital is the clinical staff's attempts to influence the family itself, either directly or indirectly.

Most commonly, the family attempts to alter the attitudes or techniques of the ward level staff in their handling of the patient/family member (particularly if it is the patient's new behavior that is the precipitant of family change) or themselves. (This is very common if the family is being directly focused upon in family treatment.) Often the result of these family interventions with the hospital is further education to promote understanding of what is being attempted in treatment. A more solid and successful therapeutic alliance between the hospital and the family may ensue. If the family is not satisfied, however, then they may decide to go up the administrative chain of command. At this point the family may want to disengage from the therapy or have the patient discharged. The family hopes to get the higher level of hospital administration or outside control agencies to change the treatment staff's attitudes. Inappropriate interventions by the hospital administration can lead to an undermining of the therapy with the result being a negative effect on the patient and family. Naturally, many situations in which the family attempts to change the hospital are not motivated by therapeutic stress nor do they result in constraints on the ward staff. The potential is always present for a positive outcome if the ward staff and hospital administration can work together to treat the patient and family in a clinically appropriate manner. Yet these family-hospital interactions are tricky and complicated; a not uncommon consequence is a situation in which the ward staff have their hands tied due to higher level administrative intervention.

The reader will notice in some of the examples given in this chapter that the families often cite as their reason for dissatisfaction a seemingly legitimate consumer complaint, such as not enough attention being paid to the patient, or need for a shorter or longer hospital stay. We recognize that psychiatric hospitals do make mistakes and at times neglect patients. In these instances, patients and families need to loudly assert their rights and corrections should be made. This chapter is not directed at the sort of family intervention with the hospital organization that we view as legitimate. The focus here is upon those family reactions to the hospital that arise when the family attempts to circumvent the therapist-patient-family relationship and which lead to a dysfunctional outcome, that is, therapeutic stalemate for the patient and family.

FAMILY REACTION TYPES

The authors have subdivided family reactions to the patient and hospital staff into three groups: the overinvolved, the uninvolved, and the pseudo-involved family. Individuals representing these family reaction types use a variety of strategies to try to change the hospital but control of the treatment process is their common goal. However, the specific demands and the motives behind the family's requests differ according to the type of family-patient-hospital relationship.

The overinvolved family is enmeshed with the patient and often the ward staff. Their motive in trying to change the functioning of the hospital is to bring about a closer relationship between themselves and either the patient or ward staff. They may try to get the hospital administration or outside control agency to allow the family more involvement in the decision making of the treatment team in order to have more control over the patient. The uninvolved group may also try to intervene with the hospital but their motivation is to increase the distance between the family and either the patient or ward staff. A family from this group often requests the hospital staff not to discharge their patient/family member. The desired goal is a closer relationship between the staff and the patient; but not the patient and family, or staff and family. A family from the pseudo-involved group presents an image of wanting to be closely involved with the patient and the treatment team. Yet when pushed for changes, their ambivalence and wish for increased separation emerges. They initially work closely and cooperatively with the staff and later intervene to get the hospital to disengage. Their motivation appears to be mixed but the consequence is usually increased separation, with the patient and hospital on one side and the family on the other. It is important for the hospital administration and other agents of control to be aware of each of these types of families because they may be approached by them to bring about change at the ward level. Likewise the ward staff, particularly the primary family therapist, should try to predict ahead of time if they have a family that may attempt to change the hospital. By observing the type of family group they are working with, they may have a better sense of what strategies will be used and why.

Research Findings

It is interesting that no one diagnostic group of patients can be found within these three types of families. For example, families of schizophrenics have been found to be overinvolved, uninvolved, or pseudo-involved with the patient and/hospital staff. Research done by Spitzer et al. have attempted to subdivide family reactions to patients and have correlated this with treatment outcome. His most recent work is reported in this volume [4]. Other researchers, such as Reiss, have tried to make predictions about how the family will react to the hospital based upon their behavior on specific laboratory tests [5]. Leff's work led to the subdividing of families into two groups depending upon the degree of emotional involvement and criticism and he has shown that the family type correlates highly with relapse rates of schizophrenic patients [6]. These research efforts are providing some support for the clinical observations that family reactions, particularly to the patient but also to others, will have a significant influence upon treatment outcome.

Overinvolved Families

This subgroup of families are usually too close to the patient and have a difficult time disengaging at appropriate points. We are aware, of course, that the family reactions to the patient are not unilateral; usually this type of family-patient relationship develops with a moderate-to-severely disabled person who is overly dependent on the family for guidance and support due to cognitive and behavioral impairments. These families frequently end up managing the patient's total life. If the patient enters the hospital, the family has a difficult time relinquishing control and moving toward partial disengagement. Consequently, these families want close contact with their hospitalized family member. They also begin to develop two types of overly enmeshed relationships with the ward staff (including the primary therapist if there is one). The first type of relationship is one of extreme dependency in which the family as a whole or certain members cling and rely on the staff for support. The second type of relationship that evolves is one in which the family tries to control the staff, becoming overinvolved in many decisions made by the treatment team concerning the patient. They may demand special privileges for the patient and want the staff to become overly enmeshed with the patient/family member, encouraging dependency on the patient's part. Families that develop either of these relationships may begin to demand that more be done for their hospitalized family member. These requests may result from some change in the patient's behavior (either in a positive or negative direction) or from some movement in the family treatment. It is this type of family that when dissatisfied with the level of their involvement with the staff or patient or with the staff's involvement with the patient may turn to other persons in the hospital hierarchy of authority, such as the physician in charge of the ward, the hospital director, a legislator, or the governor. They usually demand that these higher level administrators become intensely involved with the care of their family member. If they are successful then they may overinvolve an entire hospital staff, from the ward administrator to the top executive. In most cases this does not benefit the patient but merely soothes temporarily the family's discomfort. It also nullifies the primary therapist's attempts to change the relationships in the family.

Case 1

The following case illustrates the situation of an overly involved family. The patient, Ms. V, was a 24-year-old schizophrenic woman who had been in a private institution prior to her admission to a state mental hospital. Her family was concerned about the patient's periodic bizarre outbursts of violence and felt that they must maintain absolute control of every facet in the patient's life in order to prevent these episodes. When she was in the private institution, the family arranged to have one of that hospital's administrators see her in individual therapy concomitant to her treatment on the inpatient ward. When she was admitted to the state hospital her former therapist-administrator initially made calls to the ward staff of the hospital in order to educate them about Ms. V. Later this education became suggestions and then at times, directives for Ms. V's treatment program. The family would regularly report back to this former therapist-administrator and in this manner began to manipulate the ward staff so that Ms. V ended up under their control. The patient reacted to this with extreme ambivalence, oftentimes feeling that her parents were always watching over her, at other times feeling that this was the attention she needed. When the ward staff became fully aware of these hospital-family interactions, they began to set limits on the family and the administrator-therapist of the private institution who had referred Ms. V. This, however, was a very uncomfortable situation for the family and they began to have this same administrator-therapist call professionals higher up in the state hospital in order to "rectify some deficiencies in the patient's treatment program." The family was trying to create an overinvolved staff-patient relationship even though the patient was quite ambivalent about such an approach. The consequence of this relationship between the family and the higher echelons of the state hospital system was a constrained ward staff who felt unable to exercise their independent clinical judgement. They were always aware that the hospital administration was looking over their shoulders in a critical manner. The resolution of this pathologic hospital-family relationship occurred when the upper level administrators in the state hospital began setting limits on the inappropriate demands made by the family and her private therapist. Once these limits had been set and the family saw that further requests would not achieve anything, they became engaged in family therapy at the ward level.

In situations concerning these overinvolved families, it is essential that the hospital administration be familiar with the dynamics of their reactions. The administrator must be able to take a position which guarantees the ward staff the ability to conduct clinically appropriate treatments based on their consultation with the ward staff. Overinvolved families are a common entity in the mental health system; if both the ward staff and hospital administrators are aware of the issues, clinically appropriate limit setting and direction will take place.

Another case example points out what may happen with this type of family when they become overly dependent on the therapist and how this can influence the hospital staff.

Case 2

Ms. W was a 23-year-old single woman who had lived with her mother for the past four years during which time she had been diagnosed as suffering from chronic undifferentiated schizophrenia. The mother had become so involved in the patient's activities that she would on occasion fill in at the daughter's job when her daughter was unable to perform and even entertained boyfriends when the patient was "too sick to be available." Additionally, the outpatient psychiatrist, a female, had also developed an over-enmeshed relationship with the patient; this was overtly fostered by the mother. When the patient was admitted to the state psychiatric hospital, her outpatient psychiatrist, who also had privileges at this hospital, drove her back to the mother's apartment during leaves of absence in order to "save the mother the trouble." This overinvolvement of the psychiatrist was questioned by the hospital staff. Later, when the mother had an argument with the daughter during one of the leave of absences the daughter ran away and literally stayed in the vestibule of her outpatient psychiatrist's home for the remainder of the leave of absence. During this weekend, the mother was not concerned since she knew that the patient had been at the residence of the psychiatrist. This incident followed a turning point in family therapy which involved the mother relinquishing some of the decision making responsibility to the daughter. The problem was finally resolved when the mother, daughter, psychiatrist, and hospital family therapist met to discuss the issue of the mother's overinvolvement in the patient's life and her wish that someone could be caretaker of the patient. Further family sessions with these persons included the working through of dependency conflicts, including the mother's and daughter's enmeshment with the psychiatrist, and placing more responsibility on the patient in a gradual manner. This type of family-hospital staff alliance became detrimental to the patient because it preserved the existing dependency relation of the patient to the parent and pseudo-parent.

Uninvolved Families

This type of family-patient-hospital relationship develops most often when the family has had an extremely difficult time in previous treatment programs. In essence they have given up and desire to distance themselves from the patient. These are the families that want the patient out of their lives so that they can resume a long-hoped-for more normal way of functioning. If the ward staff go along with the family's wishes, this type of family provides little trouble. These patients and families are frequently seen in the state hospital system that has the responsibility of taking care of the patients who have been unsuccessfully treated by all other treatment modalities. The basic theme of the uninvolved family is "please take care of the patient because we cannot handle the stress."

The uninvolved family's relationship with the hospital staff can be divided into two basic subtypes. The first is the uninvolved family who wants to be totally detached from both the hospital and the patient. This family type does not concern itself with the details of how the staff are involved with their patient/family member and are usually comfortable with a custodial approach. Their major concern occurs when the patient is considered for release from the hospital. This fear is usually not based on the assumption that the patient may become violent or suicidal, but that the patient/family member may become involved again with the family. Trouble develops when the patient has improved to the point where discharge is being considered and, as is appropriate, the family is contacted for their decision. At this point the uninvolved family attempts to manipulate the various hospital hierarchical levels in order to have the patient remain in the hospital. This type of family becomes quite fearful that the patient will again be forced upon them even though a treatment plan may be developed that provides little, if any, contact with the patient's family. The fear is that the patient will again fail and the family will have the problem of a sick person on their hands. They, in their communication and relationship with the hospital administrators, attempt to put pressure on the clinical staff to reconsider the decision of discharge. They make arguments such as, the patient has never been able to live alone, or the patient has failed in the past many times. They try to convince the administrators that the patient cannot live outside the hospital in spite of any therapeutic progress during the hospital stay. This family typically is not involved in any type of family therapy during the hospital stay and is usually unaware of any progress that has been achieved. In most cases, when the hospital administrators are made aware of this situation, they are most willing to support the ward staff who are attempting to better the life of the patient. This rational and humane approach, however, may be an insufficient argument against extreme political pressures as seen in some of the examples discussed below.

Case 3

Ms. C, who was hospitalized for over fifteen years in Springfield Hospital Center (a state mental hospital), had the diagnosis of alcohol deterioration with episodic violent outbursts. The family disengaged quite early in the patient's stay at Springfield. During her long rehabilitation, the patient made progress and was able to perform the functions of daily living quite appropriately. It was then decided that she could be placed in a supervised foster care home. The family was notified weeks prior to discharge so that they could be aware of and have some part in the type of aftercare plan being formulated. The family was quite angry that the hospital would "throw out a lady that needs to be in the hospital." They began calling the various administrators in the hospital system, as well as certain officials in the local community in which she was to be discharged. The family, who had been quite outspoken during the past about their conviction that the patient would always require hospitalization, refused to participate in any type of treatment since they felt that this would achieve no solution. Thus, when plans were made for discharge, they again had the same assumption. Finally, through the skillful diplomacy of the hospital family therapist, various administrators were informed of the progress that the patient had made and of the thorough aftercare plan that was being formulated by the ward staff. The family anxiety was also handled through careful explanations and counseling concerning alternatives if the patient did not do well in the community. The family was reassured by this counseling and was also made aware that the patient would be put on an extended trial visit, i.e., she would still officially be considered a patient of the hospital even though she was living in the community in order to determine whether she could handle outpatient independence.

The second subtype of the uninvolved family is the family who desires to be disengaged from the patient and staff but wants the staff to be actively involved with the patient. They may push the staff to provide the total care and concern for the patient that they have been unable to provide. They may monitor closely how well the staff is treating the patient and become very upset with any signs of neglect or lack of attention. Yet they do not expect or desire the patient to be discharged.

Pseudo-Involved Family

The last type of patient-family-hospital relationship can be labeled pseudo-involved. This is the family who appears to be quite interested in the welfare and treatment of the identified patient. Yet, for various reasons, the family group as a whole is not able to change their behavior with the patient in such a way as to allow for discharge of the patient or for symptomatic progress to occur. The family maintains the myth of a close, caring, and supportive family but this is primarily a group defense mechanism that masks their ambivalence about themselves and having the patient home again. They engage in therapy with the ward staff if asked and are at first described as very concerned family members. What ultimately happens is that when the family realizes that they must reintegrate the patient, they become resistant to further family therapy directives or interpretations. Their argument may be that they have tried this before and it has failed, or that they are unable to provide for the needs of the patient within the family. In addition to some logical arguments given by the family there are some other ways of resisting therapeutic progress which are less direct. This indirect resistance may be revealed by a devaluation of the therapist as a professional, claiming that he is neither qualified nor competent or criticism of the therapist because he works in a facility which is not regarded highly, e.g., a state hospital. In many cases the family may start an argument with the therapist or make excessive demands in order to stall therapeutic progress. The basic theme behind this family is that they want to look like they are strong and competent but are actually unable to provide a supportive setting and do not want demands placed on them. This theme is not initially observed and is hard to ascertain in the first few interviews. When the true involvement is requested by the therapist, for example, in making changes in the family relationship, then the family moves toward manipulating the ward staff by going to the hospital administration. An excellent example of how this was handled by one family is presented as follows.

Case 4

Mr. D was a 47-year-old man with the diagnosis of a bipolar affective disorder. He had recently been involved in a buying spree and had publicly insulted his wife, a well-known figure in the community. In the initial sessions of family therapy, the wife wanted to participate fully in helping her husband overcome these difficulties. The therapist, attempting to minimize the length of hospital stay because of Mr. D's prompt response to therapy and medication, planned for an early discharge. The talk of discharge was met with great resistance on the part of the wife. She claimed that the hospital did not know what it was doing and the physician who was in charge of the patient was not fully competent to make such decisions. In spite of further assurances by the family therapist who was backed up by his supervisors, the wife stated that she did not want her husband back until he was fully "cured." She would not define what she meant by this and disengaged from therapy. During the following days she began to contact various hospital administrators and politicians in the area demanding that the patient be held in the state hospital until fully treated. The wife refused to take part in any further family sessions until the hospital guaranteed that her husband would be kept in the hospital for at least one year. It was then discovered that the wife had also been making plans to admit her husband to a local Veterans Hospital; the admitting physician contacted the state hospital staff and stated that the wife felt that her husband was in need of several years of treatment there. Additionally, the wife hired a lawyer in order to further push her point of view. The wife, a very energetic and influential woman, applied a great deal of political pressure on the ward level family therapist. Initially there were some hospital officials who recommended that this patient be kept in the hospital until the wife "calms down and is able to again talk with the family therapist." There was the additional factor of a civil hearing to decide whether the patient should be released. The hearing officer ruled that Mr. D could not be kept in the hospital as an involuntary patient. The hospital administration then decided to take a firm stand. They told the patient and family that he would be released and offered to conduct a family session which would include crisis planning for the imminent discharge. At this session, the after-care plan was formulated and supported by both husband and wife. The patient was subsequently discharged and has faithfully followed the outpatient program structured for him and his wife.

The pseudo-involved family can be extremely difficult to deal with because behind a superficial show of concern for the patient, there seems to be an underlying impulse to move toward disengagement. When these families complain to the hospital administration and other control agents, they exaggerate their concern for the patient and may form an initial alliance with these individuals for this reason. For the ward staff to resolve this alliance, they must educate the involved administrators and/or politicians in the rationale behind the therapeutic maneuvers which the patient's family is questioning. These explanations are often difficult to substantiate in view of the fact that the patient seems to have an interested family who views the therapeutic procedures as exploitive or destructive. The hospital administrators and politicians who may be involved in collusive alliances with the family should be aware of this kind of family manipulation and its potential for sabotaging a positive therapeutic outcome.

These case examples have been drawn from the authors' experiences in the state mental health system. Obviously these family-hospital dynamics are not unique to the public sector. Both general and private psychiatric hospitals are subject to these same pressures by the family to bring about some control of the clinical ward staff [1]. However, the state mental hospital system is particularly vulnerable to both administrative and political pressures as a result of family intervention. There are very few barriers that will insulate superintendents and hospital directors from consumer and political pressures. Because these hospitals spend public monies they are held accountable by numerous public agencies. Private and general hospitals also have their own boards or directors to whom they are accountable and families with influence can change these hospitals [7]. Yet the state hospitals provide a particularly rich milieu in which to learn about the dynamic interactions between hospitals and families because the hospital's boundaries are very permeable. Families use politicians to manipulate the organizational structure of hospitals. Many times the changes that families push for are positive, e.g., increased funding for therapeutic programs. Yet when families approach the hospital and/or control agencies for favors having to do with changing the therapeutic climate for their own specific patient/family member then their motives must be investigated. The directions in which they are pushing are not always in the best interest of the patient or in the long-range interest of the family.

Many families desire government officials to bring about changes that will give temporary relief from anxieties stirred by changes in the patient or the family. Families can also generate pressure on both the private and public hospital systems through other means. They may go to the press in order to embarrass a facility. Families may threaten to contact licensing bodies or may actually contact such outside regulating bodies as the Joint Commission on Accreditation of Hospitals. The authors have seen several situations in which the families threaten to do this when they did not like the direction of the treatment. No government official, hospital administrator, or ward personnel are free from such inappropriate family pressures. It is essential that professionals and administrators be aware of the motivation and rationale used by some families when they try to use political, economic, or public pressure in order to alleviate their own stress. With increased awareness and knowledge, officials will be able to screen out those families who approach them for inappropriate reasons. Consequently they will be able to pay more attention to those consumers and families who are pushing for legitimate and long-needed changes in hospitals.

REFERENCES

1. Harbin, H.T. "Families and hospitals: collusion or cooperation?" *American Journal of Psychiatry* 12 : 1496–1499, 1978.
2. Harbin, H.T. "A family oriented psychiatric inpatient unit." *Family Process* 18 : 281–292, 1979.

3. Krajewski, T. "Inpatient family therapy." *International Journal of Family Psychiatry*. In press.
4. Spitzer, S.P.; Swanson, R.M.; and Lehr, R.K. "Audience reactions and careers of psychiatric patients." *Family Process* 8 : 159–181, 1969.
5. Reiss, D.; Costell, R.; and Jones, C. et al. "The family meets the hospital: a laboratory forecast of the encounter." *Archives of General Psychiatry* 37 : 141–154, 1980.
6. Vaughn, C.E. and Leff, J.P. "The influence of family and social factors on the course of psychiatric illness." *British Journal of Psychiatry* 129 : 125–137, 1976.
7. Weintraub, W. "The VIP syndrome: a clinical study in hospital psychiatry." *Journal of Nervous and Mental Disease* 138 : 181–193, 1964.

PART II

Research Studies

8

The Effects of Family Presence and Brief Family Intervention for Hospitalized Schizophrenic Patients: A Review

IRA D. GLICK AND JOHN F. CLARKIN

The purpose of this chapter is to explore the issues of family presence and treatment for schizophrenic patients during an illness episode involving possible or actual hospitalization of the index patient. We begin with a brief discussion of the history of this concept and its implementation. A review of research on the presence of the family during hospital treatment is followed by a look at the sparse research on treatment outcome. A summary of the work to date and implications for the future concludes the chapter.

HISTORICAL REVIEW

As early as the 1950s, scientists from disparate disciplines were giving their attention to the immediate ecology—the family—of the schizophrenic for clues as to the etiology and pathogenesis of this illness. Gregory Bateson [2] and his team (which combined data from anthropology, communication analysis, psychotherapy, psychiatry, and psychoanalysis) postulated that schizophrenics' unconventional communicational habits are the result of characteristic sequential communication patterns in the family. They described the now familiar "double bind" as the classic interactional mode of consequence. Relevant to the present review is the reference Bateson et al. [3] made to the strong possibility of double-bind situations being created between the psychiatric hospital and the schizophrenic patient when the hospital staff (as the research group saw it) takes actions for the benefit of the staff while labeling them as beneficial for the patients.

During the same decade, Murray Bowen [5] was developing a general theory of family functioning using a sample of hospitalized schizophrenic patients and their families in a unique attempt to describe and understand the family ecology and its effect on the identified patient. In his extensive work with the schizophrenic and the family, Bowen described the family as a fused ego mass which lacked differentiation, and developed a controlled, intellectual approach to the family in order to further the differentiated functioning of the patient and other family members. As to the etiology of the schizophrenic condition, Bowen attributed it to the three generational process involving progressive fusion in the familial system.

Over the subsequent years, family intervention with schizophrenics and their families met with moderade-to-mediocre results. The success of phenothiazine treatment as well as research into the genetic components of the condition have led the field away from thinking of the family, whether in one or multiple generations, as having direct etiological impact. There has been difficulty in operationalizing the concept of the double bind, and thus establishing research evidence of its process and prevalence, and in fact, specificity to families of schizophrenics. Klein [18] probably best sums up the current situation by forcefully stating that psychosocial help for people with schizophrenia is appropriate for mitigating the effects of the illness, whereas psychosocial treatment for schizophrenia is ineffective. In the psychiatric hospitalization episodes themselves, there has been notable confusion and conflict about the role and importance of family intervention with the schizophrenic and his family [1].

RESEARCH

Most reviewers decry the large gap between clinical practice and research findings in general, and between family therapy and outcome research specifically [25,26,30,31]. However, a recent excellent review by Gurman and Kniskern [15] of over 200 relevant studies of marital and family therapy is more optimistic, seeing evidence for the relative efficacy of this therapeutic modality, and delineating clinical guidelines.

We will summarize findings relative to schizophrenia and the family in two areas: (1) the impact of the presence/absence of the family during a treatment episode involving hospitalization, and (2) the results of family treatment with the schizophrenic during an illness episode that includes hospitalization.

PRESENCE OF THE FAMILY
DURING AN ILLNESS EPISODE

In addition to asking whether family treatment is effective during the hospitalization of a schizophrenic, it is important to determine if the mere presence of the family is deleterious or beneficial to the patient during the crisis. This question is especially relevant in light of the recent evidence that families can be a negative influence on the post-hospital functioning of the schizophrenic patient [7].

LANGLEY PORTER STUDY

At a time when economic constraints, political pressures and the absence of good research data are forcing the disappearance of long-term hospitalization, Glick and his colleagues designed an investigation to compare the efficacy of short-term and long-term hospitalization upon the subsequent one-year and two-year adjustment of psychiatric patients, both schizophrenic and nonschizophrenic [10]. In this study, 255 patients were randomly assigned to either short-term (21 to 28 days) or long-term (90 to 120 days) hospitalization. The sample used to examine the effect of the presence/absence of the family and the effects of family therapy during the hospitalization of schizophrenic patients was composed of the 70 schizophrenic patients assigned to long-term hospitalization, since it was these patients whose length of stay afforded the possibility of sufficient family intervention to have a significant and measurable impact on the family and the patient.

Methodology

Fifty-three of the 70 long-term schizophrenic patients were assigned to one of four comparison treatment groups:

 1. Family therapy A: Patient and family seen in weekly individual family therapy for at least one month (four sessions) of the hospitalization.
 2. Family therapy B: Patient and family seen in weekly individual family therapy sessions and in weekly multifamily group therapy sessions for at least one month (four sessions) of the hospitalization.
 3. No family therapy C: Family members unavailable for family sessions, due to illness, death, or geographical distance from the hospital.
 4. No family therapy D: Family members, though physically available and in some contact with the patient during the hospitalization, not seen in family

therapy. This was usually the case because family therapy was not clinically indicated (e.g., family relationships involving elderly parents in the family of origin were not regarded as significant in contributing to the current illness episode nor in discharge planning) or because the family refused to cooperatè.

Of the 70 subjects, 17 did not fit the study criteria; 10 were excluded because they prematurely ended their hospitalization by at least one month, and another 6 subjects were not included because the family therapy they received did not fit the criteria (e.g., multifamily group therapy only).

Table 8-1 compares the four groups on the variables of sex, age, education, and length of stay in the hospital. The four groups were well matched by sex and education. The family therapy B group was in the hospital slightly longer than the other family therapy group (nonsignificant), and the family therapy B group was significantly younger than the two groups that had no family therapy.

Treatment strategy included the assessment of psychodynamics, precipitants of hospitalization, and clinical diagnosis over an initial two-to-three-week period. Treatment was oriented to a long-range psychosocial reorganization either through psychotherapy and medication, or major rehabilitative measures—change of living situation, change of job, or workshop placement—or both modalities were used. The focus was on the actual initiation of concrete change—for example, by setting up regular visits to a physician and establishing a medication regimen.

Table 8-1.   Demographic Characteristics of Patients in Two Family Therapy Groups, A and B, and Two No Family Therapy Groups, C and D

		SEX		MEDIAN	AGE		MEDIAN HOS-PITALIZATION
GROUP	N	M	F	EDUCATION	Range	Mean	(IN DAYS)
Family Therapy A	16	10	6	12	15–45	24.1	99
Family Therapy B	16	10	6	13	15–32	21.4	107
No Family Therapy C	12	8	4	12	23–37	26.6	94
No Family Therapy D	9	7	2	12	18–35	26.4	104

Family Therapy A: Patient and family seen in weekly individual family therapy for at least one month (four sessions) of the hospitalization.

Family Therapy B: Patient and family seen both in weekly individual family therapy meetings and in weekly Multi-Family Group Therapy sessions for at least one month (four sessions) of the hospitalization.

No Family Therapy C: Family members physically unavailable because of death or living too far away from the hospital.

No Family Therapy D: Family members, though physically available and in some contact with the patient during hospitalization, were not seen in family therapy.

Reprinted with permission from the editor of Family Process from Gould E. and Glick I.D. "The effects of family presence and family therapy on outcome of hospitalized schizophrenic patients." Family Process 16:503–510, 1977, p. 505.

A partially fixed drug regimen was used, and thus phenothiazine levels were kept uniformly high for all groups of patients. This was successful in that there were no clinically significant differences among groups in the amount of medication received during the first 21 days of hospitalization.

The specifics of the individual, family, and family group treatments are summarized in Table 8-2. The individual therapy was conducted by psychiatric residents.

The family therapy included all patients who had "significant others" (about half the patients). It was carried out by cotherapists, one of whom was usually the primary therapist under the supervision of an experienced family therapist. The frequency was one-to-two times per week—usually twice a week with short-term patients. For the short-term patients, the focus was on discharge planning (which usually heavily involved the family). For the long-term patients, the goals included both change in family patterns and discharge planning.

The type of family therapy intervention could best be described as pluralistic. That is, the theoretical model was based on elements of the understanding-awareness model, the strategic-behavioral model, and the experiential model [12]. The three basic techniques used were those described by Glick and Kessler [11] and included strategies that facilitated communication of thoughts and feelings; strategies that shifted disturbed, inflexible roles and coalitions; and strategies that aided family role assumption, education, and demythologizing.

In addition, other techniques were used as indicated, including educational methods to focus on the nature and consequences of the identified patient's illness and its effect on the family [23], as well as involving the entire staff in the treatment process and underlining the importance of family involvement in the identified patient's treatment. There was special emphasis on involving the family at the time of admission and engaging them in making a therapeutic contract. Symptoms (for example, delusion of being persecuted) were identified and redefined in terms of the family (i.e., was the patient being scapegoated). Where resistances were encountered, we often followed the engagement technique outlined by Harbin of telling the patient and family that the identified patient will have to leave the hospital if the family cannot arrange to come for therapy [16]. There was a focus on trying to change the family patterns during the hospitalization (not leaving this task until after discharge) and emphasis on discharge planning starting at the time of admission. Nursing staff and occupational therapy staff used a variety of techniques to involve (and change) the family during visiting hours.

No further systematic study of the family therapy given was done during the course of this sub-study (i.e., effect of family presence and family interventions), as outcome of the two types of hospitalization strategies was the primary focus of the investigation.

Table 8-2.   Description of Psychosocial Treatment Program for Short-Term and Long-Term Groups

TYPE OF TREATMENT	DESCRIPTION OF TREATMENT	FACTORS SPECIFIC TO TREATMENT MODALITY		TOTAL HOURS OF TREATMENT PER PATIENT*	
		Short-Term	*Long-Term*	*Short-Term*	*Long-Term*
Individual psychotherapy	Included all patients. Most supportive-type done by primary therapists, mostly psychiatric residents, but occasionally by a psychiatric nurse or psychology student. Frequency: 1–3 times a week for 30–60 minutes; average = 2 hours a week.	Primary goal was crisis intervention and discharge planning—little time for other goals.	Goals much more varied, such as meaning of a symptom, rehabilitation in job setting, etc.	6.0	24.0
Family therapy	Included all patients who had significant others (about half the patients). Done by cotherapists, one of whom was usually the primary therapist. Frequency: 1–2 times a week; usually twice with short-term patients. A weekly 90-minute multiple family therapy session was also conducted with about 2/3 of the long-term patients; average = 1 hour a week for long-term patients only.	Focus was on discharge planning.	Goals included both change in family patterns and discharge planning.	5.0	21.0

Table 8-2. (*Continued*)

Group therapy	Included all patients. Led by trainees in several disciplines. Frequency: 2 times a week for 90 minutes. Two groups of 8–13 patients. A transactional analysis group met once a week with an equal mix of short- and long-term patients.	No difference	4.5	18.0
Milieu therapy	Included a role play group attended by all patients, a treatment planning group consisting of all staff and patients on a particular team focusing on treatment planning and problems, and a discharge planning group focusing on discharge (all weekly); also, various activity therapy groups such as crafts, shopping, cooking, and swimming that met throughout the week. Short-term patients spent as much time with nursing staff as long-term patients during first 4 weeks.	Received more thorough discharge planning, most of which occurred in the last 2/3 of hospitalization.	60.0	240.C

*Figured on the basis of the number of hours per week of treatment modality multiplied by 3 weeks for the short-term group and 12 weeks for the long-term group.

Reprinted with permission from the editor of Family Process from: Gould E. and Glick I.D. "The effects of family presence and family therapy on outcome (` hospitalized schizophrenic patients." Family Process 16:503–510, 1977, p. 506.

Multiple-family group therapy (MFGT) was conducted by a senior member of the staff who was an experienced family therapist and two co-therapists who were trainees. Although no attempt was made to assess the quality of the therapies, there was no reason to believe that quality varied significantly from one group to another, or that quality was significantly better or worse than in other university inpatient settings.

All groups were assessed at admission, four weeks after admission, at their respective discharge times, and at one year after admission. The major instruments utilized included the Psychiatric Evaluation Form (PEF) [8], a semistructured rating of symptoms and global outcome; the Brief Follow-up Rating (BFR), dealing with job and other role functioning, social interaction, type and frequency; and the Health-Sickness Rating Scale (HSRS) [22], an independent global rating of symptoms and functioning.

Results

Analysis of the results (see Gould and Glick [14] for more detail) revealed that all three groups of patients having families available (groups A, B, and D) did significantly better than the C group patients (no available families) at a one year follow-up on global outcome as measured by the PEF. On a rating of overall functioning (BFR), patients having both families and receiving family therapy (groups A and B) also functioned significantly better than the patients without families (group C). Patients having families but receiving no family therapy (group D) also did better than patients without families (group C), but this finding was of only borderline signficance.

Both at discharge and at one year follow-up, there were no significant differences in outcomes either between the two family therapy groups A and B or between the family therapy groups A and B and the patient group D who had families, but no family therapy.

These results suggest that the presence of a family during the hospitalization of an index schizophrenic patient, and possibly following discharge, is significantly related to better post-hospital adjustment. Having a family available did not prevent hospitalization, nor did it reduce admission symptomatology—the level of psychopathology among the four groups after admission was about the same on both the PEF and BFR. Yet the presence of a family during a first or second hospitalization—early in the psychiatric history of the patient—was related to the patients' better functioning in the community following hospitalization regardless of whether family members were actively involved in treatment.

The sanguine effects of the presence of the family are worth emphasizing in light of data in the literature emphasizing the association of schizophrenia and pathological and destructive aspects of a schizophrenic's family relationships

[7,21,24]. Although it appeared that in many cases the family relationships were less than optimal, they may be better than having no family (unless the schizophrenic patient finds a workable placement elsewhere as in a foster home). This is consistent with the fact that schizophrenic patients themselves rated informal contact with their families (visits, passes) as much more important and useful in their overall treatment program than did staff [14].

The meaning of the lack of impact of the family therapy itself is unclear and inconclusive. Perhaps the outcome measures were not sensitive to important changes in the family, or possibly there was not significant attention given to certain subgroups of schizophrenics and families so that treatment effects washed out in group means. Attention to results of family treatment in the section to follow may shed more light on this issue.

TREATMENT OUTCOME STUDIES

Esterson et al. treated 42 adult (ages 15-to-35) schizophrenic inpatients with family therapy during 6-to-12 weeks of hospitalization [9]. Only 17 percent of the patients treated with family therapy were readmitted in the following year, as opposed to a 52 percent readmission rate for a large group of similar patients.

Bowen treated seven families with a schizophrenic member during inpatient stays of up to 35 months [6]. As rated by the therapist, three were improved in terms of family functioning while four remained unchanged. In addition, Bowen saw another seven families in long-term outpatient family therapy, and five were reported as improved and two as essentially unchanged.

Laquer et al. treated 80 families of hospitalized patients, most of whom were schizophrenic, with multiple-family (four-to-six families) group therapy of long duration [20]. According to ratings by therapists, 62 percent of the families were improved in communication and understanding. As rated by the families themselves, 67 percent reported improvement.

Lack of control groups makes these studies difficult to interpret.

Langsley and his colleagues did a partially controlled comparative investigation of family crisis intervention begun at the brink of hospitalization compared with traditional hospital treatment [19]. From a pool of 300 families who sought psychiatric assistance during a crisis, half were randomized to one of the two treatment approaches. Inpatient care, which lasted an average of 28.6 days, consisted of individual, group and milieu therapy, and pharmacotherapy. The family crisis intervention consisted of a small number of office and home visits and pharmacotherapy over three weeks. On follow-up evaluation 6, 12, and 18 months following treatment, family crisis therapy patients were less frequently rehospitalized (and for shorter duration). Social adjustment was not different for the two groups. Although this study has many often-cited positive attributes, including randomization, large sample size, and investigation of a crucial decision point; it has been criticized for not having a real control group since the hospitalized patients received a variety of non-family therapies [15,30]. In addition, it is unclear as to which aspect of the outpatient intervention—its crisis nature, family focus, greater medication compliance, or simple avoidance of the more drastic step of hospitalization—was responsible for its comparative efficacy. Rittenhouse, in a partial replication study, contrasted ambulatory family therapy with hospital treatment of the identified patient [27]. The family treatment was superior to the hospital treatment on patient global improvement and readmissions, while there was no difference on family pathology or community adjustment. These two investigations suggest that family therapy can be effective in preventing hospitalization for schizophrenics but reveal no additional advantage in terms of increasing social functioning in the community (a dimension notoriously difficult to alter).

In what has been called one of the most impressive comparative studies to date [15] Ro-Trock et al. compared family treatment to individual treatment during a brief hospitalization of adolescent patients about 50 percent of whom were diagnosed as schizophrenic [28]. The 28 patients were randomly assigned to the two modes of brief (10 sessions) treatment. Outcome measures included self-report, family performance on a problem solving task, community adjustment, and rate of rehospitalization. At three month follow-up, the family therapy group was significantly superior in rate of rehospitalization (0 percent as opposed to 43 percent) and a shorter period needed for return to functioning in the community. Given the focus of this review, i.e., schizophrenia, it is important to know by what criteria adolescents were diagnosed as schizophrenic and if the results for the schizophrenic patients were in line with the results for the group as a whole.

Goldstein et al. investigated the effects of chemotherapy and brief (six sessions) family therapy for schizophrenic patients during their after-care immediately following a brief (average of 14 days) first or second hospital admission [13]. One hundred and four schizophrenics with a mean age of 23.4 years were assigned by stratified random method to one of four treatment conditions: (1) high dose fluphenazine, family therapy; (2) high dose fluphenazine, no family therapy; (3) low dose fluphenazine, family therapy; and (4) low dose fluphenazine, no family therapy. Premorbid adjustment, specific to males and females, was used to stratify the samples. The family therapy is described as crisis-oriented with emphasis on acceptance by the patient and family of the psychotic episode, mutual identification of precipitating stresses, and planning on the avoidance of future similar stresses. Outcome measures included relapse rate and clinical ratings with the BPRS at admission, discharge, six weeks, and six months follow-up. In general, the results support differential effects of the treatments by sex and premorbid adjustment. During the six-week treatment phase, ten patients deteriorated clinically; these were concentrated largely in the group with minimal medication and an absence of family intervention. (In seven out of eight contrasts, the family therapy group was rated as less withdrawn and affectively flattened than the no-therapy group.) At the six-month follow-up, there was not a single relapse in the high-dose therapy group, while nearly 50 percent of the low-dose, no-therapy group had had some form of relapse. These data argue for the efficacy of chemotherapy and family therapy in effectively reducing relapse rates both during the active treatment phase and in the subsequent five months.

While relapse data support an interpretation of a major drug effect and significant drug-therapy interaction, symptom ratings (BPRS) support the efficacy of family therapy that shows independently of drug level during the six-week treatment phase, and is sustained over the following six months only in the group that received an adequate drug dosage.

Premorbid adjustment and sex were also significant in the outcome variance. *Good premorbid males* showed negligible relapse and a positive level of response to family therapy sustained over six months, independent of drug dose level. *Good premorbid females* showed a marked responsiveness to family therapy but required a higher dose to sustain the therapy gains over the follow-up period. Those with reduced dose plus no family therapy were particularly vulnerable to relapse. *Poor premorbid females* responded most favorably to high doses with family therapy; they readily relapsed in the low-dose condition whether or not family therapy was present. *Poor premorbid males* (i.e., the group with the worst prognosis) are the most confusing group. While they show high-dose sensitivity, with family therapy they show gains initially but reverse during the follow-up. The authors suggest that this "toxic" effect of family therapy with this group possibly reflects the brevity of the therapy or increased contact with noxious family members.

CONCLUSIONS AND IMPLICATIONS

The state of the art for process and outcome research for the family model has improved. Gurman and Kniskern have provided a helpful listing of criteria for outcome research in the area of family intervention [15]. These include the usual design requirements for outcome studies plus one that is unique to family intervention: presence of outcome measures for not only the identified patient, but also other family members.

Family therapy is a format of treatment (patient and family present for all or most of the sessions) as opposed to a specific type, (e.g., dynamic, behavioral, etc.) of intervention. Thus, it remains the burden of future researchers to more closely define the nature of the family intervention being used. Other reviews of outcome research in psychotherapy have argued cogently that comparisons between various psychosocial treatments will only yield specific answers when the treatments themselves are defined very concretely and specifically [17]. In the major outcome studies (Glick [10], Langsley [19], Ro-Trock [28], Goldstein [13]) on family treatment with hospitalized acute schizophrenics reviewed here, one can infer a growing consensus about the type of family treatment that is considered beneficial with this population. These researchers seem to be emphasizing a focused, goal-directed approach that places importance on stress reduction and management and family facilitation of concrete functioning in the daily life of the schizophrenic. Such an approach is in line with recent theoretical writings about the need for emphasis on communication enhancement rather than affectional-motivational factors [25], teaching families and schizophrenics to tolerate each other and to anticipate and prevent future stress that could precipitate other psychotic episodes [4].

The issue of the family presence and its impact on the schizophrenic family member is a complicated one that requires further scrutiny and research. This issue has an obvious impact on the practical matter of where the schizophrenic should live following hospitalization. Family contact can be defined by two parameters: (1) extent of contact (living with family or living apart from family; amount of hourly contact with family members), and (2) quality of family contact (emotional tone, communication, etc.). Since schizophrenics are by definition disabled and dependent on support systems, the extent and quality of family contact prior to, during, and following psychiatric hospitalization is important to adjustment. Although the Langley Porter data, discussed at some length in this chapter, show a positive correlation between some form of family contact and better adjustment following hospitalization, unfortunately neither the extent (even whether living with family or not) nor the quality of family interaction were measured.

While there are those who argue that for young unmarried schizophrenics the goal of family intervention should be to help the family deal with separation from their afflicted young member [25], we are less definitive for practice and theoretical reasons. In many cases there is no viable alternative living arrangement to returning to the family of origin. On more theoretical grounds, the Brown, Birley and Wing data strongly suggest that while there are households characterized by emotional, hostile overinvolvement with the patient that are correlated with relapse, a large percentage of homes (55 percent) were low on the destructive variables investigated [7]. For those 55 percent, a return to the home environment may be the most viable move. For the other 45 percent, either placement outside the home or focused family intervention with the goal of reducing the destructive interactions may be indicated [1].

Future research in the family treatment of schizophrenia should follow the lead of Goldstein in differentiating treatment response for subgroups of schizophrenics [13]. His attention to the differential effects of the sex and premorbid adjustment of the schizophrenic member, and the interaction of these variables with differential treatment outcome is very valuable. While variables relating to the index patient are important to outcome, it is also very likely that different dimensions of the family itself—and its interaction with the patient—may be highly important to the treatment outcome. Likely family dimensions would include the level of social and occupational functioning of key family members, level of expressed emotion [7], communication style [29], and family resources.

Any modality of psychosocial treatment may be useful and effective in producing immediate change (typically measured at the end of the treatment period), but may or may not be effective in maintaining the change over the follow-up period. There is often a neglect in attending to the difference between the two, with the subtle implication that a treatment that initiated change but that does not show maintenance of change on follow-up, is no good. Of the other major psychosocial approaches to treatment (i.e., individual or group), it is possible that family therapy—because it deals directly with the ecology of the patient—may offer the most direct approach to maintenance effects with the patient. In family treatment, there is the possibility of directly changing the family and thus the daily parameters for the patient when he lives with or stays in contact with the family (the usual case). More attention should be given to how family treatment can increase patient function outside of the hospital. Furthermore, attention should be given on follow-up measures to how the family maintained or failed to maintain its change.

It is clear that family treatment offers a promising, but as yet untested modality for preventing hospitalization, promoting recovery after an acute episode, and preventing rehospitalization, as well as increasing patient function and thus reducing family burden. At the same time, for some families the modality can be toxic, for example, increasing both patient and family dysfunction and promoting the need to extrude the patient in order to regain family homeostasis [13].

REFERENCES

1. Anderson, C.M. "Family intervention with severely disturbed inpatients." *Archives of General Psychiatry* 34 : 697–702, 1977.
2. Bateson, G.; Jackson, D.D.; and Haley, J. et al. "Towards a theory of schizophrenia." *Behavioral Science* 1 : 251–264, 1956.
3. Bateson, G.; Jackson, D.D.; Haley, J. et al. "A note on the double bind—1962." *Family Process* 2 : 154–161, 1963.
4. Beels, C.C. "Family and social management of schizophrenia." *Schizophrenia Bulletin* 13 : 97–118, 1975.

5. Bowen, M. "A family concept of schizophrenia." In D.D. Jackson (ed) *The Etiology of Schizophrenia.* New York: Basic Books, 1960, pp. 346–372.

6. Bowen, M. "Family psychotherapy." *American Journal of Orthopsychiatry* 31 : 40–60, 1961.

7. Brown, G.W.; Birley, J.L.T.; and Wing, J.K. "Influence of family life on the course of schizophrenic disorders: a replication." *British Journal of Psychiatry* 121 : 241–258, 1972.

8. Endicott, J. and Spitzer, R.L. "What! Another rating scale? The psychiatric evaluation form." *Journal of Nervous and Mental Disease* 154 : 88–104, 1972.

9. Esterson, A.; Cooper, D.; and Laing, R. "Results of family-oriented therapy with hospitalized schizophrenics." *British Medical Journal* 2 : 1462–1465, 1965.

10. Glick, I.D. and Hargreaves, W.A. *Psychiatric Hospital Treatment for the 1980s: A Controlled Study of Short versus Long Hospitalization.* Lexington, Massachusetts: Lexington Press, 1979.

11. Glick, I.D. and Kessler, D.R. *Marital and Family Therapy* (2nd ed). New York: Grune and Stratton, 1980.

12. Glick, I.D.; Kessler, D.R.; and Clarkin, J.F. "Different approaches to family therapy." In H.K.H. Brodie (ed) *American Handbook of Psychiatry*, Volume VII, New York: Basic Books, 1981.

13. Goldstein, M.J.; Rodnick, E.H.; Evans, J.R. et al. "Drug and family therapy in the aftercare of acute schizophrenics." *Archives of General Psychiatry* 35 : 1169–1177, 1978.

14. Gould, E. and Glick, I.D. "The effects of family presence and brief family intervention on global outcome for hospitalized schizophrenic patients." *Family Process* 16 : 503–510, 1977.

15. Gurman, A.S. and Kniskern, D.P. "Research on marital and family therapy: progress, perspective and prospect." In: S.L. Garfield and A.E. Bergin (eds.) *Handbook of Psychotherapy and Behavior Change: An Empirical Analysis* (2nd ed.). New York: John Wiley, 1978.

16. Harbin, H.T. "A family-oriented psychiatric inpatient unit." *Family Process* 18 : 281–302, 1979.

17. Kazdin, A.E. and Wilson, G.T. *Evaluation of Behavior Therapy: Issues, Evidence and Research Strategies.* Cambridge, Massachusetts: Ballinger, 1978, Ch 4.

18. Klein, D.F. "Psychosocial treatment of schizophrenia, or psychosocial help for people with schizophrenia?" *Schizophrenia Bulletin* 6 : 122–130, 1980.

19. Langsley, D.G.; Pittman, F.; and Swank, G. "Family crisis in schizophrenics and other mental patients." *Journal of Nervous and Mental Disease* 149 : 270–276, 1969.

20. Laquer, H.P. and LaBurt, H.A. "Family organization on a modern state hospital ward." *Mental Hygiene* 48 : 544–551, 1964.

21. Lidz, R. and Fleck, S. "Family studies and a theory of schizophrenia." In: T. Lidz, S. Fleck, and A. Cornelison (eds.) *Schizophrenia and the Family.* New York: International Universities Press, 1965.

22. Luborsky, L. "Clinicians' judgments of mental health." *Archives of General Psychiatry* 7 : 407–417, 1962.

23. May, P.A. "Schizophrenia: overview of treatment methods." In: A.M. Freedman, H.I. Kaplan, and B.J. Sadock (eds.) *Comprehensive Textbook of Psychiatry* (2nd ed.) Baltimore, MD: Williams & Wilkins, 1975, pp 923–938.

24. Mishler, E.G. and Waxler, N.E. *Family Process in Schizophrenia.* New York: Science House, 1968.

25. Mosher, L.R. and Gunderson, J.G. "Group, family, milieu and community support systems treatment for schizophrenia." In: L. Bellak (ed.) *Disorders of the Schizophrenic Syndrome.* New York: Basic Books, 1979, pp 399–452.

26. Olson, D.H. "Marital and family therapy: integrative review and critique." *Journal of Marriage and the Family* 32 : 501–538, 1970.

27. Rittenhouse, J. "Endurance of effect: family unit treatment compared to identified patient treatment." Proceedings, 78th Annual Convention of the American Psychological Association: 535–536, 1970.

28. Ro-Trock, G.K.; Wellisch, D.K.; and Schoolar, J.C. "A family therapy outcome study in an inpatient setting." *American Journal of Orthopsychiatry* 47 : 514–522, 1977.

29. Singer, M.T. and Wynne, L.C. "Thought disorder and family relations of schizophrenics." *Archives of General Psychiatry* 12 : 187–212, 1965.

30. Wells, R.A.; Dilkes, T.; and Trivelli, N. "The results of family therapy: a critical review of the literature." *Family Process* 7 : 189–207, 1972.

31. Winter, W. "Family therapy: research and theory." Current Topics in Clinical Community Psychology 3 : 95–121, 1971.

9

Measuring the Effects of Family Involvement on a Psychiatric Inpatient Unit

DAVID J. WITHERSTY AND E. RAYMOND KIDWELL

"Happy families are all alike; every unhappy family is unhappy in its own way."
Leo Tolstoi, *Anna Karenina*, 1875

One would assume that hospitalizing a person on a psychiatric unit would not only have an effect—beneficial, it is hoped—on the identified patient, but would also have some impact on the patient's family. The degree and significance of that impact depends upon a number of factors: the relationship between patient and family, the severity of the psychiatric illness, the level of understanding possessed by the family, the circumstances surrounding admission, as well as a variety of factors—both tangible and intangible. It might be possible to begin to measure the effects that psychiatric hospitalization has on the family by means of questionnaires and taped interviews. One might also follow members of the patient's family longitudinally and observe for changes that might occur in their attitudes or knowledge if repeated hospitalizations were necessary. The task would not be an easy one, but one could hypothesize an appropriate research design.[*]

If hospitalization has an effect on a patient's family, one might also assume that a patient's family could have some effect on the therapeutic outcome for the

---

[*] An instrument for measuring the effect that psychiatric hospitalization has on families has been developed and the interested reader is referred to descriptions of studies utilizing the Family Evaluation Form (FEF). They can be found in Herz, Endicott, and Spitzer. "Brief versus standard hospitalization: the families." *American Journal of Psychiatry* 133 : 795–801, 1976, and also in Herz, Endicott, and Gibbon. "Brief hospitalization—two year follow-up." *Archives of General Psychiatry* 36 : 701–705, 1979.

identified patient. It would be particularly reasonable to assume an effect if the family involvement occurred during therapy and was an integral part of the psychotherapy.

Many practitioners in the mental health field do seem to believe that family involvement in patient care is generally apt to be of value. The prominent position of family therapy in the field of psychotherapy is convincing evidence of this fact. Communication and general systems theorists have provided a conceptual base for family involvement. Therapists oriented toward individualized treatment usually welcome, at least, the additional information provided by a family. Many physicians look to families to increase compliance with medical treatment. Even if family psychopathology is in part responsible for symptomatic behavior, it may be argued that such a contribution can go unrecognized, undelineated, and untreated without some involvement of the family itself. Nonetheless, tangible supporting evidence for such assumptions remains minimal at best, especially in specific areas of family participation. There have been noteworthy exceptions, however, and the attempts made by those concerned with the family therapy movement to measure the effects that this particular approach has had on therapeutic outcome is referred to below.

This chapter addresses two issues: First, whether family involvement which occurs at times in a patient's psychiatric hospitalization, other than psychotherapy, affects the final therapeutic outcome; and second, whether it is possible to quantify, in some manner, how this "family involvement" that is not "family therapy" affects outcome measures. For example, is it important for the family to accompany a patient to the hospital? Is it of any consequences, therapeutically, whether or not a patient's family goes through the admitting process with the patient? Is it beneficial that a patient receive visits from the family? Is it of value that the family contribute to the establishment of a treatment contract, or that steps are at least taken to insure their understanding of it?

After a review of literature findings that address the question of how family involvement affects outcome variables, the authors' describe an inpatient psychiatric unit and a research project that attempted to assess and quantify the effects of family participation. Research findings and implications are also discussed.

"FAMILY THERAPY" VERSUS "FAMILY INVOLVEMENT"

In an overly simplified hypothesized course of events one might suggest the following steps occurring prior to, during, and following psychiatric hospitalization. An individual undergoes a stress which results in the disruption of his normal adaptive pattern. At some point following this disruption the decision is made, either voluntarily or involuntarily, in favor of hospitalization. The patient is taken to or goes to a hospital and is evaluated; some form of psychotherapy and perhaps organic intervention as well is begun. During hospitalization the patient comes in contact with and interacts with people who are actively involved in his treatment (physicians, nurses, psychologists, social workers, etc.) as well as those who do not have direct responsibility for his care (technicians, other patients, support personnel). During the hospitalization, the patient's family may call or visit the staff in search of progress reports. Family members may also visit the hospitalized patient on either a steady or sporadic basis. The family may be asked to come in on a regular basis and to take part in the therapy, either as formal family therapy, as part of a group therapy program, or in a less formalized treatment paradigm. After some period of time, the decision is reached as to whether sufficient improvement in functioning has occurred to warrant discharge, or if long-term hospitalization is the preferred course of action. If discharge is to occur, follow-up arrangements are made.

For the purpose of this chapter, family will be used in the empirical manner suggested by Block, "Practically this often indicates who (in the household) is actually available for therapeutic work" [3]. Family therapy will be identified as that period of time that the family members engage in a program of treatment at the suggestion of a therapist, usually with both the therapist and with the identified patient present and with the focus ultimately on relationships. Family therapy effectiveness in either inpatient and outpatient settings is not discussed in this chapter. The interested reader is referred to the excellent reviews of the literature by Gurman and Kniskern [20], Wells et al. [20], Wells and Dezen [21], Masten [15], or the chapter by Glick and Clarkin in this book.

In this chapter, family involvement will be used to refer to family participation at various "steps" in the schema above other than that identified as family therapy.

LITERATURE SURVEY

If it is difficult to define "precisely or consensually what marital-family therapy is" as suggested by Gurman and Kniskern [10], and family therapy is a subset of family involvement, the task of comprehensively reviewing the literature of studies reporting the effects of "family involvement" becomes an impossible one, or at least a difficult one. But studies have been reported that demonstrate the effect that significant others can have on a hospitalized patient. While the following study does not deal with psychiatric inpatients, it does demonstrate that outcome variables, e.g., psychiatric symptoms, can be influenced positively by family involvement. The study is important in another way in that it uses measurable outcome variables in order to demonstrate the effects of specific types of family participating. Chatham reports that by training wives how to interact with their husbands in an intensive care unit after the men had undergone open heart surgery, specific manifestations of postcardiotomy psychosis could be decreased. Wives were taught to include more eye contact and frequent touching and verbal orientation to time, place, and person during visits with their husbands. As a result of these specific behaviors, the experimental group "were more oriented to time, person and place, were more appropriate and less confused as shown by speech and behaviors, had fewer delusions, and had longer periods of sleep as compared to subjects in the control group" [6]. Although reports of this nature are difficult to find in the literature, the authors' recently reviewed in a comprehensive manner studies dealing with irregular discharges from psychiatric units [13]. Some of these articles did suggest that family involvement influenced the type of discharge that might terminate the hospitalization.

A study by Miles et al. concluded that family involvement or lack of participation was a critical factor that affected the type of discharge (discharges against or with medical advice) that occurred from voluntary psychiatric units [16]. They found that three different groups could be identified:

In summary, then, one should be alert to the increased possibility of an AMA discharge in all patients with a poor treatment response, and specifically in: The somewhat older, neurotic woman with a hostile-dependent relationship with a significant other, usually her husband, who contrives to be hospitalized to influence the significant other. The younger patient, usually single and schizophrenic, with significant others, usually parents, who either oppose hospitalization or use it to reject the patient. The socially isolated schizophrenic patient who appears to find the interpersonal aspect of the ward environment particularly threatening. . . . For patients in groups I and II the need for family involvement before and during hospitalization was apparent. For many of those patients the involvement of the significant others was a case of too little, too late. One of the contributing causes of the insufficient involvement was a lack of sufficient supervision available for family interviews. That meant that the sessions were often postponed until several days after the patient's admission. By that time, hitherto unrecognized family factors in the patient's hospitalization had often reached crisis proportions.

Of major significance was the follow-up finding by those same authors that "since the completion of this study, increased involvement of significant others before and during hospitalization has contributed to a marked decrease in the rate of AMA discharges, from 16.7 percent in 1972 to 7.7 percent in 1975" [16]. Thus it would seem from this particular study that family involvement or lack thereof, as well as the timing of such participation, had a significant effect on the type of discharge and the number of AMA discharges that occurred following psychiatric hospitalization.

A study which addresses one of the questions raised in this chapter was conducted by Bowen and Twemlow [4]. These authors' postulated that alcoholic patients who were accompanied to a hospital with family members would have a lower dropout rate from the treatment program than those alcoholic patients who did not have family members accompany them. They were also interested in the issue of nonfamily members' (caseworkers, Alcoholics Anonymous sponsors, friends, neighbors) influence on dropout rates. The authors' were quick to point out the practical benefit of having an alcoholic patient, who might be in an intoxicated state at the time of admission, accompanied by another individual. They state that the other individual obviously can "provide social history data. The relative's presense gives staff an opportunity to begin any needed work with the family and helps indicate the degree of family support for the patient." Their study showed that "of the three hundred sixteen patients whose relative accompanied them to the hospital, only seventy-six , or 24 percent dropped out." It is interesting to note that "however, the dropout rate for those accompanied by a community caretaker—fifty-nine patients, or 37 percent—was similar to the rate for those who came alone—two hundred five patients for 34 percent. The difference in drop-out rate between those accompanied by a relative and those who came alone or with a community caretaker is statistically significant." An additional finding pertinent to the question of family involvement was the fact that "not only is the patient whose relative accompanies him to the hospital more likely to complete the program, but his relative is also more likely to attend the family workshop."

A final point made in this study which has significance to the study which the authors' present later in this chapter is the authors' comment that, "The implications of these findings for treatment are considerable. The point at which relatives are first seen is a critical one, the time at which hospital programs were explained, information given about the family workshop, and addresses established for future contact. For many relatives, the decision to attend the workshop is made at admission."

Although the studies cited above might suggest that family involvement during a patient's hospitalization will usually have a beneficial result, continued survey of the AMA discharge literature suggests that this is not always true. Fabrick, Ruffin and Denman reviewed psychiatric hospital discharges by means of a questionnaire sent to 250 patients discharged from their hospital [9]. Along with other factors, they found that patients who were discharged against medical advice "reported more coercion to enter psychiatric treatment than did other patients. This finding was significant beyond the 0.05 level." Although one might postulate that the coercion was from family members, coercion on the part of a therapist or a community caseworker cannot be ruled out.

This same study did go on to note, however, that "the patients who left the hospital against medical advice reported a lower level of functioning in terms of their degree of personal adjustment, employment capability, and *personal relationships with their families*." The emphasis is ours (DJW & ERK) and not the other authors.

In the same vein, a study by Daniels, Margolis and Carson, resulted in the following explanation of the dynamics of AMA process [7]: (1) inadequate preparation and referral of the patient and of the family; (2) threatening aspects of the ward environment; (3) difficulties in the patient-therapist or therapist-supervisor relationship; (4) interference from significant family members. In terms of inadequate preparation and referral of a patient and of the family, the authors' note, "Since hospitalization means that family members lose the emotional support previously provided by the patient, an emotional realignment may be necessary. These families need help in getting support and gratification from new sources that can substitute for the old sources."

The authors' also found that interference could occur from significant family members when "there was a sudden threat to the families' equilibrium or when the patient's progress or goals were out of keeping with the families' desires and expectations. In the first instance the discharge of the patient serves to keep the family stable in a time of crisis. In the second instance either too little or too much progress on the part of the patient provoked the family to action. The goals of the patient and therapists need to be related to the goals of the family if the patient plans to return to his original family setting. Thus ongoing contact with the family is an essential part of the treatment process for both the patient and the hospital staff."

As a result of their studies the authors' made several changes in their therapeutic approach. One of the changes that relate to the role of the family member in the treatment program was to evaluate the family more thoroughly before and during admission. Earlier and more extensive contact with the family by members of the inpatient staff was initiated and often included visits to the ward even before admission. Again one notes the emphasis on early contact with the family.

A study of 54 voluntary patients discharged from the Payne Whitney Psychiatric Clinic against medical advice found that the attitude of relatives was significantly related to that particular type of discharge. Kohl found that "when relatives are over dependent upon the patient, fear his retaliation, feel guilty and responsible for his illness or feel themselves threatened by the patient's treatment, they may proceed to give into his demands and remove him against medical advice" [14]. The author concludes, "therefore, it is important for the therapist to establish early contact with relatives, to keep them informed of the therapeutic progress, and to educate them about the nature of the patient's illness. The degree of contact between the patient and his relatives through correspondence, telephone calls and visits should also be given due consideration in the total plan of treatment."

Another study which looked at outcome variables in terms of improved functioning of alcoholic and drug abusing patients was that conducted by Webb et al. [19]. Although this study did not address the issue of family involvement during the period of hospitalization, it did document the significance that the family plays in outcome of treatment programs. Thirty-six patients involved in the treatment program were followed, 19 of whom were alcoholics and 17 drug users. Patients were divided into three groups in accordance with their pretreatment residential settings. Patients were administered the Social Dysfunction Rating Scale (SDRS) as well as the Hopkins Symptom Distress Checklist both before treatment and after treatment. Findings were significant in that "those who had lived alone or with non-relatives prior to admission changed the most, becoming significantly less dysfunctional and symptomatic. Those coming from parental families showed the least improvement, while those who had lived with their spouses showed moderate improvement. Findings were consistent for both drug and alcohol patients. Results indicate that the type of home environment from which substance abusers come before engaging in treatment significantly influences their receptivity to rehabilitation."

Recidivism has been used as an outcome to determine the effect that family involvement has on psychiatric treatment. Esterson et al. have described a study wherein 20 male and 22 female schizophrenics were treated by conjoint family and milieu therapy in two mental hospitals [8]. This study is included here because the treatment program outlined in the article did not appear to be formal family therapy but rather family involvement as we have defined it. The authors' state, "We try to help the patient and his family to be less disturbing to each other by intensive work with the whole family, including the patient during his stay in the hospital. By the time patients' are discharged they will perhaps have learned to understand one another a little better and have come to feel there is someone else who understands them. They are encouraged to feel that in any crises they can refer back to us for an emergency family consultation either at hospital or, where hospital arrangements have allowed, in their own home."

All of the patients in the study were discharged within one year after admission. The average length of stay was three months. Recidivism findings revealed 17 percent were readmitted within one year from time of discharge in contrast to the previously reported figures of 40 to 50 percent: "Seventy percent of the others were sufficiently well adjusted socially to be able to earn their living for the whole of the year after discharge."

Recidivism was also the outcome parameter used in the study by Barrett et al. [2]. When an emergency situation brought about a release of a large number of chronic patients from a state psychiatric hospital the authors studied a random sample of these patients to determine how many would remain out of the hospital when the emergency was over. The authors report that "of the original study sample, twenty-nine percent were in the community six months later. Of this group seventeen percent had been out of the hospital continuously, and twelve percent had returned, usually only once, then discharged, and then had subsequently remained in the community. Of the group who had initially remained out for four weeks, sixty-two percent were still in the community six months later."

In terms of family involvement the authors found that a patient was more likely to remain out of the hospital if he was actively involved with the family to whom he was discharged: "If the patient 'always' contributed to the family he remained out of the hospital, whereas if he 'never' did he was more likely to return. If a patient helped with household chores, helped with child care, or helped support the family financially, he was more likely to remain out of the hospital."

In a somewhat related study by Brown et al. using recidivism as an outcome measure, they too found that the "emotional environment within the family" correlated significantly with readmission [5]. The interested reader is referred to the original data for an explanation of "emotional environment" as defined by the research teams.

WVU FAMILY INVOLVEMENT RESEARCH STUDY

In 1974–75 a research project was designed and carried out at the West Virginia University Psychiatric Inpatient Service in order to attempt to measure the effects that family participation on the unit had in terms of recidivism and return to home and job responsibilities one year after the patient had been discharged. What follows is a description of the unit in which the study was conducted; a description of the treatment philosophy utilized on the psychiatric inpatient unit; and finally, the research project design and findings.

Facilities

The inpatient service in the Department of Behavioral Medicine and Psychiatry consists of 32 beds and serves both as a training facility for a variety of disciplines within the health field [18,22,23,24] as well as a referral treatment center.

Inpatient services are staffed by two psychiatrists, one assigned on a full-time basis, plus a faculty social worker. Psychiatric residents, third-year medical students, social work graduate students, and nursing students make up the remainder of the treatment team. The unit is totally open. There are no seclusion rooms, no locked doors, no elevators that require keys to operate. All patients are first evaluated by a physician within the department prior to admission. Patients admitted to the unit represent all of the various psychiatric diagnostic categories and all admissions are voluntary. Patients are usually fifteen years of age or older.

Program Description

When a family member anticipating admission comes to the emergency room, the inpatient program is discussed. The family and designated patient are told that responsibility for one's behavior rests on each individual member of the family and that changes in the family situation will occur only if each and every member of the family is willing to accept the responsibility for making changes within his own behavioral repertoire. The concept of relearning new behavioral patterns is described to both patient and family. All patients are told that many behavioral patterns are learned phenomenon and that the admission to our unit indicates that their patterns of relating to family members and to other individuals within their environment now appears to be ineffective. They are further told that it is expected that they will accept responsibility for their own behavior and that they are expected to learn or relearn more effective patterns. Once admitted, the patient is oriented to the unit and assigned to a private or semiprivate room. Soon after admission the patient is evaluated medically. Physical exam is performed and a history and biography taken. The physical examination is conducted by a third-year medical student and the student is supervised by a psychiatric resident. Medications, if necessary, are often started at this time. Group, milieu, and crisis intervention principles are utilized in the program, with family participation emphasized throughout. Early studies of the effectiveness of the unit appeared to indicate that in terms of recidivism and return to home and job responsibilities that the unit was an effective treatment modality [18,12,25].

The Learning Approach

The therapeutic method used on the inpatient service is behaviorally oriented and based on social learning theory. The setting provided for this relearning process consists of a total milieu designed for learning with participation of the patient and his family.

Since the inpatient service functions both as a training ground for students as well as a treatment modality for patients, it has proven beneficial to conceptualize this service as a "learning laboratory" [18,12,25]. All participants in the inpatient service (students from various disciplines, faculty members, house staff, nurses, and patients and their families) are considered to be students of human behavior. Students and faculty are advised that they need to learn more about human behavior and to improve their interpersonal functioning in order to better themselves as professionals. "Patient students" are advised that they too have a need to relearn patterns of relating interpersonally in order to avoid hospitalization or to be better able to deal with situations similar to the one which resulted in their hospitalization. All students are advised that they can learn or relearn patterns of communicating by interacting with one another. Interaction with members of the nuclear family is especially encouraged.

The primary setting for this learning process is the group. It is not at all uncommon to have groups of 15 to 25 "students" wherein "patient students" and their family members are outnumbered two to one by "professional students." The purpose of the group sessions is to allow people to interact with one another as people and not in accordance with rigid role definitions. The inpatient setting is designed to allow all participants to analyze and to learn from the interactions that occur at the moment whether the interchange is between two professionals, two "patient students," or a "patient student" and a "professional student." Behavioral patterns which appear to be effective are noted and reinforced. Those behavioral patterns which appear to be nonproductive are likewise noted and negatively reinforced.

Research Design

In order to determine the effect that family involvement had on the outcome of psychiatric hospitalization a comparison was made between psychiatric inpatients who had family members involved with them during their treatment and patients who did not. The specific hypothesis for the investigation was that family involvement would result in lower recidivism rates and higher rates of return to responsibilities.

Between February 21 and April 22, 1974, 153 (57 males, 96 females) were admitted to the unit. Age range was from 14 to 78 years old with a mean of 42 years. Diagnoses at time of discharge encompassed the usual spectrum for a psychiatric inpatient population. Psychotic disorders were primary or secondary diagnoses in 19.9 percent. Other major categories of primary diagnosis were neuroses (39.1 percent), transient situational disturbances (17.9 percent), nonpsychotic organic brain syndromes (5.8 percent), drug dependence (3.8 percent), mental retardation (1.3 percent), and psychophysiological disorders (0.6 percent). The average length of hospitalization was approximately two weeks.

Attempting to measure something as illusive as family involvement presents obvious difficulties, especially so in any qualitative sense. Therefore, several different quantitative parameters were examined. First, all patients were observed as to whether members were present with them at each of five times: (1) initial contact with the Psychiatry Department (usually in the Emergency Room); (2) admission to the inpatient unit; (3) group therapy sessions; (4) staffing, when the treatment contract was negotiated; and (5) visiting hours (both family visits in the hospital and the patient's leaves of absence with family members were reported).

Second, attempts were made to determine and quantify the degree of family involvement in the unit's primary therapeutic modality, e.g., group therapy. At the end of each group session, treatment team members were asked to report how verbal family members had been (0 = no participation, 1 = one to three sentences, and 2 = four or more sentences). If several family members were present, they were treated as a unit for the purpose of rating their verbal participation.

Third, in order to account for the numerous unscheduled contacts that treatment team members had with family members, a daily list was kept for each patient. A "conference" was defined as a conversation with family lasting five minutes or longer. Each conference that a treatment team member engaged in with family members was reported at the beginning of the next day. The number of conferences could equal the number of days of hospitalization. Thus, the percentage of conferences held with the treatment team was felt to be another indication of the amount of family involvement.

A follow-up survey was made one year after discharge. Of the initial 153 patients, 123 (80.4 percent) were contacted by phone or mail by a work-study student not involved in the original data collection. Information regarding rehospitalization and return to former responsibilities at work and at home was obtained and then compared with the original data of patients who had family involvement and those that did not.** Chi-square analyses were performed with the .05 level required for significance.

The only statistically significant relationship found (p = .01) was between patients who had family members' with them in the emergency room and those who did not: The former were less likely to have been hospitalized during the year following discharge. There was no statistically significant relationships between family members presence in the emergency room and the eventual return to home and job responsibilities. Further, there were no significant relationships between family presence and any of the four other stages of treatment or between degree of participation in group sessions or unscheduled conferences and outcome measures.

** Kotin and Schur have investigated the question of whether comparable information could be obtained from discharged psychiatric patients by questionnaire as well as by home interview, with a tentative conclusion that this was indeed the case.

Kotin, J. and Schur, J.M. "Attitudes of discharged mental patients toward their hospital experiences." *Journal of Nervous and Mental Disease* 149 : 408–414, 1969.

DISCUSSION

Outcome may be defined as the overall success of a treatment program. The question was raised whether family involvement on a psychiatric inpatient service might affect outcome. Although the evidence is certainly not overwhelming, both the literature review as well as our own research project would seem to suggest that family involvement can in fact influence a number of outcome parameters and that these parameters can be measured.

In our own research project at the West Virginia University Hospital we also asked the question whether or not it was possible to begin to quantify the amount of family involvement. Although admittedly our first attempts at quantifying the amount of family involvement were crude, the answer to this question was definitely yes.

Recidivism and return to former responsibilities are only two areas which lend themselves to study as represented within our research project. Certainly other parameters of outcome also lend themselves to quantitative examination:

1. Patient and family approval or disapproval of a treatment facility.
2. Patient compliance with outpatient follow-up.
3. The patient's need for post-hospitalization medication as well as compliance with such treatment.
4. The length or duration of hospitalization.
5. The type of discharge (AMA versus medical approval).
6. The degree of organic treatment required during hospitalization.
7. The period of time between discharge and rehospitalization (if any).
8. Suicide and homicide attempts, whether successful or not.

It is important to note that the amount of family participation does not provide sufficient information as to the quality of the participation of the family members. Many authors have noted that active participation by the family in a treatment inpatient setting may be either positive or negative in its effects. Harbin, in his descriptions of the interaction between families and psychiatric hospital units, points out that "these transactions between the hospital and families are complex; they are extremely important to recognize because they can undermine the family and individual psychotherapy" [11].

The potential for negative consequences from family involvement was also pointed out by Tengari: "Unless they are understood, the same stresses, conflicts and difficulties in the family that lead to the patient's hospitalization may recur, even though he may show dramatic improvement when he leaves the hospital. To the extent that family involvement is an intrinsic part of the total treatment effort, the chances of recurrence may diminish" [17].

With the realization of the importance of family interaction both in terms of quantity and quality, methods are currently being offered that will aid mental health professionals increase the level of family participation [1]. Review of the literature as well as our own study would also seem to indicate that the timing of family involvement is a crucial factor. It would appear that early involvement of the family with the psychiatric treatment team would seem to lend itself to beneficial outcome results.

Finally, it is necessary to point out that not only is there a need for examination of multiple outcome factors, but the meaning of positive finding must be closely scrutinized to ascertain their significance. Findings may have marked different meanings for various subpopulations of psychiatric patients. In short, correlation according to diagnostic groupings needs to be done. For example, although one might consider rehospitalization occurring only a short time after discharge as being a negative outcome parameter, such an occurrence in a schizophrenic patient who had earlier refused acceptance of hospitalization when it was necessary might indicate a positive finding and an actual improvement in his condition.

In summary, it is important to note that family involvement does appear to effect treatment modalities and that this assumption made by many mental health professionals can begin to be supported by research projects that review various outcome parameters. From the limited number of such studies, as well as the difficulties involved in conducting them, it should be obvious that a considerable amount of additional work needs to be conducted in this area.

REFERENCES

1. Anderson, C.M. "Family intervention with severely disturbed inpatients." *Archives of General Psychiatry* 34 : 697–702, 1977.
2. Barrett, J.E.; Juriansky, J.; and Gurland, B. "Community tenure following emergency discharge." *The American Journal of Psychiatry* 128 : 958–964, 1972.
3. Block, D.A. "The family of the psychiatric patient." In S. Arieti (ed.) *American Handbook of Psychiatry* (2nd Ed., Vol. I). New York: Basic Books, 1974, pp. 179–201.
4. Bowen, W.T. and Twemlow, S.W. "People who accompany alcoholics to the hospital as a predictor of patient dropout." *Hospital and Community Psychiatry* 28 : 880–1, 1977.
5. Brown, G.W.; Birley, J.L.T.; and Wing, J.K. "Influence of family life on the course of schizophrenic disorders: a replication." *British Journal of Psychiatry* 121 : 241–258, 1972.
6. Chatham, M.A. "The effect of family involvement on patients' manifestations of postcardiotomy psychosis." *Heart and Lung* 7 : 995–999, 1978.
7. Daniels, R.S.; Margolis, P.M.; and Carson, R.C. "Hospital discharges against medical advice." *Archives of General Psychiatry* 8 : 120–30, 1963.
8. Esterson, A.; Cooper, D.G.; and Laing, R.D. "Results of family-oriented therapy with hospitalized schizophrenics." *British Medical Journal* 2 : 1462–1465, 1965.

9. Fabrick, A.L.; Ruffin, W.C.; and Denman, S.B. "Characteristics of patients discharged against medical advice." *Mental Hygiene* 52 : 124–128, 1968.

10. Gurman, A.S. and Kniskern, D.P. "Research on marital and family therapy: progress, perspective, and prospect. In S.L. Garfield and A.E. Bergin (eds.) *Handbook of Psychotherapy and Behavior Change: An Empirical Analysis* (2nd Edition). New York: John Wiley and Sons, 1978, pp. 817–901.

11. Harbin, H.T. "Families and hospitals: collusion or cooperation?" *American Journal of Psychiatry* 135 : 1496–1499, 1978.

12. Jacobs, M.K. and Trick, O.L. "Successful psychiatric rehabilitation using an inpatient teaching laboratory." *American Journal of Psychiatry* 131 : 145–148, 1974.

13. Kidwell, E.R. and Withersty, D.J. "Compliance and the irregular discharge." In D.J. Withersty; J.M. Stevenson; and R.H. Waldman (eds.) *Communication and Compliance in a Hospital Setting.* Springfield, Illinois: Charles C Thomas, 1980, pp. 147–175.

14. Kohl, R.N. "Termination of Treatment Against Medical Advice." *Psychiatric Quarterly* 33 : 498–505, 1959.

15. Masten, A.S. "Family therapy as a treatment for children: a critical review of outcome research." *Family Process* 18 : 323–335, 1979.

16. Miles, J.E. et al. "Discharges against medical advice from voluntary psychiatric units." *Hospital and Community Psychiatry* 27 : 859–864, 1976.

17. Tengari, A. "Family involvement in the treatment of a psychiatric inpatient." *Hospital and Community Psychiatry* 25 : 792–794, 1974.

18. Trick, O.L.; Jacobs, M.; and Spradlin, W.W. "Inpatient laboratory as a milieu force." In A. Jacobs and W. Spradlin (eds.) *The Group as an Agent of Change.* New York: Behavioral Publications, 1974, pp. 43–62.

19. Webb, N.L.; Pratt, T.C.; Linn, M.W.; and Carmichael, J.S. "Focus on the family as a factor in differential treatment outcome." *The International Journal of the Addictions* 13 : 783–795, 1978.

20. Wells, R.A.; Dilkes, T.C.; and Trivelli, N. "The results of family therapy: a critical review of the literature." *Family Process* 11 : 189–207, 1972.

21. Wells, R.A. and Dezen, A.E. "The results of family therapy revisited: the non-behavioral methods." *Family Process* 17 : 251–274, 1978.

22. Withersty, D.J. "Training for community mental health service." *Journal of Medical Education* 49 : 998–1000, 1974.

23. Withersty, D.J. "Psychiatric residents provide extra manpower for rural community agencies." *Hospital and Community Psychiatry* 26 : 270–271, 1975.

24. Withersty, D.J.; Linton, J.; and Quarrick, E. "Implementing personal development in a medical clerkship—an evaluation." *Journal of Medical Education* 50 : 632–636, 1975.

25. Withersty, D.J. "Effectiveness of an educational approach in treating psychiatric inpatients." *Social Science and Medicine* 12 : 27–29, 1978.

10

Family Reactions and the Career of the Psychiatric Patient: A Long-Term Follow-Up Study

STEPHAN P. SPITZER, RAYMOND M. WEINSTEIN, AND HERBERT L. NELSON

The term "career" refers to the sequence of movements from a position in any particular network of social relations to another position in the same or in a different social network, as well as the individual adjustments accompanying the movement. The concept of career has received a wide variety of applications, for example, in the analysis of organizational adjustment [18], medical education [15], marijuana use [1], and mental illness [10]. Our investigation is addressed to this last type of application. According to Goffman, the career of the psychiatric patient has three distinct phases: a prepatient phase (the person in the community prior to hospitalization), an inpatient phase (the person in hospital treatment), and a postpatient phase (the person back in the community after hospitalization). In describing the patient career, Goffman focuses on the consequences of being labeled as psychiatrically deviant, accommodating to institutional life, and forming alignments with other patients and hospital personnel.

The career of the psychiatric patient—the movement from one phase to another and the length of time spent in each phase—is greatly affected by the reactions of family members. In the prepatient phase, the family plays a major role in the identification of psychiatric symptoms [9,19,21,29], determines the type of help sought [24,40,41], and provides socialization into the sick role [26,35]. Family characteristics and behavior in the inpatient phase often affect the type of commitment [12,17], course of hospitalization [5,23], and timing of discharge [13,32]. In the postpatient phase of mental illness, the reactions of family members can contribute to the patient's feelings of alienation and stigma

[4,30], erect barriers to community reintegration [25,33], and lead to rehospitalization [6,31].

Different types of career patterns develop among psychiatric patients. Some persons are hospitalized shortly after the appearance of psychiatric symptoms while others do not receive treatment for many years. Some patients have relatively short hospital stays whereas others with similar levels of symptomatology are discharged after much longer periods. Also, recidivism is characteristic of some patients; others are more successful at remaining in the community. The particular directions in which psychiatric careers evolve are closely tied to the structure and attitudes prevailing in the patient's family. Two "sensitizing concepts" or family attributes associated with career paths may be identified: *Level of Expected Performance* and *Propensity for Action*. Each concept reflects a constellation of characteristics of particular families, and are summary predictors of attitudes toward the sick role, mental illness, and psychiatric treatment.

Level of expected performance refers to what the family requires of its members in various dimensions—economic, interpersonal, community relations, conformity, and so forth. In short, what behavior does the family expect for participation and membership? When Freeman and Simmons explored in detail the performance levels of former patients, they found that the family set up certain expectations in terms of stability of employment and associative patterns [7,8]. Performance level expectations were higher among middle class and conjugal families, in comparison to working class and parental families, and accounted for their higher recidivism rates. In another investigation, performance level expectations were observed to be associated with the former patient's family position; higher performance levels were set for persons having a key role in the family [20]. Studies of the prepatient phase of mental illness also bear on the concept of performance levels. Gordon's research on the sick role disclosed marked variations in expectations regarding the rights and obligations to be assumed once this role was ascribed [11].

A family's propensity for action refers to its differential readiness to impute the psychiatric label and seek hospital treatment for one of its members. What is regarded as mental illness in one family is not necessarily regarded as such in another. Investigations concerned with the process of recognizing psychiatric problems disclose noticeable variations among families [3,16,22,29]. Families also differ in their tolerance for accepting deviation from normative patterns before taking action. Myers and Roberts found that permissiveness was greater in lower than middle-class families [24], Clausen and Yarrow reported large differences in the degree to which family members were willing to support and tolerate deviance [3], and Mechanic indicated that nonconformity is tolerated depending upon the seriousness of the deviation's consequences [22]. Moreover, even within a given family, tolerance limits established for different family members tend to vary [14]. Finally, families differ in ability to withstand stress. Parsons and Fox believe that the American family is prone to reject deviant members, since deviance disturbs family equilibrium [26]. On the other hand, in some families the deviant serves an integrative function by providing, for example, a convenient outlet for personality difficulties [38], a means for resolving conflicts [21], or a role needed to maintain stability [2]. Hence some families are able to tolerate considerable stress before initiating plans for action.

This chapter is concerned with the impact of family reactions on the careers of psychiatric patients. More than a decade ago, the histories of 79 first admission patients with functional mental disorders at a university hospital were examined [36,37]. A fourfold typology of family reactions based on the family's expected level of performance and propensity to take corrective action was developed. Clinical and survey data were utilized to describe families with different performance levels and propensities for action, and predictions concerning the particular directions in which the psychiatric career should evolve in conjunction with these two variables were made. Recently, a follow-up study of the original cohort of patients was conducted in order to examine the tenability of the original model. These data are used to examine the career outcomes for persons in the original cohort and to update the case histories in the earlier reports [34,36,37].

A TYPOLOGY OF FAMILY REACTIONS

Any given family may be viewed as either high (Hi) or low (Lo) on the dimensions of Level of Expected Performance (LEP) and Propensity for Action (PA). As shown in Fig. 10-1, four "ideal types" of families emerge from the cross-classification of these two different variables. The *anticipatory-prohibitive* (HiLEP-HiPA) type of family has high expectations for performance and tends to prohibit deviance, in part, by seeking hospital treatment for members who deviate. The *anticipatory-tolerant* (HiLEP-LoPA) family similarly holds high performance expectations but generally tolerates deviant behavior and is unlikely to hospitalize one of its members. The *detached-prohibitive* (LoLEP-HiPA) type of family envisions very little from its members with respect to performance but has a proclivity to restrict deviant behavior and to initiate hospitalization if compliance is not obtained. The *detached-tolerant* (LoLEP-LoPA) family, in contrast, is characterized by satisfaction with a low level of performance and, while not actually oblivious to psychiatric deviance, has an indifferent or apathetic response to such behavior.

Because families are characterized by properties in addition to those on which the typology is based, within-category distinctions are made for three of the four family types. Attitudes toward psychiatric hospitals and mental health professionals, concepts used to understand human motivation and the etiology of psychiatric disturbance, and styles of interpersonal conduct are among the additional dimensions on which families tend to vary, and as such, serve as bases for differentiating among the Fig. 10-1 family types.

Level of Expected Performance

Propensity for Action		High	Low
		Anticipatory-Prohibitive	Detached-Prohibitive
High		Assertives Altercasters	Authoritarians
		Anticipatory-Tolerant	Detached-Tolerant
Low		Stoics Poltroons	Pacifists Stumblers Do-Nothings

Figure 10-1 Four "Ideal Types" of Families of Psychiatric Patients

Anticipatory-Prohibitive Families

Assertives

Members of the Assertive type of family are willing to inform the deviant that he or she might be mentally ill and point to which behaviors are disruptive to them. Because of their value orientations, the patient is expected to perform at a high level. Deviance is intolerable on the basis of principle or because it is threatening to family integration. Moreover, the family may believe that, in the interests of the patient's welfare, illness should be treated as soon as possible. Attempts are made to evoke conformity through interpersonal pressures, but, as it becomes evident that attainment of conformity is improbable, the deviant is presented with the ultimatum of "shaping up or shipping out." If this threat does not produce the desired result, arrangements are made for psychiatric treatment.

Assertive family members are not overly concerned with the prepatient's attitudes toward them, since warning of the consequences of continued deviation have been given. In addition, they can subscribe to the moral justification that hospitalization would benefit both the patient's health and the family's welfare. They hope that psychiatric treatment will be successful, but they anticipate returning the postpatient to the hospital if problems recur after discharge.

Case 1 For as long as he could remember, Richard had been punished by rejection and humiliation for not living up to an ideal standard. His parents feared that his boyish misdeeds might blemish the family's reputation, and most of Richard's precollege years were spent with a relative in another city, in a camp for problem children, and a military academy. Because he did not do well at a local college and would not participate in the family's active social life, arrangements were made for psychiatric hospitalization. He was admitted in 1966 at the age of 20 with the diagnosis of Chronic Undifferentiated Schizophrenia. In the hospital his behavior was described as exceedingly hostile and his adjustment as poor. His parents informed several staff members as well as Richard that he would not be allowed to return home until he had become more "respectable." Richard was discharged four months later with the understanding that he would seek employment and obtain outpatient psychiatric assistance. However, since he assumed neither one of these obligations, the family arranged for commitment to a state psychiatric hospital. He was discharged after several months and returned home. He was hospitalized again on two additional occasions during the next two years. Two more rehospitalizations occurred in 1970 and 1979.

Altercasters

In this type of family, expectations for performance and propensity to initiate action are also high. Altercasters are inclined to avoid direct confrontation with the deviant and often go to great lengths to conceal their responsibility for his or her removal from the family. However, they are less threatening than Assertives. Rather than forming an active coalition with the family physician or psychiatrist, they may present the help source with the deviant (along with a detailed summary of the deviant's transgressions), casting the help source into the position of making a treatment decision. A case in which a family shopped around for a suitable physician and then employed a moral obligation to their advantage is described as follows.

Case 2   Shortly after his election to the school board Mr. S began to show signs of despondency and suspiciousness, claiming that people were talking about him and impugning his motives for community participation. Responsibility for managing and working the farm became too much for him. He was unable to sleep and vacillated between periods of depression and agitation.

The first physician which his wife and brother consulted recommended medications but a second volunteered to arrange for commitment. Mr. S was informed by the family that, much to their regret, the matter had passed out of their control and that he would have to undergo hospitalization. Upon arriving at the hospital it was discovered that the commitment papers had not preceded their arrival, but by stressing their obligation to carry out the physician's orders, the family persuaded Mr. S to admit himself voluntarily. Mr. S made a fairly good adjustment in the hospital and was discharged as much improved several weeks later. He was seen on an occasional outpatient basis for the next few months. He was not admitted to inpatient status during the next 14 years.

Another Altercaster pattern is one in which the family endeavors to convince the prepatient that his symptoms are indicative of mental illness. If the prepatient internalizes a definition of self-as-sick he is likely to seek out a professional help source. Similarly, if the prepatient accepts the obligations attached to the sick role, he is also likely to seek out professional assistance. Hence, the family may accomplish the same end as if the patient had been taken to the help source directly. Often what appears to be a self-made decision to seek psychiatric treatment is actually an outcome of the altercasting process. In such cases, rehospitalization is self-perpetuating.

Case 3   During the two years prior to hospitalization, Miss T's behavior was a source of embarrassment to her family. Her mother described her as a rebellious girl who failed to live up to responsibilities, showed disrespect for the mother's wishes, and spent most of the time daydreaming or engaging in other frivolous activities. Her parents also expressed concern for her grades.

Miss T's mother had suspected a psychiatric problem for some time. Almost daily, the daughter was urged to see a psychiatrist. However, the mother neither offered to make any arrangements nor suggested how to proceed. Although passive most of the time, the father sided with the mother when forced to voice an opinion regarding the status of the daughter's psychological health.

Miss T appeared at the hospital alone and without an appointment. In response to the question of why she had come, she stated that she was mentally ill and wished to have herself hospitalized. She was admitted with the diagnosis of Adjustment Reaction to Adolescence. After two months she was discharged as much improved and with an excellent prognosis. She returned home but reappeared at the hospital a month later with the explanation: "They think I'm crazy." Since then Miss T has checked in periodically whenever she "needs fixing." She has had six readmissions between 1966–80.

Anticipatory-Tolerant Families

Stoics

The stoic family is characterized by a "philosophical" outlook on life. Propensity for action is low when deviation of a family member is observed. Stoics have a high tolerance level for deviant behavior and a marked ability to withstand stress. They believe that painful experiences can be endured and that mental illness does not necessarily lead to progressive deterioration. Expectations for performance are high but demands on the deviant are minimal. Stoics are exceptionally silent and uncomplaining.

Stoics rarely play a major part in initiating psychiatric treatment for their deviant members. The deviant often comes to the attention of outsiders, who may come to play an active role. In such instances family tolerance limits are finally exceeded and plans for treatment are initiated. During the inpatient phase, family members visit the patient frequently but do not attempt to influence his or her attitudes and behavior in any appreciable way. They may temporarily accept a psychiatric definition of illness, but during the postpatient phase they tend to revert to their old behavior patterns. Although family members may be disappointed that the postpatient fails to perform at a satisfactory level, their demands remain low. Action is rarely initiated for hospitalization, although it may come about at the urging of outsiders.

Case 4 By age six, Robert's awkwardness and inability to perform at the level of his age-mates was obvious to all who knew him. When he began to stutter at age eight his mother suggested seeking professional assistance, but his father argued that Robert would outgrow his difficulties if left alone. Although his high school grades were far below average, both Robert and his family made extensive plans for him to attend a large midwestern university. When his application was rejected, the family became somewhat despondent but encouraged Robert to apply to other colleges.

Because of a suspicion of brain damage, interpersonal difficulties at school, and the obvious discrepancy between family aspirations and the young man's abilities, a school counselor attempted a revision in career plans. The advice was rejected by both Robert and his parents. Referral to a vocational rehabilitation office led to a referral for psychiatric evaluation and subsequent hospital admission at age 17.

Upon discharge from the hospital, Robert was accepted by a local community college. At the end of the year his grades were so poor that his advisor suggested that he "make a more suitable career choice." He managed to gain entry to a small southern college but continued to experience a great deal of difficulty with his grades. His parents maintained that they were confident that he could graduate if he just worked a little harder. He did not reappear for hospital treatment.

Poltroons

Although the necessity of removing a deviant member is acutely felt, the Poltroon family is reluctant to undergo a direct confrontation. Because of a desire to avoid strains in their relationship with the deviant their ability to tolerate stress is high. Fear of stigma associated with mental illness contributes to a reluctance to take immediate action. Although slow to respond to deviance, once action is initiated, the strategy is to operate behind the prepatient's back. Under false pretenses (such as getting a routine physical checkup or having some minor ailment looked at), the deviant is urged to visit the family physician who has been secretly asked to recommend psychiatric hospitalization. Or in the event that the family physician declines to fulfill their expectations, arrangements may be made for the deviant to see some other help source who has been similarly coached. Sometimes a member of the extended family, such as an uncle or cousin, may be recruited to act as "complainant," either in making an admissions appointment or signing commitment papers at the courthouse.

Once the prepatient is hospitalized, Poltroons align themselves with the treatment authorities, offering their full cooperation. Once the patient is discharged, and the necessity for readmission arises, action on the part of the family becomes less duplicitous. Family members can now justify initiating a readmission proceeding on the basis of their obligation to the hospital and/or the postpatient's personal welfare. Consequently, persons from this kind of family have a fairly high potential for readmission.

Case 5   Mr. Z is married to a well-educated but domineering woman who inherited the family farm, runs the household, and unilaterally makes all important decisions. This has contributed to Mr. Z's feeling that he is not needed and has served to support the belief that his wife and others are plotting against him. During the last four years Mr. Z had several severe attacks of depression, with the most recent one complicated by a prostate problem. Although his wife and daughters tried to dissuade him of his allegations, he has grown increasingly suspicious and jealous, accusing his wife of having an affair with the local feed salesman.

During a rather bizarre attempt to keep the salesman off the farm, he experienced what was thought to be a heart attack and was taken to the local hospital. His wife drew Mr. Z's suspiciousness to the attention of the administering physician, who agreed to commit Mr. Z to a psychiatric hospital. Rather than taking Mr. Z back to the farm where he believed he was returning, the ambulance delivered him to the psychiatric hospital. Even when being seen by the intake psychiatrist, he was unaware that his wife was actually at the hospital providing information to a psychiatric social worker, and assumed that the physician at the local hospital was responsible for having the commitment papers drawn.

During his hospitalization he continued to believe that the family was not responsible for his internment, complaining frequently that he was being held against his will. The diagnosis was Paranoid Reaction. At the time of discharge his wife attempted to get Mr. Z's psychiatrist to accord her the responsibility of reporting any further instances of paranoid behavior to him. However, the psychiatrist placed Mr. Z into outpatient treatment and also induced him to agree to contact the hospital if his jealousy reappeared rather than directing accusations at his wife.

Although Case 5 was not readmitted during the follow-up period, a more typical Poltroon family outcome is Case 6.

Case 6 At age 14 Donna developed a religious fervor and a preoccupation with death. She began to call the rectory several times daily and became increasingly aggressive when asked to stop. At age 15 she ran away but was located the next day. The following day her mother approached the priest and asked him to contact the family physician in order to arrange for inpatient psychiatric treatment. Moreover, the mother made it clear that she did not want her daughter to know she was involved in the treatment decision.

Donna indicated that while her mother and the priest were the persons who first noticed something unusual about her behavior, the decision to hospitalize was made solely by the clergyman and physician. Donna was given an intake diagnosis of Adjustment Reaction to Adolescence and was discharged in 17 days. One month later she was admitted to a nearby state psychiatric hospital and discharged four months later. This was followed by three additional hospitalizations during the next four years in state and municipal psychiatric hospitals.

Detached-Prohibitive Families

Authoritarians

This type of family presents a severe, stern, and harsh image. Even slight deviations are intolerable. While Authoritarians usually present the deviant with only one or a few requirements, on those occasions when a series of expectations are enumerated, family members actually anticipate superficial performance on the specified dimensions. In regard to propensity for action, they adhere rigidly to the medical model of illness. More often than not, hospitalization functions less to benefit the deviant or to preserve integration of the family than it does to punish the deviant member.

Little indecision or remorse is shown when Authoritarians arrange for hospitalization. The patient is often committed without forewarning. Occasionally family members dispose of the deviant through the same techniques used by Altercasters or Poltroons, but they act more out of convenience than temerity. However, to the extent that their stipulations are mere bluster and to the extent that the deviant adopts ways of "making out" in this restrictive atmosphere (an easier task than in Assertive or Altercaster families since the probability of norm violation varies directly with the available number of norms potentially violated), family reactions may progress no further than a decision to utilize psychiatric treatment *if* and *when* necessary. But once the decision to implement the treatment decision is made, persons are moved into treatment rapidly from this type of family and rehospitalization becomes quite probable.

Case 7   At the time of Carolyn's admission, 892 lacerations were counted on the back and lower extremities of this 16-year-old girl who was referred for evaluation in connection with child abuse charges pending against her parents. Her battered condition was first noticed by school authorities when she appeared one morning covered with blood. Since her claim to have fallen on barbed wire was unconvincing, she was referred to the child welfare bureau, which, in turn, referred her to the psychiatric hospital. Upon extensive questioning, Carolyn reluctantly admitted that her mother had beaten her with a nail-studded paddle on at least two occasions. The abuse followed her smoking and drinking, a violation of two of her parents' norms. Otherwise Carolyn indicated that her parents were almost totally indifferent to what she did.

The parents are characterized as rigid and compulsive personalities who neither admitted nor denied administering the beatings. The recommendation of family therapy was rejected without a second thought. Carolyn was admitted with no specific diagnosis. Because it was felt that she had neurotic tendencies which would be aggravated in such a home environment, she was released to a foster home. Because she adjusted poorly there, she was eventually returned to the parental home. Although an agreement had been reached that there would be no more smoking and drinking, Carolyn was caught smoking. Her mother attempted unsuccessfully to have her readmitted to University Psychiatric Hospital shortly thereafter.

Case 7 was not rehospitalized between 1966–80, although her mother made several attempts to commit her. Another case from an Authoritarian family is described below.

Case 8   Since early childhood, B's parents stressed the value of an advanced university degree. Not only would an advanced degree provide him with a sense of pride, but it would also assure him of financial security and community respect. During grade school, B considered becoming a physician, but during his high school years he wanted to be a physician or a lawyer. By the end of his second year of university study, he had changed his undergraduate major several times and ultimately received a B.A. in English. Halfway through his first year of graduate work in a Ph.D. program, he panicked, fled from the university and found himself 200 miles away with no recollection of how he got there.

His parents came to pick him up and during the ride home he was bombarded with reprimands and admonishments. How could he fail to appreciate how easy they had made life for him? Hadn't they provided room and board, tuition, a car, and a generous allowance? And what was expected of him?

Nothing, except for him to complete his studies. Anybody else would be eternally grateful! B returned to the university but lost interest in his classes. Soon he stopped attending altogether. However, B maintained the pretense of continuing his studies by commuting to the university on a regular basis. Knowing that he would eventually have to provide an accounting for his academic failure, he was overcome with anxiety and attempted suicide. Although the exact circumstances are unclear, he was discovered in a semisomnambulent state and was rushed to a municipal hospital where he was treated for a barbituate overdose.

Highly distressed that their vicarious aspirations had been jeopardized again, his parents insisted that B seek psychiatric treatment. He was admitted with the diagnosis of Character Disorder, passive-dependent personality, and discharged a month and a half later with the diagnosis of Psychotic Depressive Reaction. During the next year B was twice admitted to the psychiatric unit of a county hospital. When not hospitalized he lived at home with his parents.

Detached-Tolerant Families

Pacifists

While the necessity for obtaining professional help for a member might have been considered in the past, this type of family has come to accommodate itself to the deviant member. Pacifists have lowered their expectations for performance and have become resigned to having a deviant in the home. At one time they tried to evoke conformity by a variety of techniques such as begging, nagging, threatening, withdrawal of rewards, pointing out the deleteriousness of deviance for the family, etc. But once it is realized that their efforts to control have proved to be relatively ineffective, the situation is redefined so as to be seen as not so severe that rejection of the deviant is an absolute necessity. While this response accords the deviant an even greater latitude for deviation and may, thus, result in additional problems, the degree of family integration is such that accommodation is the lesser of two evils. Although there may be concern that the deviant's "illness" may grow progressively worse, this is counterbalanced by the hope that deviance may be "outgrown" or that spontaneous recovery might occur. Initial hospitalization of the family member is often precipitated by a critical event which disrupts the accommodative process. Rehospitalization is relatively improbable, but if it does occur, an extended latency period between discharge and readmission is likely to be observed.

Case 9   William showed a pronounced personality change (increased inattentiveness, insomnia, confusion, apathy, singing, and mumbling) following a truck accident in which he received a hard blow to the head. A neurological examination failed to disclose evidence of brain damage. He was referred to Psychiatry where examination disclosed a long history of abnormal behavior. At age 14 his grades dropped precipitously and at age 16 he became very rebellious. Since that time there were numerous instances of extremely poor judgment. He abused two cars beyond repair, seriously damaged several pieces of expensive farm machinery through misuse, and repeatedly caused other unnecessary inconveniences and expenses to the family. Later he recklessly drove and overturned a truck known to have defective brakes and, although the oil had drained out, drove it home, burning out the engine. This was followed by a series of obscene remarks directed at a female neighbor and an episode where he was found masturbating and striking his penis against the living room wall.

While once holding expectations consonant with the patient's age, both parents had lowered their expectations. The father had "given up" on William and subjected him to continuous depreciatory comments. The mother resorted to treating William as if he were seven years old.

William disappeared during preadmission screening but returned four days later. The mother, who visited daily, was described as overprotective and seductive by the nursing staff. After confiding how homesick he was to his mother, he walked out a second time. He was returned the next day and discharged a week later with the diagnosis of Schizoid Personality. He was maintained on drugs and seen on an occasional outpatient basis for one year. During this period, William's mother described his home adjustment as satisfactory in spite of several additional "incidents." Four years later he was readmitted to inpatient status.

Stumblers

In another variation of the detached-tolerant family, members recognize departure from normal functioning, are ready to seek clarification of the problem, and inadvertently stumble into psychiatric treatment. Deviance is invariably interpreted as resulting from physical causes. Contact is made with a medical practitioner who is likely to recognize the problem as psychiatric. Because these family members are generally uninformed about psychiatric interpretations or intimidated by the high status of physicians, they act upon the professional judgment. Arrangements for psychiatric hospitalization are frequently made without consulting the family.

Since psychiatric treatment is not what the Stumbler family had envisioned, they are dismayed to discover that the situation has passed out of their control. At first, the patient may be urged to do whatever the treatment authorities deem necessary, but later, the activities of the family may become directed toward facilitating the deviant's release from the hospital. In any event, the concept of psychiatric deviance is not readily understood or actually denied. Consequently, the family is unlikely to attempt to persuade the patient to accept the attitudes and orientations of the psychiatric staff.

The directions in which the patient career evolves for persons from Stumbler families are twofold. One direction results from an uncritical acceptance of the professional definition. Although the family members still have not come to understand the concept of psychological motivation, any further deviation on the part of the postpatient is cause to seek out the old authority for clarification and advice. In such instances rehospitalization is fairly likely to occur. A second more prevalent course of direction results from learning what took place during the initial experience. Stumblers may tend to avoid seeking medical treatment, may exercise more discretion in disclosure of information to medical practitioners, or assert the right to forego psychiatric treatment if such a recommendation is made. Rehospitalization for psychiatric disorder under such circumstances is highly unlikely.

Case 10   Mrs. E (age 46) was treated as a medical patient for inflammation of the lower extremities and then transferred to Psychiatry to explore techniques to reduce an anxiety reaction resulting in a condition of obesity. The patient weighted 380 pounds at admission. After admission, Mrs. E's diagnosis was Personality Trait Disturbance, mild anxiety resulting in extreme impairment (obesity). She and her husband were seen at a staff conference at which time a three-month-stay for relief of the symptoms of anxiety and implementation of a medically controlled diet was recommended. Neither Mrs. E nor her husband agreed with the recommendations. Mr. E refused to recognize obesity as a problem. Nor did he identify Mrs. E's anxiety as a problem in his relationship with her or as interfering with her functioning as a housewife and mother. One week later the patient was released at her husband's insistance, on the condition that Mrs. E be placed on a diet and given medications to relieve the anxiety. This was agreeable to both husband and wife on grounds that this type of treatment was directed toward a physical problem. Mrs. E was not hospitalized again during the next 14 years.

Do-Nothings

In the Do-Nothing family, psychiatric deviance may or may not be recognized, and in some instances classified under another rubric, e.g., troublemaking, crime, alcoholism. If the deviation is recognized as indicative of mental illness, utilization of psychiatric treatment is not considered as a possible remedial action. Sometimes the family may be opposed to psychiatric care but indifference is the predominant pattern. Accordingly, expected level of performance is extremely low, perhaps requiring no more than sporadic contributions to the economic needs of the family, carrying out of occasional household tasks, or merely refraining from interfering with the everyday operations of the family.

The prepatient is rarely moved out of the home by members of this kind of family. Since social control within the family is absent, the deviant is not constrained from acting in an increasingly aberrant fashion. As frequency and intensity of deviation increases, it becomes more and more salient to the outside community. Usually, the career begins because of the intervention of some outside agency or person. If a recommendation for psychiatric treatment is made to the family, little or nothing is done to facilite treatment. Do-Nothings may endorse the decision to utilize psychiatric care, but acquiescence is the general rule.

Because of a rapid transition from unrecognized to recognized deviance, a carry-over of an attitude of indifference, or little or no socialization for the events that are beginning to occur, the family is both slow and reluctant to accept a psychiatric definition of the situation. Thus, the Do-Nothing family remains uninvolved during the course of hospitalization. Once the patient returns home whatever minimal psychiatric definition that developed quickly fades into the background. Consequently, the likelihood that the family will initiate rehospitalization is very low, although the possibility of outside intervention still remains.

Case 11   Although Mr. G had a 20-year history of alcoholism and intermittent employment, it was not until about eight years ago that he became highly irritable and began to suffer from a variety of physical problems. Conflict relating to his excessive drinking, intermittent employment, and an emergent pattern of family violence eventually led his wife to assume a separate residence in the small town where they both lived. During the months that followed, Mr. G continued to drink heavily, experienced further complications with his health, and developed pronounced depressive symptoms. The local physician recommended inpatient psychiatric treatment to several family members, including an adult daughter from a previous marriage. However, no action was taken until the sheriff picked up Mr. G for loitering in a nearby town. Upon notification of this event, the daughter contacted the outpatient clinic of University Psychiatric Hospital and made a vague inquiry about treatment. On his own initiative the sheriff took Mr. G to Inpatient Admissions at the hospital. He was admitted and discharged one month later with the diagnosis of Passive-Dependent Personality, depressive reaction, chronic alcoholism.

Mr. G returned to his home town, moved in with his ex-wife, but continued to abuse his current spouse and young son, particularly during his drinking episodes. However, no one made any attempt to get Mr. G to resume treatment. Four months later, he was picked up by the sheriff in a state of intoxicated depression and taken back to Inpatient Admissions. Although he was refused admission, a referral was made to the closest state psychiatric hospital where he was driven by the sheriff and admitted. During the next three years Mr. G was picked up twice again and taken directly to the state hospital where he was treated and released on each occasion.

A totally apathetic family is described in Case 12.

Case 12 Since the age of seven, Ray had been involved in numerous antisocial activities such as theft, breaking and entering, assault and battery, and truancy. At age 17 he attempted to force a young woman into a car at knife-point. As a result he was referred by court services for psychiatric evaluation. Diagnosis at admission was Sociopathic Personality Disturbance, antisocial type.

Not only did the mother condone Ray's antisocial behavior, but she consistently withheld information from the father and interfered when the father attempted to discipline the boy. Although the mother had been hospitalized for psychiatric disorder, neither she nor the father regarded Ray's behavior as indicative of psychiatric deviance. Moreover, it appeared that the mother derived vicarious pleasure from the boy's behavior (particularly the event that resulted in the pregnancy of Ray's girl friend) and used the boy as a husband substitute.

The charge of assault was held in abeyance with the stipulation that Ray would undergo outpatient treatment. Although he missed half of the appointments, his probation officer reported that Ray's family and school adjustment was satisfactory. He obtained a part-time job and intended to enter the military service after graduation from high school, hoping to specialize in underwater demolitions. He was not readmitted to inpatient status again.

METHODS

The sample of 79 patients was obtained from the University of Iowa Psychiatric Hospital, Iowa City. All first admission cases with functional disorders entering the hospital between 4 April and 2 December, 1966 were selected for inclusion. This cohort of patients represents 85 percent of the hospital's first admission cases during this 9-month interval; the remaining 15 percent of these cases were not included because they were admitted under emergency conditions or during evenings or week-ends when an interviewer was not available. Patients in the sample ranged in age from 15 to 62, 35 percent were diagnosed as psychotic, and 46 percent were male. The typical patient was white, Protestant, of Germanic descent, married, 39-years-old, a high school graduate, living in an urban area, of lower middle-class status, and diagnosed as having a personality disorder.

Data on patients and their families were collected via interview schedule and hospital records, two different but complementary methods. Each patient and his/her primary significant other was interviewed as early as 30 days prior to hospitalization. (The primary significant other was almost invariably a nuclear family member who accompanied the patient at the request of the hospital.) Since the interviews took place during "preadmission screening," less than 30 percent of the patients or significant others had knowledge of if or when hospital admission would actually occur. In order to reconstruct the events prior to hospitalization, the prepatient phase of the psychiatric patient career was trichotomized according to the major milestones that individuals passed on the road to hospital entry: Definition and Appraisal of Psychiatric Deviance, Decision to Utilize Psychiatric Help, Implementation of Psychiatric Care. For each of these subphases, both the prepatient and the family member were questioned separately with respect to *what* it was that was recognized and responded to, *when* this psychiatric deviance occurred, and *who* was involved in the decision-making process. Information was also sought on the relative influence of various family members during each step of the way.

Data from hospital records were used to supplement information obtained by personal interviews. Records compiled during "preadmission screening" contained a psychiatric evaluation of the prepatient, a social work evaluation of the family member, and the results of an interdisciplinary staffing. Inpatient records contained evaluations and other reports by psychiatric staff, nursing staff, and social workers on patient symptomatology, ward behavior, and family visitations. From these, we could determine how prepatients and family members responded to the initial definition of psychiatric deviance, how each patient accommodated to institutional life and therapy, and how the family responded to the general situation.

Working with both the interview and hospital record information, but without any knowledge of case outcome, four independent judges were instructed to eliminate those cases for which our family reactions model was inappropriate and to assign the remaining cases to the one of the four family types (and subtypes) which it most closely approximated. Two cases were eliminated because the patient either had no family or was separated from the family before the onset of psychiatric disturbance. Setting the criterion for "agreement" as consensus among at least three of four judges resulted in the immediate classification of 60 cases. In 17 cases judges were divided between two categories or subcategories but did not show any greater degree of disagreement. Differences in opinion were resolved without undue difficulty by group discussion. Thus, while not all cases fit the taxonomy perfectly, there was sufficient correspondence between the characteristics of the observed cases and the "ideal" types that 77 cases could be classified with substantial agreement.

In predicting the career outcomes of first admission cases, rehospitalization was chosen as the major dependent variable. However, three other dependent variables are also of interest in examining the career outcomes of psychiatric patients: number of readmissions, length of time between initial hospital discharge and first readmission (latency period), and outpatient treatment. To gather information on these four variables, records were checked at University Psychiatric Hospital, the four public psychiatric hospitals serving different quadrants of the state of Iowa, and a large private psychiatric hospital in Cedar Rapids. These follow-up data were collected during July 1980, approximately 14 years after patients in the original cohort had been discharged from University Psychiatric Hospital.

Analysis of the records of the six target hospitals revealed that 30 of the 77 cases (39 percent) had undergone at least one rehospitalization in the period from 1966–80. Five of the 30 cases were readmitted to a psychiatric facility other than one of the six hospitals. For these five the dates of readmission had to be estimated based on the requests for "evaluation summaries" and "records releases" from the other inpatient facilities. Patients in the original cohort who were rehospitalized in facilities that did not request information from the hospitals whose records we checked are not included in our measures of recidivism. Data on outpatient treatment were collected only at University Psychiatric Hospital. These records were often ambiguous as to whether such care was at the behest of the institution, so we decided to exclude those cases in "continuous treatment." Thus the data are based on cases in which the time lapse between hospital discharge and outpatient care was three months or more.

RESULTS

In the original study knowledge of each of the two independent variables, a family's Level of Expected Performance and Propensity for Action, permitted general predictions about the outcome of psychiatric patients' careers [36,37]. We anticipated that postpatients would tend to be rehospitalized more frequently if they came from families characterized as high LEP. Families with a high and not-low PA would similarly be more likely to rehospitalize their deviant members. Via the cross-classification of these two variables, more specific predictions were possible. It was suggested that readmission rates would be highest among patients in the anticipatory-prohibitive (HiLEP-HiPA) type of family, and lowest in the detached-tolerant (LoLEP-LoPA) type. Anticipatory-tolerant (HiLEP-LoPA) and detached-prohibitive (LoLEP-HiPA) families were expected to have readmission rates falling somewhere between these extremes.

Presented in Table 10-1 are the "main effects" of the two independent variables on the four dependent variables. From these data it is clear that a family's LEP and PA are related to the career outcomes of psychiatric patients. Both independent variables affected three of the four dependent variables in a manner consonant with our general predictions. Patients from families whose

LEP is high were readmitted to a psychiatric hospital more often during the 14-year-period following their discharge, had a higher number of readmissions, and received outpatient treatment more often than did patients from low LEP families. When PA is high the readmission rate is higher, the latency period much shorter, and the outpatient treatment rate higher than when PA is low. Moreover, the data indicate that of the two independent variables PA is the more important for determining recidivist patterns, as its high-low differences are greater than those for LEP. For example, almost twice as many high PA families (52 percent) as low (28 percent) are rehospitalized, whereas readmissions for high LEP families are only one-third greater than for low (44 percent vs. 33 percent).

Data for the four dependent variables in terms of the typology of family reactions are given in Table 10-2. Here our predictions concerning case outcome were realized for the major dependent variable, readmission rate. Anticipatory-prohibitive families had the highest proportion of readmissions between 1966–80, more than twice as many as detached-tolerant families (55 percent vs. 25 percent). Both of these types of families are "polar opposites" according to the typology and, ostensibly, should be at opposite extremes. The anticipatory-tolerant and detached-prohibitive types, as anticipated, occupy intermediate positions; that the latter proved to have the higher readmission rate merely reflects the greater influence of PA over LEP on case outcome. For the other three dependent variables there is a strong tendency for the anticipatory-prohibitive family to lead the others on recidivist characteristics, but the detached-tolerant type is not positioned at the opposite pole.

A comparison of the data in Tables 10-1 and 10-2 suggest that the predictive abilities of the two independent variables are greater when they are correlated with the dependent variables separately rather than in combination with one another. The dichotomization of a family's LEP and PA yielded more consistent relationships with patients' career patterns than did the fourfold typology. However, the four ideal types of family reactions appear especially useful when considering variations within, instead of between, types. A number of predictions made in the original study concerning family subtypes are largely substantiated by Table 10-2 statistics. This is particularly evident when Stoic and Poltroon families are examined. These two subtypes differ substantially from one another on all outcome indicators, and the directions of the recidivist differences are consistent with our theoretical expectations. The Stoic family's ability to withstand stress is underscored by their low rate of patient rehospitalization, few subsequent rehospitalizations, rather long time (more than four years) before the first readmission occurs, and small number receiving outpatient treatment. By contrast, Poltroon's faintheartedness and irresoluteness account for their higher number and proportion of readmission cases, much shorter latency period (1½ years), and much higher rate of posthospital care. Assertive and Altercaster families also differ substantially; the former, as anticipated, showing higher scores on all four recidivist measures.

Table 10-1. Effects of Independent Variables on the Career Outcomes of Psychiatric Patients

INDEPENDENT VARIABLES	READMISSIONS N	N	%	MEAN NUMBER OF READMISSIONS*	MEAN LATENCY (IN MONTHS)	OUTPATIENT TREATMENT N	%
Level of Expected Performance							
High	41	18	44	2.9	18.9	14	34
Low	36	12	33	1.9	19.3	10	28
Propensity for Action							
High	34	18	52	2.7	9.4	13	28
Low	43	12	28	2.2	33.5	11	26

*Based on readmitted cases only.

Table 10-2. Career Outcomes of Psychiatric Patients by Type of Family

TYPE OF FAMILY	N	READMISSIONS N	%	MEAN NUMBER OF READMISSIONS*	MEAN LATENCY (IN MONTHS)	OUTPATIENT TREATMENT N	%
Anticipatory-Prohibitive	22	12	55	3.3	10.3	10	45
Assertive	12	7	58	3.6	8.9	5	42
Altercaster	10	5	50	3.0	12.4	5	50
Anticipatory-Tolerant	19	6	32	2.0	35.8	4	21
Stoic	9	3	25	1.7	53.3	1	8
Poltroon	10	3	42	2.3	18.3	3	43
Detached-Prohibitive	12	6	50	1.5	7.5	3	25
Authoritarian	12	6	50	1.5	7.5	3	25
Detached-Tolerant	24	6	25	2.0	31.2	7	29
Pacifist	7	1	14	1.0	60.0	1	14
Stumbler	7	2	29	1.5	31.0	1	14
Do-Nothing	10	3	30	3.0	21.7	5	50
Total	27	30	39	2.4	21.1	24	31

*Based on readmitted cases only.

Several predictions were made in the original study regarding detached-tolerant family subtypes. We claimed that Pacifists were not likely to rehospitalize their deviant members, but when they do, it would probably not be before an extended period of time. Data in Table 10-2 certainly substantiates this. Pacifists have the lowest readmission rate (14 percent), the longest latency between discharge and first readmission (five years), and the second lowest rate of outpatient care (14 percent) of all eight family subtypes. We also claimed that Stumblers would be relatively low on recidivst measures and this too appears to be borne out by the data. In comparison to the other subtypes, Stumbler families are among those with the lowest readmission rate, lowest number of readmissions, longest latency period, and lowest posthospital treatment rate. Persons from these families were as adroit as we anticipated in learning to avoid stumbling onto pathways of treatment again. Our records analysis disclosed that both readmitted cases returned to the hospital as a direct consequence of a psychiatric referral.

The data in Table 10-2 reveal that Do-Nothing families are more recidivist-prone than Pacifist; they are more likely to undergo repeated admissions, remain in the community for a shorter length of time, and enter outpatient facilities. However, Do-Nothings, compared to the eight subtypes of families, are less polar on the dependent variables than might be expected. It will be recalled that most persons from Do-Nothing families came to the hospital via community rather than family reactions. Once activated, these secondary group mechanisms of social control are probably operating again after the patient's return to the community. An inspection of the hospital records of the three Do-Nothing cases who were rehospitalized uncovered that it was the direct result of police intervention for two of them. The reactivation of formal community controls may also help to explain the exceptionally high proportion of postpatients from Do-Nothing families who underwent follow-up treatment.

These findings dealing with readmission rates—the major dependent variable of this investigation—would be limited if they were affected by patients' social and psychiatric characteristics. If, for example, males were rehospitalized five times as frequently as females, then the correlations of LEP and PA with recidivist measures would be biased by sex. This issue of data limitation was therefore examined. We discovered that the readmission rate did not vary greatly when the sample was subdivided according to age, sex, marital status, religion, education, occupation, and urban-rural residence. Differences between patient groups on these social factors were less than six percentage points. Similar results were obtained with psychiatric characteristics of patients or illness (Table 10-3). Group differences are relatively small, eight percentage points at most. As might be expected, psychotic patients and those with an unfavorable prognosis returned to the hospital slightly more often than the nonpsychotic and those evaluated favorably. Surprisingly, patients thought to have improved in their hospital

Table 10-3. Readmission Rates of Psychiatric Patients by Characteristics of Illness

		READMISSIONS	
CHARACTERISTICS OF ILLNESS	N*	N	%
Diagnosis[1]			
Psychotic	28	12	43
Nonpsychotic	51	18	35
Prognosis[2]			
Favorable	35	12	34
Unfavorable	33	13	39
Hospital Adjustment[3]			
Improved	35	13	37
Unimproved	37	11	30
Length of Hospitalization[4]			
Short-term	39	16	41
Long-term	38	14	37

*Information not available for all 79 patients in sample.
[1] As listed on patient's intake record.
[2] Based on attending psychiatrist's final evaluation.
[3] Based on ward nurse's notes.
[4] A dichotomization of the sample at the median length of hospital stay, 40 days.

adjustment had a somewhat higher readmission rate than the unimproved. Viewed as a whole, the data suggest that various attributes of patients do not substantially affect their likelihood of rehospitalization.

DISCUSSION

The findings presented in this chapter indicate that our fourfold typology of family reactions, and dichotomization of the variables it is composed of, are useful devices for predicting the career patterns of psychiatric patients. Knowledge of a family's Level of Expected Performance for its members and Propensity for Action in hospitalizing and rehospitalizing members who deviate from such expectations helped explain its standing on various recidivist measures. We observed that whether or not a postpatient is readmitted to a psychiatric hospital within 14 years of discharge, the number of such readmissions, the time lapse between discharge and first readmission, and if outpatient treatment was received are all largely determined by his/her family's high or low LEP and PA. Family types (differentiated by performance expectations and predilection to utilize societal controls to curb deviant behavior) and subtypes (differentiated by attitudes toward mental illness and psychiatric institutions) were also found to be important predictors of career outcomes. Social and psychiatric characteristics of patients, in contrast to our typology of family reactions, had little to do with recidivism.

Studies of family reactions to psychiatric disorder over the past quarter-century have been giving greater attention to the milieu from which the hospital patient comes and returns. At times the focus was on the stages through which families pass in recognizing and adjusting to deviant members [3,17,27,29]. Other researchers sought to identify the social variables that differentiate families on the basis of their responses to psychiatric deviance and the consequences of such responses [13,28,39]. In these latter studies, typologies were developed to classify families. Greenley used three categories, based on whether the family wants the patient released, retained, or is ambivalent about hospital stay [13]. Reiss et al. created four types via the cross-classification of two independent variables: a family's level of configuration (use of each other's observations and ideas to solve problems) and degree of coordination (interpretation of problem-solving activities) [28]. Voiland and Buell relied on the criteria of pathology and social functioning to categorize families as perfectionist, inadequate, egocentric, and unsocial [39]. Like our own typology, these three classificatory schemata successfully predicted certain outcomes of psychiatric treatment.

Our typology of family reaction serves theoretical, empirical, and clinical purposes. First, a typology should sensitize the social scientist to alternative ways of conceptualizing a particular phenomenon. Case outcomes, before the seminal work of Freeman and Simmons, were generally thought of as being determined by the effects of psychiatric factors on patients [7,8]. These researchers demonstrated that the probability of readmission was largely a function of posthospital performance standards set by the family. Another team of investigators approached the question of readmission determinants more directly [6,20]. They found that the posthospital family milieu and the socioeconomic status of the patient were fairly accurate predictors of case outcome, while various psychiatric variables were relatively unimportant in assessing recovery potential. Thus, the incorporation of different types of family reactions into our framework highlights in a theoretical way the importance of nonpsychiatric factors for patient careers. The typology draws attention to the manner in which disturbed behavior among postpatients is connected to familial processes. The four ideal types of families also serve to "set the stage" for empirical research. Levels of expected performance and propensity for action need to be considered because they predict psychiatric case outcome better than patient characteristics. This is especially true for long-term follow-up studies. We observed that the period of time intervening between discharge and first readmission varied markedly according to family types. Now, even though 14 years have passed, patients in the original cohort are still appearing and reappearing at inpatient psychiatric facilities, albeit in progressively smaller numbers.

The use of our typology for clinical purposes is both possible and feasible. Hospital staff cannot become intensively involved with the families of all psychiatric patients. A more practical course of action for mental health professionals would be to make an initial appraisal of each family's situation and then select those cases which are in most need of services [37]. By classifying families according to LEP and PA, patterns of reactions to a deviant member can be predicted and clinicians could more appropriately direct their efforts toward the realization of treatment goals. The hospital seeks to reduce the family's resistance to inpatient, outpatient, and crisis intervention services, and knowledge of family types and subtypes can make these tasks easier. The clinical and objective data contained in this report may assist mental health professionals to more fully understand the process of patient adjustment after hosptalization, and to deal more effectively with families on a variety of levels during that time.

In the original study we observed that staff-family contacts are infrequent and unsystematic. During the prepatient phase families were seen only once, for information gathering purposes, rather than for intervention in the on-going family process. During the inpatient phase, only one family in the entire sample was the object of continuous intervention activities. The parents of Carolyn, Case 7, were monitored for three years following her hospitalization. The other 78 families were limited to unscheduled contacts with the nursing staff and occasional consultations with psychiatrists. Contacts with social workers were virtually nonexistent. During the postpatient phase the situation was no different. At University Hospital and the other target facilities, few staff persons contacted the patient or his/her family. Our follow-up results thus reflect how the careers of psychiatric first-admissions cases evolve in the *absence* of concerted hospital initiatives at intervention. Data on readmissions and outpatient treatment presented here may serve as points of comparison for empirical research on the effectiveness of family-oriented intervention programs. The success of such programs may be measured by the degree to which follow-up data on the recidivism of similar cohorts of psychiatric patients in comparable treatment settings deviate from our baseline findings (Tables 10-1 and 10-2). Such comparisons may also have implications for mental health policy.

All patients face certain posthospital adjustment problems: finding suitable employment, maintaining contacts with therapists, residing with family members or board-and-care facilities, coping with feelings of stigma, worrying about the recurrence of symptoms, and so on. The patient who leaves the hospital for return to the community is typically not "cured" of the problems which initially led to hospitalization [23]. Our data on career outcomes of psychiatric patients actually say little about the kind of problems different types of families are likely to encounter. However, the data do suggest that many patients may be having serious problems of adjustment, since 39 percent of our patient sample returned to the hospital, most within one year of discharge. Families with high LEP or high PA especially need to be counseled by hospital personnel. In order to circumvent a premature rehospitalization an oft-tried technique is to encourage family members to view the patient as an individual with strengths as well as weaknesses. A collaborative review of the patient's social history could function as a point of departure to engender latent empathic abilities. Reflective discussion of the implications of interactions with the patient for family dynamics are an important step in the socialization process.

Helping families accept the possibility of rehospitalization is perhaps the most difficult task for the staffs of psychiatric hospitals. Families of patients with chronic illnesses—such as schizophrenia—in which there is continual remission and exacerbation of symptoms, are hit especially hard with the reality of multiple readmissions. Our results indicate that Stoics and Pacifists need to be forewarned and prepared for this occurrence more than any other type of family. These families have an exceptionally long time span between patients' discharge and first readmission, completely out of balance compared to other families. This suggests that Stoics and Pacifists may be holding patients back unnecessarily from needed treatment. Community agency cooperation may be considered in order to help motivate members of these types of families to take necessary remedial action. Direct confrontation with such family members during the inpatient phase might serve to dispel apathy, but the success of this technique is probably dependent upon continuing education about mental illness and increased involvement with psychiatric hospital goals and functions.

In closing, it may be stated that a typology of family reactions such as ours may help mental health professionals consider families, like persons, as unitary cases. Research by Reiss et al. also points in this direction [28] They provided evidence of their classificatory scheme's successful prediction of a family's response to a family-oriented treatment program. Families could be classified before treatment begins in an effort to predict their responses and to formulate the best psychiatric treatment program. In future research studies it might be possible to associate other variables (e.g., family structure, patient symptomatology, family class status) with specific reaction patterns. Establishing the degree of association between family variables and reaction patterns would allow greater predictability of case outcomes and better determination of intervention activities. Further investigation might also test whether the use of our typology does make a difference in the attainment of certain goals in behalf of the patient.

ACKNOWLEDGMENTS

We would like to express our appreciation to the directors of the Iowa Mental Health Institutes at Mt. Pleasant, Independence, Clarina, and Cherokee, and to the administrator of Saint Luke's Methodist Hospital in Cedar Rapids for providing access to their records. George Winokur, M.D., Chairman, Department of Psychiatry, State Psychiatric Hospital, University of Iowa, permitted us access to records and also provided other helpful assistance. We also thank Ms. Ida Swearington for her careful reading of an earlier version of this manuscript.

REFERENCES

1. Becker, H. "Becoming a marijuana user." *American Journal of Sociology* 59 : 235–242, 1953.
2. Bursten, B. and D'Esopo, R. "The obligation to remain sick." In T.J. Scheff (ed.), *Mental Illness and Social Processes*. New York: Harper & Row, 1967, pp. 206–218.
3. Clausen, J.A. and Yarrow, M.R. "The impact of mental illness on the family." *Journal of Social Issues* 11 : 2–11, 1955.
4. Cumming J. and Cumming E. "On the stigma of mental illness." *Community Mental Health Journal* 1 : 135–43, 1965.
5. Deasy, L. and Quinn, O.W. "The wife of the mental patient and the hospital psychiatrist." *Journal of Social Issues* 11 : 49–60, 1955.
6. Dinitz, S.; Lefton, M.; Angrist, S.; and Pasamanick, B. "Psychiatric and social attributes as predictors of case outcomes in mental hospitalization." *Social Problems* 8 : 322–28, 1961.
7. Freeman, H.E. and Simmons, O.G. "Mental patients in the community: family settings and performance levels." *American Sociological Review* 23 : 147–54, 1958.
8. Freeman, H.E. and Simmons, O.G. "Social class and posthospital performance levels." *American Sociological Review* 24 : 345–51, 1959.
9. Glassner, B.; Haldipur, C.V.; and Dessauersmith, J. "Role loss and working-class manic depression." *Journal of Nervous and Mental Disease*, 167 : 530–41, 1979.
10. Goffman, E. "The moral career of the mental patient." *Psychiatry* 22 : 123–142, 1959.
11. Gordon, G. *Role Theory and Illness*. New Haven: College and University Press, 1966.
12. Gove, W.R. and Fain, T. "A comparison of voluntary and committed psychiatric patients." *Archives of General Psychiatry* 34 : 669–676, 1977.
13. Greenley, J.R. "The psychiatric patient's family and length of hospitalization." *Journal of Health and Social Behavior* 13 : 25–37, 1972.
14. Gurin, G.; Veroff, J.; and Feld, S. *Americans View Their Mental Health*. New York: Basic Books, 1960.
15. Hall, O. "The stages of a medical career." *American Journal of Sociology* 53 : 327–336, 1948.
16. Hollingshead, A.B. and Redlich, F.C. *Social Class and Mental Illness*. New York: John Wiley, 1958.
17. Horwitz, A. "The pathways into psychiatric treatment: some differences between men and women." *Journal of Health and Social Behavior* 18 : 169–78, 1977.
18. Hughes, E. "Institutional office and the person." *American Journal of Sociology* 43 : 404–413, 1937.
19. Larkin, W.E. and Loman, L.A. "Labeling in the family context: an experimental study." *Sociology and Social Research* 61 : 192–208, 1977.
20. Lefton, M.; Angrist, S.; Dinitz, S.; and Pasamanick, B. "Social class, expectations, and performance of mental patients." *American Journal of Sociology* 58 : 79–87, 1962.
21. Lidz, T. et al. "Patients and their siblings." *Psychiatry* 26 : 1–18, 1963.

22. Mechanic, D. "Some factors in identifying and defining mental illness." *Mental Hygiene* 46 : 66–74, 1962.
23. Moore, K.B. and McCravy, N., Jr. "Family interaction as a factor in prolonging hospitalization." *Journal of Nervous and Mental Disease* 136 : 485–91, 1963.
24. Myers, J.K. and Roberts, B.M. *Family and Class Dynamics in Mental Illness*. New York: John Wiley, 1959.
25. Omark, R.C. "The dilemma of membership in Recovery, Inc.: a self-help ex-mental patients organization." *Psychological Reports* 44 : 1119–25, 1979.
26. Parsons, T. and Fox, R.C. "Illness, therapy, and the modern american family." *Journal of Social Issues* 8 : 31–44, 1952.
27. Raymond, M.E.; Slaby, A.E.; and Lieb, J. "Familial responses to mental illness." In C.E. Munson (ed.) *Social Work With Families*. New York: Free Press, 1980, pp. 418–427.
28. Reiss, D.; Costell, R.; Jones, C.; and Berkman, H. "The family meets the hospital: a laboratory forecast of the encounter." *Archives of General Psychiatry* 37 : 141–154, 1980.
29. Sampson, H.; Messinger, S.L.; and Towne, R.D. *Schizophrenic Women*. New York: Atherton Press, 1964.
30. Schwartz, C.C.; Myers, J.K.; and Astrachan, B.M. "Psychiatric labeling and the rehabilitation of the mental patient: implications of research findings for mental health policy." *Archives of General Psychiatry* 31 : 329–34, 1974.
31. Serban, G. and Gidynyski, C.B. "Significance of social demographic data for rehospitalization of schizophrenic patients." *Journal of Health and Social Behavior* 15 : 117–26, 1974.
32. Simmons, O.G.; Davis, J.A.; and Spencer, K. "Interpersonal strains in release from a mental hospital." *Social Problems* 4 : 21–28, 1956.
33. Spiegel, D. "The ex-mental patient." In D. Spiegel and P. Keith-Spiegel (eds.) *Outsiders U.S.A.: Original Essays on 24 Outgroups in American Society*. San Francisco: Rinehart Press, 1973, pp. 298–325.
34. Spitzer, S.P. "Determining pathways to psychiatric treatment by family reactions to deviance." Unpublished report. Iowa City, Iowa: Iowa State Mental Health Authority, 1968.
35. Spitzer, S.P. and Bealka, R.J. "Family influences on psychiatric patient performance." *Child Welfare*, 48 : 545–51, 1969.
36. Spitzer, S.P.; Swanson, R.M.; and Lehr, R.K. "Audience reactions and careers of psychiatric patients." *Family Process* 8 : 159–81, 1969.
37. Spitzer, S.P.; Morgan, P.A.; and Swanson, R.M. "Determinants of the psychiatric patient career: family reaction patterns and social work intervention." *Social Service Review* 45 : 74–85, 1971.
38. Vogel, E.F. and Bell, N.W. "The emotionally disturbed child as the family scapegoat." In N.K. Bell and E.F. Vogel (eds.) *Modern Introduction to the Family*. Glencoe, Ill.: Free Press, 1960, pp. 382–97.
39. Voiland, A.L. and Buell, B. "A classification of disordered family types." In C.E. Munson (ed.) *Social Work With Families*. New York: Free Press, 1980, pp. 196–208.
40. Wood, E.C.; Rakushin, J.M.; and Morse, E. "Interpersonal aspects of psychiatric hospitalization, I: the admission." *Archives of General Psychiatry*, 3 : 632–41, 1960.
41. Yarrow, M.R.; Schwartz, C.G.; Murphy, H.S.; and Deasy, L.C. "The psychiatric meaning of mental illness in the family." *Journal of Social Issues* 11 : 12–24, 1955.

11

The Patient's Family and Length of Psychiatric Hospitalization

JAMES R. GREENLEY

One of the many ways that a psychiatric inpatient's family influences the patient's treatment course is through their impact on the length of hospitalization. This chapter presents data from a study that examines the magnitude of this influence and from subsequent studies that confirm these findings. The relationship of family attitudes toward continued hospitalization of their patient member are then examined in relation to broad styles of family involvement with the patient and treatment staff during hospitalization.

Clinicians, administrators, researchers, and others have a variety of reasons for wishing to better understand how families may have an impact on length of hospitalization. Correlates of length of hospitalization are sought because length of treatment is often taken as a crude measure of therapeutic effectiveness. Long periods of hospitalization are felt to undesirably "institutionalize" patients, and the size of the patient population and thus the cost of care are as dependent on length of stay as the number of admissions.

The actions and attitudes of families relevant to length of hospitalization may have an impact on such diverse aspects of the psychiatric treatment experience as the timing of the initial identification and hospitalization [31], the choice of a patient's placement in the community [25] and the chances for and time of rehospitalization [4,9,12]. Also, it has long been recognized that family members may play a crucial role in the etiology, treatment, and recovery of the patients. Therefore, in this chapter, the relationship of family desires and length of hospitalization are explored, alternative explanations are examined, and implications of our findings are discussed.

Numerous observers have argued for a causal link between family desires concerning release and discharge timing. Some suggest that the presence of relatives who do not desire a loved one released can delay the release

[13,17,20,24]. A few imply that a family who wishes to speed a release can do it [23]. Several have noted that family interest in release may aid the patient's recovery [7,14,20].

Negative attitudes on the part of the family may deprive the psychiatrist of an adequate placement for the patient in the community. Despite these numerous and careful observations, for the most part, substantive research into this factor has been lacking. The desires of the family may be influential for a variety of reasons or might only be spuriously related to length of hospitalization due to several other factors long thought to be determinants of discharge decisions.

From a medical perspective, the type and severity of the patient's psychopathology should be a useful indicator of when the patient will be released. On the whole, the relevant research supports this view, although there are some inconsistencies. Clinical observers have argued that the timing of discharge depends on the type and severity of the patient's illness [16]. Diagnostic categories signifying more severe impairment, e.g., schizophrenia and organic disturbances, are associated with longer hospital stays [13,27]. Clinical assessments of psychiatric impairment have shown that more impaired patients tend to stay hospitalized longer [11,22,27]. However, the observations of clinical teams in one study indicated that only in rare instances did discharge decisions relate to psychopathology [23]. Similarly, a small study of schizophrenics could not distinguish those discharged from those retained on the basis of mental status examinations or observations of ward behavior [5]. Three studies, including the one just cited, employed psychiatric rating devices but did not find that those patients who tested as more psychiatrically impaired stayed longer [2,5,8]. Thus, while psychiatric diagnoses are found to be related to length of hospitalization, other estimates of impairment give conflicting results.

Psychiatric institutions are often seen as "social control" agencies as well as medical facilities [21]. As such, mental health professionals have been thought to base their release decisions in part on the consequences to the community [2,18]. There is considerable speculation in the literature that patients may be kept hospitalized when their behavior cannot be adequately controlled, such as through outpatient care [30] or through placement with a family who agrees to assume responsibility [7]. Surprisingly, one study of criminally insane patients transferred to civil state mental hospitals found that past dangerous behavior was not related to length of hospitalization, although assaultiveness during the civil hospitalization did have some predictive value [26,27]. Because the dangerous patient may remain hospitalized longer, in part because of the fearful family's refusal to accept him back in the home, the patient's destructiveness to himself or others requires careful examination.

THE NEW ENGLAND STUDY

A study of adult admissions to a New England state psychiatric hospital forms the basis of most of the research described in this chapter. The setting and methodology of this study is briefly but carefully described here.

The research site is a six-ward "unit" of a large New England state mental hospital serving a defined geographical area. Extensive informal observations were made of day-to-day contacts among patients, psychiatrists, and nursing staff. From thirty to several hundred hours were spent in each of a variety of settings: nursing stations; patient-patient interaction at meals and on the ward; records room; nursing supervisor's office; staff dining room; staff coffee lounge; truck landing where patients informally congregated; central lobby of the hospital building; and staff conferences concerning patients. Private, semistructured interviews were conducted with most administrative personnel on this unit, several social workers, and most of the psychiatrists.

The psychiatric staff of this unit includes: (1) consulting psychiatrists from both the community and a local prestigious eastern university who supervise residents and handle intake and disposition staffings; (2) resident psychiatrists, most of whom are foreign-born and foreign-trained; and (3) nonpsychiatrically trained M.D.s who are often in administrative positions and typically have been working with psychiatric patients for years. All three categories are represented in the interviews with and observations of the psychiatrists described below.

This hospital is by reputation neither exceptionally good nor exceptionally poor in the quality of patient care given. The staff is conscientious (even though normally harassed by an overly large patient load) and generally views the hospital with pride. Extensive use of pharmacological treatment was supplemented by an active occupational therapy unit, some group therapy, and a very small amount of individual psychotherapy. A number of the staff recognized the importance of involving families in the treatment process but, due to limited time and staff resources, only an occasional patient received any form of family therapy.

The research involved gathering information from the patient, his psychiatrist, his family, and the ward staff during the hospitalization and relating this information to the timing of patient's discharge. A total of 342 structured interviews were obtained from the patients, families, and psychiatrists involved in 125 psychiatric admissions from a New England city with a population of about 140,000, plus virtually all its suburbs. The "cases" chosen for study were consecutive admissions between May and September 1969, 21 to 65 years old, and not primarily suffering from drug addiction, alcoholism, or senility.

As a group, 72 percent of the patients in the study group were white and 51 percent were female; 41 percent were under 30 years of age and only 9 percent were 50-years-old or older. About one-third (34 percent) were married, 30 percent were single, and the remainder were widowed, divorced, or separated. Educationally, 15 percent had some college education, an additional 28 percent were high school graduates, and 25 percent had not attended high school. The largest occupational group were unskilled workers or unemployed (39 percent), but 16 percent were white-collar workers, and 13 percent were professionals, small businessmen, and so forth. While 29 percent had never been psychiatrically hospitalized previously, 45 percent had been hospitalized three or more times.

With few exceptions, interviews were obtained with the psychiatrist and the patient during the first week of hospitalization. After three weeks, the patient and his psychiatrist were reinterviewed and, at this time, the patient's family was also interviewed. Interviews were again obtained before the patient was released from the hospital and the patient's hospital record was searched for further relevant information.

Thirty-nine percent of the attempted initial interviews with the psychiatrists were not obtained because they refused to participate, regardless of who their patients were. Because patients were assigned to psychiatrists by intake personnel on a rotational basis, there is no reason to suspect a systematic bias to result from the loss of these cases. A second interview was sought from all patients and psychiatrists from whom initial interviews were obtained. Refusal rates for the second interviews with psychiatrists, for both the interviews with patients and for the family interviews, ranged from 0 to 11 percent. Because each interview schedule administered resulted in a different completion rate, various maximum numbers of cases were available for and used in different statistical analyses. Chi-square goodness-of-fit tests were done individually for each schedule to determine if the completed cases differed from the 125 originally selected admissions on the following characteristics: sex, age, marital status, religion, occupation, education, social class, and previous admission to a psychiatric hospital.* In no instance did any completed group of cases differ significantly from what would have been expected on the basis of the original 125 cases.

The major dependent variable—the outcome of the release decision—is measured behaviorally in terms of when the patient actually left the hospital,

---

*The categories of control variables used here and throughout this study are as follows: Age: 21–30, 31–40, 41–50, 51–65; Race: white, black (3 of the 125 cases were eliminated from this analysis because they were Puerto Rican); Religion: Protestant, Catholic (11 of the 125 cases were dropped from this analysis because they listed themselves as "none," "Jewish" or "other"); Marital Status: married, single, divorced, widowed, or separated; Education: less than 7 years, 7–9 years, 10–12 years, some college, completed college, graduate work; Occupation: Seven categories used as given in Hollingshead's Two Factor Index of Social Position; Social Class: Five categories used as computed by Hollingshead's Two Factor Index of Social Position.

rather than being based on a report or opinion concerning what decision was made. Patients left the hospital in five relatively distinct groups. The first group, the "Rapid Exit Group," consists of those patients leaving at or very near the time of their "intake staffing." The intake staffing is a formal 15-to-30 minute review of the patient's condition conducted by a senior consulting psychiatrist heading a team of psychiatric residents, nurses, social workers, aides, and auxiliary personnel (occupational therapists, music therapists, etc.). Those patients leaving after the intake staffing, but before a "review" staffing is scheduled, form a distinct group to be called the "Attenuated Stay Group." The third group are those patients who are released from the hospital near the time of their review staffing (21-to-36 days from admission). These patients, being proportionately the most numerous, are called the "Modal Stay Graoup." The fourth group, the "Extended Stay Group," are those patients leaving the hospital between 37 and 100 days from admission, that is, clearly after the period of their review staffing but before the staff begins to lose hope and interest in them. After 100 days of hospitalization the probability is 3-to-1 that a patient will remain over 200 days. This last patient group, experiencing a sharply reduced chance of exit, is called the "Long Stay Group." Only by treating length of hospitalization in terms of these five ordered groups can the realities of this hospital's organization and staff attitudes be taken into account.

Desires of the patient's family were assessed in interviews with the patient's "closest relative," as defined by the patient. Forty-two percent of closest relatives were spouses; 4 percent children; 40 percent parents; and 13 percent other relatives, mainly siblings. One friend of a patient was interviewed. Interviews were conducted in the homes of family members in order to minimize the chance that the family member would attempt to please the hospital staff with his response. In addition, it was made clear that the interviewer was not on the hospital staff and responses would not be made available to the hospital staff. During these interviews, family members were asked straightforwardly whether they wished their relative to remain hospitalized. Generally, their responses were direct and unequivocal. In only 5 of 80 cases (6 percent) could the family's response be considered "neutral," "undecided," or "ambivalent." These five cases were scored as being neither definitely in favor of nor against release but as somewhere between these extremes. Other measures are more usefully described as they are encountered in the presentation of the results.

RESULTS OF THE NEW ENGLAND STUDY

Family desires concerning release are strongly associated with the length of time each patient remained in the hospital, as shown in Table 11-1. This relationship remains statistically significant and substantial in each category of the following

Table 11-1.   Family Desires and Length of Hospitalization

	FAMILY DESIRES		
EXIT GROUP	Family Wants Patient Released % (N)	Family is Neutral or Ambivalent % (N)	Family Wants Patient Retained % (N)
Rapid Exit Group	32 (5)	0 (0)	2 (1)
Attenuated Stay Group	31 (5)	80 (4)	7 (4)
Modal Stay Group	25 (4)	20 (1)	29 (17)
Extended Stay Group	6 (1)	0 (0)	30 (18)
Long Stay Group	6 (1)	0 (0)	32 (19)
Total	100%	100%	100%

Gamma = .78, $p < .001$, N = 80

control variables: age, sex, race, religion, marital status, education, occupation, and social class. A "medical model" view of discharge, as discussed above, suggests that release decisions should be based on psychiatric impairment. Thus psychiatrist's evaluations of the patient's psychiatric impairment were examined to see if they related to length of hospitalization and therefore might, in some way, account for the relationship between family desires and length of hospitalization. Family desires, for instance, might simply reflect what family members felt the psychiatrist thought best on clinical grounds.

Each patient's psychiatrist was asked during the private interview, "How psychiatrically impaired is this patient now?" Six response categories were supplied ranging from "very severely impaired" to "no visible impairment." It is admittedly difficult to tell what factors were most determinant of the psychiatrist's responses. Comments made by psychiatrists at the time of their response indicated that they took into account, among other things, prognosis, diagnosis, present behavior, past behavior, and availability of treatment. Yet these comments give no indication as to which factors were more salient in the minds of the psychiatrists. In any event, their responses are strongly related to the timing of the patient's exit, as shown in Table 11-2, with those patients rated most impaired remaining longer.

A patient who is dangerous to himself or others may be hospitalized longer. To the extent psychiatric hospitals serve a social control function, a dangerous patient may be retained longer simply because the hospital's task includes protecting the community from such persons [18]. As a patient dangerous to others is very different from one who is only a threat to himself, each of these possibilities requires separate treatment.

Table 11-2. Length of Hospitalization Associated with Psychiatric Impairment, Dangerousness, and Professional Judgments

INDEPENDENT VARIABLE	LENGTH OF HOSPITALIZATION		
	Gamma	Level of Significance	N
Psychiatric Impairment (psychiatrist's assessment)	.44	**	62
Dangerousness Assaultive, Destructive, and Homicidal Tendencies	.10	NS	125
Suicidal Tendencies	− .32	*	125
Potential Dangerousness (psychiatrist's prediction)	.05	NS	59
Need of Hospitalization (psychiatrist's judgment)	.53	*	63

*** Indicates $p < .001$, ** indicates $p < .01$, * indicates $p < .05$, NS indicates $p > .05$

A patient's danger to others is measured here by whether he is assaultive, destructive, or homicidal. On the basis of behavior both during and before hospitalization, each patient is listed in the hospital records as either being or not being "assaultive," "destructive," or "homicidal." Reference to a patient's classification is taken from statements in the hospital records. Employing hospital records, despite their notorious reputation, is probably useful in assessing these patient characteristics. If a patient is not assaultive, destructive, or homicidal, it is unlikely he would be recorded as such. And if he had a history of this type of behavior, especially homicidal behavior, it is reasonable to assume that in most cases such information would be found in records. Yet, whether a patient is recorded as possessing none, one, two, or all three of these behavior patterns is essentially unrelated to the length of his hospitalization as shown in Table 11-2. There is only a slight tendency for patients threatening to others to remain longer. These findings are somewhat surprising in the face of consistent claims by psychiatrists that release depends relatively heavily on the patient's dangerousness [29].

Suicidal behavior is the form of dangerousness-to-self that is often given as a reason for initial hospitalization and continued hospitalization. Thus, suicidal patients are examined to see if they remain hospitalized longer. A patient is considered to be suicidal if registered as such in the hospital records. The hospital staff is motivated to keep somewhat accurate records of this due to the possibilities and consequences of a patient actually commiting suicide while at the hospital. Yet, despite the numerous times that suicidal tendencies are given by psychiatrists as reasons for denying release, patients listed in the records as suicidal leave significantly earlier, as shown in Table 11-2. As might be expected, suicidal patients exit sooner as a group because they tend to be concentrated in those diagnostic categories (the neuroses and transient situational disturbances) with shorter average hospitalization. The negative relationship between suicidal behavior and length of hospitalization disappears within diagnostic groups. Yet, even within diagnostic groups, the suicidal patient tends to remain no longer than the nonsuicidal patient. Danger to self, measured in this manner, does not appear as a factor helping explain why some patients exit sooner than others.

As an additional measure of dangerousness, each patient's psychiatrist was asked: Is this patient potentially harmful to himself or others? Five response categories were supplied ranging from "definitely yes" to "definitely no." This question is concerned not only with the patient's past behavior, as were the other measures of dangerousness, but also with future behavior. What the patient will do is possibly more important in the decision to release than are his past actions. Yet even with this further consideration, length of hospitalization is not found to be associated with whether the psychiatrist views the patient as harmful. Thus, dangerousness of the patient, whether measured in terms of past behavior or a professional prediction of future behavior, is not associated with the timing of the patient's release.

According to the medical model as described by Goffman [10], the psychiatrist is the expert who makes treatment-related decisions such as when to release a patient. The psychiatrist uses much more information in his recommendation about discharge than simply the patient's psychiatric impairment and dangerous tendencies. He judges the totality of the relevant information, evaluating the meanings of various patterns of signs and symptoms. Thus each patient's psychiatrist was asked to make a global assessment of how much their patient was in need of further hospitalization, and they were given five ordered-response categories. This question allowed the therapist to assess both considerations of psychopathology and dangerousness. Furthermore, it allowed him to incorporate in his judgment such diverse factors as availability of a placement in the community and ability of the hospital to care for or help the patient. And, as would be expected, those patients seen as most in need of further hospitalization remain hospitalized longer (see Table 11-2). Yet this relationship is much weaker than that between length of hospitalization and family desires.

Family desires are thus more strongly associated with length of hospitalization than are measures of dangerousness or professional judgment used here. Family wishes may be only spuriously related to length of hospitalization. The family may desire further hospitalization ony because the patient's psychiatrist has recommended it and the patient may remain because of the psychiatrist's decision. Therefore the family desires and length of hospitalization relationship is examined controlling for the above indicators of dangerousness and professional judgments. As shown in Table 11-3, in no case does the control variable appear to account for any substantial part of the relationship. None of the partial Gammas differ significantly at the .05 level

Table 11-3. Length of Hospitalization and Family Desires Relationship Controlled by Psychiatric Impairment, Dangerousness, and Professional Judgments

	LENGTH OF HOSPITALIZATION AND FAMILY DESIRES	
	Gamma	*N*
Zero Order Relationship	.78	80
Control Variables	Partial	
	Gammas	N
Psychiatric Impairment		
(psychiatrist's assessment)	.74	42
Dangerousness		
Assaultive, Destructive and Homicidal Tendencies	.76	80
Suicidal Tendencies	.85	80
Potential Dangerousness		
(psychiatrist's prediction)	.60	40
Need of Hospitalization		
(psychiatrist's judgment)	.87	42

from the zero order Gamma. Thus despite the influence of dangerousness and psychiatrist's evaluations, family desires appear to have a strong impact on the timing of the patient's exit.

Exploring Explanatory Hypotheses

None of the findings presented so far suggest a clear mechanism or "causal" process by which family desires may influence the timing of release. Although the data are limited, several possibilities are examined here.

Family influence, although appearing strong, may be of little practical significance if the influence on release occurs for patients neither extremely pathological nor impairment-free. A large number of patients may obviously not require or desperately need hospitalization, and more discretionary psychiatric decisions concerning release or retention of these patients may be "tipped" by an expression of family desires. In this situation, family desires may be highly related to release timing, even controlling for psychiatric impairment, but the degree of family influence may be more apparent than real. To examine this possibility, release timing and family desires are examined among two groups: (1) patients psychiatrically rated as severely ill and whose families wanted release, and (2) patients assessed as having little pathology but whose families wanted extended hospitalization. Although only six such cases occur in this sample, the tendency even among these extreme cases is for the family influence to be more important than the psychiatric condition (Gamma = ±.20, NS, N = 6).

A second possibility is that positive family attitudes toward release may aid recovery and this leads to earlier release. To examine this proposition, a measure of relative patient improvement was devised by comparing the psychiatrist's original impairment estimate with one he made three weeks later. The psychiatrist's second estimate of impairment is subtracted from his first estimate (the response categories being numbered one to six). The resulting "improvement" score, ranging from -5 to $+5$, is used with the original impairment estimate employed as a control variable in each instance reported. This is done because the more impaired a patient was initially, the more he could and the more likely he did improve according to this measure. There is no relationship between family desires and patient improvement measured in this manner. From the families' point of view, patients reported as "better now" than when they were hospitalized are only slightly more likely to be wanted home (Gamma $= 11$, NS, $N = 47$). No evidence could be found suggesting that family attitudes accelerate release by speeding recovery.

A third explanation is suggested by results showing that a family may be able to have release occur in the face of opposition by the psychiatrist. The desires of the psychiatrist for release or retention are themselves strongly associated with length of hospitalization (Gamma $= +.58$, $p < .001$, $N = 79$). In those cases in which the psychiatrists' desires are opposite the wishes of the family, the timing of the patient's exit most closely corresponds to the family's desires (Gamma $= +.81$, $p < .01$, $N = 9$). When the family wants the patient to remain but the psychiatrist wishes the patient discharged, in three cases the patient remains beyond the Modal Group and in only one case does he leave before it. But when the family wants the patient discharged and the psychiatrist wishes the patient to remain, two patients leave before the Modal Group and none after it. The family's ability in these cases to secure the patient's release or retention when the patient's psychiatrist wishes otherwise suggests a direct influence explanation in which powerful family influences are not able to be resisted by the psychiatrist.

Families may be able to pressure a psychiatrist into granting a release or keeping a patient. To explore this possibility, psychiatrists placed each patient's family into one of four ordered categories through a series of four questions. The first category are those families whose patient's psychiatrist did not even know whether the family wished release or retention of the patient. Second category families are those whose desires were known to the psychiatrist but who never confronted the psychiatrist with these desires. Third are those families who went out of their way to explicitly tell the psychiatrist what they wanted. In the fourth category are those families who made the psychiatrist feel "pushed" by the family to decide in favor of release or retention. This variable is not associated with how long a patient remains hospitalized, (Gamma = +.01, NS, N = 33) and, more importantly, patients are not significantly more likely to leave in one of the more extreme exit groups when the psychiatrist feels the family is more aggressively "pushing" for release or retention (Gamma = +.11, NS, N = 33). Thus family desires are probably not associated with length of hospitalization simply because some families actively use what power and influence they have to effect a decision to their liking.

In summary, the major finding from this New England study is that the desires of mental patients' families are strongly related to how long patients remain hospitalized. The relationship is not spurious due to other variables traditionally thought to influence the release decision, such as psychiatric impairment, dangerousness, or clinical judgments concerning need for hospitalization. Neither is the relationship due to differential patient improvement or overt pressure placed on the psychiatrist by the family. Before discussing other possible mechanisms linking family desires and length of hospitalization, subsequent studies of this relationship are briefly reviewed.

OTHER STUDIES OF FAMILY DESIRES AND LENGTH OF HOSPITALIZATION

Since the original New England research reported here, several other studies have examined the importance of family desires and length of hospitalization. In each study, family desires have appeared as an important predictor of the timing of release.

The Texas Study

In the Texas Study, researchers attempted to predict which patients would be released from Texas state mental hospitals [22]. In 1966, a random sample of 1537 patients were surveyed in detail through psychological testing, independent physical and psychiatric examinations, laboratory tests, social work interviews, record reviews, and questionnaires completed by relatives. In 1971, these patients were resurveyed to determine their psychiatric treatment history.

The purpose of the study was to discover variables which discriminated between "chronic" patients—defined as those who were continuously hospitalized during the five-year follow-up period—and "nonchronic" patients—defined as those who had been released during the follow-up period and never readmitted. Patients who died were readmitted, or were resident in another institution, such as a nursing home, were omitted from the analyses.

Sufficient data were available to allow comparison of 393 "chronic" patients with 170 "nonchronic" patients.

Relatives' attitudes toward release were measured on a four point scale from "unqualified positive" to "unqualified negative." Table 11-4 shows that relatives' attitudes were strongly related to release (Gamma = .63, N = 563) [22].

The discriminant analysis revealed only one variable—length of hospitalization at the time of the 1966 survey—to be a better discriminator between the "chronics" and the "nonchronics" than relatives' attitudes. In addition to these two variables, a "conceptual disorganization" measure and a social adequacy scale both significantly improved the discriminant prediction. Unfortunately, the discriminant analysis measure does not allow examination of possible spuriousness between relatives' attitudes and continued hospitalization due to, for instance, level of psychiatric impairment. The results show, however, that relatives' attitudes were an extremely strong predictor of release over a five-year period.

The New York Studies

Investigations in the New York studies report findings on a special group of 239 male New York state mental hospital patients who had been transferred in the mid-1960s to civil mental hospitals from hospitals for the criminally insane [26]. Patients who were released from the civil state mental hospital (N = 116) were compared to patients who were never released (N = 123) with regard to expressed family interest in the patient's release. Hospital records were used to classify patients into three groups according to family support: (1) those who had friends or relatives in the community who expressed an interest in the patient's release by their willingness to sponsor them for home visits or home care; (2) those who lacked sponsors but who had some extra hospital contact through letters, telephone calls, or visits; and (3) those who had no contact with individuals in the community.

Table 11-5 shows a strong relationship between release and the family's expressed interest in the patient's release as measured in this study (Gamma = +.67, p < .001, N = 239). The authors conclude, "as documented in previous studies of non-criminal civil mental patients, the presence of interested families and friends in the community was found to be the most important factor in release." [26]

This study is limited in that it does not include multivariate statistical tests for spuriousness of "causal" mechanisms, and it includes no measures of dangerousness or psychiatric impairment. Also, while the patients may have been previously confined to hospitals for the criminally insane, officials of these

Table 11-4. Relatives' Attitudes and Release [22]

RELATIVES' ATTITUDE TOWARDS RELEASE	CONTINUOUSLY HOSPITALIZED FOR FIVE YEARS		RELEASED WITHIN FIVE YEARS AND NOT REHOSPITALIZED	
	%	(N)	%	(N)
Unqualified Positive	8	(31)	45	(76)
Qualified Positive	19	(77)	25	(42)
Qualified Negative	47	(184)	21	(36)
Unqualified Negative	26	(101)	9	(16)
Totals	100	(393)	100	(170)

F for the difference between group means equals 98.42, $p < .001$

hospitals had decided they were appropriate for transfer to a civil hospital, suggesting that they were unusual in some respect, such as having particularly good prognoses or having exhibited little violent or otherwise dangerous behavior in the past.

A second, more extensive study of New York state mental hospital patients overcomes almost all of these possible limitations. In this study, patterns of release from civil mental hospitals of a group of male patients transferred from institutions for the criminally insane because of a court ruling were examined [27]. These patients, known as the "Baxstrom" patients following the legal case of this name, were transferred as a group to the civil mental hospitals by the New York State authorities as a means of complying with the court's decision. As such, they were not transferred because they were psychiatrically select or had unusual criminal histories. The authors were particularly interested in whether release would be influenced by the histories of violent criminal behavior, possessed by many of these men.

Table 11-5. Family Expressed Interest in Discharge and Release of "Criminally Insane" Patients from New York State Mental Hospitals [26: Table 4]

RELEASE STATUS	EXPRESSED FAMILY INTEREST IN THE PATIENT'S RELEASE					
	None		Letters, Calls, and Visits		Sponsors	
	%	(N)	%	(N)	%	(N)
Never Released	71	(81)	59	(26)	20	(16)
Released	29	(33)	41	(18)	80	(65)
Total	100	(114)	100	(44)	100	(81)

Chi-square = 48.83, df = 2, $p < .001$

No substantial or statistically significant relationship was found between release and any of five measures of a patient's dangerousness, including commission of violent crimes and assaultiveness while in the hospital (but not including suicidal tendencies). They did find that release was significantly less likely if the patient was evaluated as more psychiatrically impaired, less improved psychiatrically while in the criminal hospital, or diagnosed as a catatonic schizophrenic. Thus mental condition was related to the probability of release.

Civil hospital record data were gathered for each patient on whether a family member had expressed any interest in the patient, particularly with regard to any expressed desire to have the patient released. Patients whose families expressed such an interest in them were significantly more likely to have been released (Gamma = .83, N = 174). See Table 11-6.

Multivariate analysis of family-expressed interest was significantly associated with release, controlling for psychiatric impairment and other measures of mental condition. Furthermore, family-expressed interest was the most important predictor of release in this study.

In summary, all the known studies find family desires to be a strong predictor of the timing of release. While the studies are limited to state mental hospital patients, the findings are consistent across several states and, in the case of the criminally insane, in a population of patients in which considerations of violence might be expected to be a particularly important issue in release decisions. Multivariate analyses do not find the association between release and family desires to be spurious due to dangerousness or psychiatric condition.

FAMILY INVOLVEMENT IN THE HOSPITALIZATION

Clinicians, administrators, and others are often concerned with involving the patient's family in the hospitalization process. Family involvement in the patient's hospitalization has been seen as a means of reducing chronicity [19], facilitating effective treatment, and bridging the gap between the hospital and the community. Data from the New England study will be presented here which examine the relationship among family involvement, family desires for the patient's release, and length of hospitalization.

The New England state mental hospital study, as noted above, only involved a very occasional patient in any form of family therapy. Attempts at involving families were usually limited to gathering intake and background information from the patient's relatives or making some minimal discharge plans, often done by a social worker over the telephone. Thus, most contacts between the family and the psychiatrist or other hospital staff were initiated by the family, as were family visits of the patient at the hospital.

In terms of the amount of family involvement, at one extreme are the patients who have no family. Similar to these cases are those in which a family

Table 11-6. Release by Expressed Family Interest in the Patient [27: Table 7.6]

RELEASE STATUS	NO FAMILY INTEREST EXPRESSED		EXPRESSED FAMILY INTEREST	
	%	(N)	%	(N)
Never Released	57	(73)	11	(5)
Released	43	(56)	89	(40)
Totals	100	(129)	100	(45)

Chi-square = 27.90, df = 1, $p < .001$

exists but is essentially inactive, neither visiting the patient nor in any way contacting the hospital staff. Next in terms of increasing amount of involvement are families who merely visit their hospitalized relatives. These cases are followed by those in which the families contact the hospital staff, even though they do not visit the patient. The most active category of patients' families are those who both visit the patient and contact the hospital staff.

Patients with no families do not leave the hospital either significantly earlier or later than patients with families. The pattern of exits of patients with families who do not become actively involved in the hospitalization is similar to the distribution of exits for patients with no families. These two groups in turn differ from patients who do have families actively involved in that those with more active families tend to fall into the more extreme exit categories. Patients in the Rapid Exit Group, as defined above, are somewhat more likely to have involved families than patients in the Modal Stay Group (Gamma = .26, p < .04, one-tailed, N = 66). At the same time, patients in the Long Stay Group also tend to have more involved families than patients in the Modal Stay Group (Gamma = .13, p < .19, one-tailed, N = 75). In sum, there is a slight curvilinear relationship with patients with more involved families tending to cluster in the shortest *and* longest length of hospitalization categories. This relationship is explored by examining family involvement separately among: (1) patients who leave before the modal period, and (2) patients who are released after the modal period.

Patients Who Exit Before the Modal Period

As noted, patients who leave before the modal period are more likely to have involved families than those who leave during the modal period. This is true whether one uses family visits to the patient or family contacts with the patient's psychiatrist as the measure of involvement. As also has been seen, family wishes for an early release are positively associated with a shorter length of hospitalization.

Examination of family desires and involvement during the first weeks of hospitalization shows that, regardless of the measure of family involvement, the sooner the family wants the patient out of the hospital, the more involvement the family has (for similar findings see [3,27]). Only 35 percent of the families who want their relatives to remain "indefinitely" visit the hospital at all during the first three weeks of hospitalization, while 77 percent of the remainder of the families visit the patient during this time at least once (see also Table 11-7). Similarly, the more the family wishes the patient's release, the more contact they have with the hospital staff.

The relationship between family involvement and the length of hospitalization is examined to see if what the family desires is "causing" the relationship. The relationship between family visiting and length of a patient's hospital residence is seen to fall sharply when family disposition desires are controlled (Zero-order Gamma = .256, and the partial Gamma = .038). Similarly, the relationship between family-staff contact and length of hospitalization essentially disappears when what the family wants is controlled (Zero-order Gamma = .236, and the partial Gamma = .027). The relationship between measures of family involvement in the early weeks of hospitalization and the length of time the patient remains an inpatient is the result of what the family desires.

The mechanisms producing such a pattern are suggested by the case of Mr. R, who felt that his thin blond wife should never have entered the hospital. He was told not to worry because she would have a review staffing at the end of three weeks. In this manner he realized that the hospital staff did not intend to discharge her in a few days. When Mr. R became aware of this, he escalated his involvement from visits to his wife to telephoning and visiting her psychiatrist in an attempt to secure her release. Because the hospital is organized—as was described above—such that the modal patient moves in, through, and out in about 30 days, if a family member desires his relative to leave the hospital earlier, he must take the initiative, contact the hospital staff, and make his views known.

The example suggests that families may contact the hospital staff because they perceive themselves disagreeing with the hospital staff. To tap this feeling families were asked, "Do you feel pushed?" It is clear that those who feel this way experienced more contact with the hospital staff as measured by the family-staff contact index (Gamma = .49, p < .05, N = 49). This examination of the relationship between family participation and feelings of being "pushed" shows that families who wish the patient to leave do, to some extent, contact the hospital staff when they feel in disagreement with them. Yet, regardless of what brings families to contact the hospital, when they want their members out, these families do take this step and their members exit earlier. This strongly reinforces the contention that the relationship between family involvement in the early weeks of hospitalization and the timing of release is due to what the family wants.

Table 11-7. Family Visits to Patients and Family Desires

NUMBER OF FAMILY VISITS IN THE FIRST THREE WEEKS OF HOSPITALIZATION	FAMILY DESIRES					
	Family wants the Patient to Leave Soon or Immediately N =		Family wants the Patient to Stay for a Certain Period N =		Family wants the Patient to Remain Indefinitely N =	
Family visited the hospital five or fewer times.	41%	(9)	90%	(19)	100%	(8)
Family visited the hospital six or more times.	59%	(13)	10%	(2)	0%	(0)
Total	100%		100%		100%	

Gamma = .410, $p <$ .01, N = 51*

*Gamma and probability computed with number of visits and family desires uncategorized, i.e., the table above is a collapsed form of the one on which computations were done.

Patients Who Exit After the Modal Period

The desires of families who become involved later in their member's hospitalization are examined here to see if their wishes account for why the longest hospitalizations are also associated with greater family involvement.** The interview data indicate that by the beginning of the Modal Exit period most, if not all, families who want the patient released have contacted the hospital staff (see Table 11-8). Few families who want their members to remain tell the staff what they wish during this early stage in the hospitalization. This strongly suggests, as do other observational data, that families who become involved later in the hospitalization desire their relatives to remain hospitalized.

After the initial three weeks, families who wish the patient retained become involved through a pattern which the following example may make clearer.

Mrs. E was the wife of a patient who, after several weeks of hospitalization, was led to believe he would be discharged within another week. As his wife did not wish his release, when she learned of his expectations she contacted her husband's psychiatrist to explain how difficult it would be to have him home and how much hope she had for his improvement with continued hospitalization. She was prompted to contact the hospital because the staff had intentions of discharging the patient before she wanted the discharge to occur. Mrs. E and

**While the previous discussion is based largely on material from interviews with families, information in this section comes mainly from cases followed personally, through contacts with psychiatrists and social workers, and through a review of hospital records. It deals with that time, the Modal Stay period and after, for which no interview data exist.

Table 11-8. Family Desires and Family Contact with the Hospital Staff
by the End of Three Weeks

	FAMILY DESIRES			
FAMILY CONTACT WITH THE HOSPITAL STAFF	*Family wants the Patient to Remain N =*		*Family wants the Patient Discharged N =*	
Family has not contacted the staff	81%	(33)	0%	(0)
Family has contacted the staff	19%	(8)	100%	(14)
Total	100%		100%	

Gamma = 1.0, *p* <.005, Fisher's Exact Test, N = 55

others like her probably do contact the hospital staff and visit the patient more often only when prompted by the appearance of an unwanted release plan.

Not until the period of review staffing, between 21 and 30 days after admission, are many families confronted by the hospital staff or patients with a possible undesired discharge. At admission, psychiatrists do not plan on having many patients leaving during these first weeks; psychiatrists estimate that 47 percent of the patients leave in the Modal Group while only 19 percent are expected to leave in the first two weeks. Not only do psychiatrists not have in mind discharging patients this soon, only 24 percent of families who have not contacted the psychiatrists in the first three weeks heard, through the patient or otherwise, of any disposition plan whatsoever. Thus, families not desiring release are rarely faced with an imminent discharge in the initial three weeks, and they rarely become involved.

Yet, when confronted with an unwanted discharge plan, families begin participating. For example, five families said they wanted the patient in the hospital, but, nevertheless, reported having talked with the patient's psychiatrist. One was a young male patient's family, whose LSD-disturbed son telephoned his separated mother after he had been in the hospital about one week and said, "I'll be home." As his mother said later, she was "used to following doctor's orders" and, therefore, had not been in touch at all with the hospital staff. Yet, after her son telephoned, she "called the doctor to check," telling him that she did not "want to rush the patient."

Another young male patient slashed his wrists in order to be transferred to the hospital from the jail he was in. Two days after arriving at the hospital, he obtained the psychiatrist's permission and began pressing his father to have him transferred to a private psychiatric hospital. This prompted his father to call the psychiatrist and request that his son be kept "there at least until evaluated."

In two additional cases, wives wanted to be rid of their husband-patients semipermanently. Neither wife contacted the hospital until the hospital made clear its plans to discharge, at which time they both telephoned the hospital staff.

The fifth patient had a criminal case against him stemming from the use of heroin. His wife, on the advice of his lawyer, wanted him to spend several months in the hospital for the "good of his case." Despite the patient's desire to remain in the hospital, she learned that the hospital wanted to "send him back to jail." Then she made an appointment to see his psychiatrist and told the psychiatrist that the patient "would commit suicide if sent back to jail." In none of these cases did the family initiate contact with the psychiatrist before learning of unwanted discharge planning. In every case the contact occurred shortly after the family member learned of an imminent release.

Where the family had not contacted the psychiatrist, 15 out of 19 families knew of no existent plan for the patient's release. Of the plans that were known, not all were for immediate release. It is highly unlikely that those families who contacted the psychiatrist did so independently of their knowledge of a release plan, as shown in Table 11-9. Thus, when the family wants the patient kept in the hospital, feelings of being "pushed" by the hospital staff probably account for much of the family's involvement in the hospitalization process.

Hospital Staff Reactions to Family Involvement

The New England state mental hospital described here is probably typical of many hospitals with an overworked staff and no family-oriented treatment philosophy resulting in systematic or aggressive attempts to involve families in treatment. In such hospitals, for understandable reasons, hospital staff may avoid initiating family contact and may resist family-oriented treatment efforts.

As the data presented above show, those families most likely to contact the hospital staff have definite desires about the timing of release. They are also likely to make these desires known in an attempt to influence release decisions. These then are the families that the staff of such a hospital sees and to which they react. One consequence is that the staff sees families that are to them complicating factors, and thus views family contacts as likely to harbor disruption to the normal flow of work and routines of treatment.

Not contacting a family may be a "rational" work-related coping behavior on the part of the hospital staff. If the staff wish a patient released rather early, they probably realize from experience that if the family has not become involved by the end of two weeks of hospitalization that the family most likely will resist release. Of those families who want the patient out, for instance, 87 percent have visited their relatives six or more times by this time. Thus, those families with whom the staff would most likely need to initiate contact are probably not going to favor release. Similarly, after the first few weeks of hospitalization, if the staff favors release, most likely contacting a family will reveal a family desiring a longer hospitalization.

Table 11-9. Family Knowledge of Release Plan and Family Contact with Psychiatrist
for Families Who Want the Patient to Remain

FAMILY KNOWLEDGE OF A RELEASE PLAN	FAMILY CONTACT WITH THE PSYCHIATRIST	
	Family Spoke to Psychiatrist	Family Did Not Speak to Psychiatrist
Family did not know of release plan	0	15
Family did know of release plan	5	4

Gamma = 1.00, $p < .005$, Fisher's Exact Test, N = 24

Contacting a family may, furthermore, result in the staff's discharge plan not being carried out, while noncontact may result more often in the plan's success. If the family is contacted about a decision before action is taken, the family may balk and undermine the decision. Thus, while it was informal hospital policy that social workers would contact families to discuss impending discharges, social workers would often tell the patient he was discharged and give him permission to call his family and have them pick him up. The effect of allowing the patient to "spring" a *fait accompli* discharge on the family is to make it extremely difficult for the family to refuse the patient. The potential, longer term, negative consequences of such activity are clear, as are the work pressures favoring their adoption.

A hospital staff in such a situation has little desire to seek out families and actively share information with them. The consequences are varied, including, no doubt, the staff's limited openness to family therapies and the families' often negative reactions to the staff's resultant appearance of defensiveness and withholding of information [6]. Because families selectively involve themselves, those families who would be the most responsive to the hospital staff are largely hidden from view. Perhaps aggressive attempts to integrate families in the treatment process would help counter possibly existing negative staff perceptions of families by bringing staff into contact with a wider and potentially more helpful and agreeable set of families.

Family Involvement and "Medical" and "Social Control" Models

From a medical perspective, the relatively more extreme the patient's pathology, the greater may be the family involvement. On the one hand, family-patient contact may be associated with lesser degrees of pathology because contact speeds the patient's recovery [3,7,19]. On the other hand, higher family-patient contact might be related to greater psychiatric problems if the contact perpetuated the social interaction that brought the patient to the hospital in the first place [4,18].

Yet, in the New England study, family visiting of patients is not significantly related to psychiatric improvement, as measured using the difference between the psychiatrist's ratings of the patient's psychiatric impairment at the first and second interviews (Gamma = $-.09$, N = 49). Other measures of family involvement are also not significantly related to this measure of improvement. Family involvement is not related to the patient's change either for the better or worse. This study provides no evidence that family involvement is related to length of hospitalization because it is associated with greater improvement or deterioration of the patient's condition.

With regard to social control explanations, measures of family involvement are not associated with indicators of past dangerous behavior or the psychiatrist's estimates of potential dangerousness. Thus the social control perspective is not helpful in explaining the relationship between length of hospitalization and family involvement.

DISCUSSION

The research reviewed here shows that the desires of mental patients' families are strongly related to how long patients remain hospitalized. Evidence is presented that this is not a spurious factor; other variables traditionally thought to influence release decisions are not determinant of both length of hospitalization and family desires. Neither is the relationship due to differential patient improvement or overt pressure placed on the psychiatrist by the family. Involvement of the family in the hospitalization is higher for families who have definite opinions concerning release and want to make their wishes known. Involvement of the family is related to release timing because of its link to family desires and not because involvement promotes or hinders recovery or because involvement is related to psychiatric impairment or dangerousness. Unfortunately, the evidence from these studies does not adequately suggest a mechanism by which family desires and length of hospitalization are linked.

Informal observations of family-psychiatrist interaction do indicate that family desires may be closely related to the timing of discharge because psychiatrists consider family wishes very seriously when making release decisions. There are several possible reasons why psychiatrists in this inpatient setting may be influenced by the families' preferences. First, the psychiatrist is much more likely to successfully place the patient in the home if the family supports his return. The family who wants the patient released is likely to be supportive and to help the patient reintegrate into the community; the reluctant family may undermine the plans of the psychiatrist, exacerbate the patient's symptoms, and drive the patient back to the hospital. Rational planning of treatment decisions, such as discharge, may demand seriously taking into account the desires of the family.

A psychiatrist in court expressed this view when assessing whether Johnnie Baxstrom, the central figure in the "Baxstrom" case, should be detained in a civil hospital:

I think one of the outstanding things about him that I noticed in the record is that he has a person who is interested in him and who has maintained contact with him for many years, and has been a tremendous support to him, sent him money and written him regularly and has offered her home to him. This is his sister in Baltimore, who . . . is willing to make a home for him. It seems to me that the record does show that he's got this stable force in the community to go to, and I sincerely believe that this would be a good way to start his rehabilitative return to the community. [27]

Despite these views of psychiatrists and other mental health professionals, there is little or no evidence suggesting that patients whose families want them home are less likely to relapse or be rehospitalized. Steadman and Cocozza did not find that expressed family interest in release was related to whether the "Baxstrom" patients released from civil hospitals were rehospitalized within six months of release [27]. A four-year follow-up of the released New England study patients found that patients with family members who originally did not want the patient to return home were rehospitalized significantly earlier on the average and tended to experience more readmissions during the follow-up period [12]. However, these relationships appeared spurious when statistically controlled for other family attitudes. Nevertheless, psychiatrists working with the New England study patients may sense from experience that families' positive attitudes toward release are good indicators of family situations beneficial to rehabilitation. Clearly, more research would be welcome in this area.

Second, and possibly more important, the psychiatrist may follow the wishes of the family to avoid a range of possible family actions. At one extreme, the family may use the judicial system in seeking release or further retention. The psychiatrist may wish to avoid a hearing or other courtroom processes because they have a damaging impact on the patient, or consume a considerable amount of his time and effort. The therapist may prefer to discharge the patient "Against Medical Advice" or to hold a patient while seeking a nonfamily placement in the community. Families may also place psychiatrists in awkward positions by taking their questions and demands to unit chiefs, department heads, or superintendents of the institution involved. Institutional leaders both expect and easily tolerate a few such complaints. Yet, if such complaints multiply beyond a scattered few, these leaders may come to question not the assertive families, but the accused psychiatrists. This may give a family considerable leverage of which even it is unaware. Most commonly, a family's persistent questions and demands constitute a significant nuisance to the psychiatrist himself. In the state hospital study the work load was so heavy that a moderately interested and aggressive family could cause a substantial and disruptive drain on the psychiatrist's available time and energy. Under the pressure of too many patients, the psychiatrist appears to welcome the family which wishes to remove the patient from the hospital and the responsibility for him from the psychiatrist. On the other hand, if the family resists the patient's return, the over-worked psychiatrist often redirects his limited energies toward patients whose return to the community seems more likely, thus continuing the hospitalization of the unwanted patient. Finally, the psychiatrist may seek to please the family because he feels it to be as much his client as is the patient himself. The family is often the complainant, the patient often only its symptom.

In general, psychiatrists may follow family wishes as a means to cope with the exigencies of their jobs. Their response to family desires may be one means of stretching limited resources into maximum patient care. It may also signify that psychiatric hospitals give high priority to avoiding complaints from its nonpatient community. Unfortunately, a mental hospital which simply avoids stirring waves of public protest is often seen as adequate. In order to best serve and protect the institution, himself, and his patients, the psychiatrist may bow to the wishes of the patients' families. This view does not assume that families in any sense make decisions. The psychiatrist decides when the patient will leave, often without the active participation of the family. Nevertheless, family desires may be even larger determinants of length of hospitalization than the psychiatrists' own preferences. Investigations are needed to determine if this is in fact the link between family desires and length of hospitalization.

These findings suggest than an exploration of the origins of family desires would be useful. The above results do indicate family desires may be less dependent on the patient's psychopathology or potential dangerousness than on other factors. Our interviews with family members reveal that family wishes are typically based on factors beyond the knowledge and even interest of the hospital staff. Relatively few families have their relative's health as the primary concern. They may want the patient retained or released for a wide variety of reasons including: availability of housing; plans to move to a new home or state; the timing of a vacation; the loss or gain of income from job, welfare agency, disability payments, or relatives; the need for help with child care; fear of being attacked; pressure on the part of municipal authorities; consequences for a coming court appearance; loneliness; guilt; shame; past experiences with mental hospitals; and a death in the family. Because family desires appear important in release timing, it would be useful to empirically explore those factors leading to various family attitudes toward release. At the same time, further assessment is needed of the impact of other variables such as social class, marital status, and race.

Whatever the determinants of family wishes concerning release, the therapist needs to be aware of their potential impact on his desires and the eventual outcome. For rational therapy decisions to be made, such as when to discharge a patient, the crucial role of family preferences needs to be made overt. Unseen and unrecognized pressures often are largely unmanageable, having consequences, benign or not, which cannot be sought or avoided. Making them conscious factors may facilitate their manipulation through treatment strategies, such as how to approach a family. Thus psychiatrists may benefit from a fuller consciousness of the nature and extent of the impact of patients' families on their decisions.

REFERENCES

1. Barry, John R. and Fulkerson, Samuel C. "Chronicity and the prediction of duration and outcome of hospitalization from capacity measures." *Psychiatric Quarterly* 40 : 104–121, January 1966.
2. Brim, Orville G. and Wheeler, Stanton. *Socialization After Childhood: Two Essays*. New York: John Wiley, 1967.
3. Brown, George. "Social factors influencing the length of hospital stay of schizophrenic patients." *British Medical Journal* 2 : 1300–1302, December 1959.
4. Brown, G.W.; Birley, J.L.T.; and Wing, J.K. "Influences of family life on the course of schizophrenic disorders: A replication." *British Journal of Psychiatry* 121 : 241–258, 1972.
5. Bullard, Jr., Dexter and Hoffman, Barbara R. "Factors influencing the discharge of chronic schizophrenia patients." In: *Research Conference on Therapeutic Community, Manhattan State Hospital, Wards Island, New York, 1959*. Springfield, Illinois, Charles C Thomas, 1960, pp. 215–228.
6. Deasy, L.C. and Quinn, O.W. "The wife of the mental patient and the hospital psychiatrist." *Journal of Social Issues* 9 : 49–60, 1955.
7. Dunham, H.W. and Weinberg, S.K. *The Culture of the State Mental Hospital*. Detroit: Wayne State University Press, 1960.
8. Ellsworth, Robert B. and Clayton, William H. "Measurement of improvement in 'mental illness.'" *Journal of Consulting Psychology* 23 : 15–20, February 1959.
9. Freeman, Howard E. and Simmons, Ozzie G. *The Mental Patient Comes Home*. New York: John Wiley, 1963.
10. Goffman, Erving. *Asylums: Essays on The Social Situation of Mental Patients and Other Inmates*. Garden City, New York: Anchor Books, 1961.
11. Greenley, J.R. "The psychiatric patient's family and length of hospitalization." *Journal of Health and Social Behavior* 13 : 25–37, March 1972.
12. Greenley, J.R. "Family symptom tolerance and rehospitalization experiences of psychiatric patients." In: Roberta G. Simmons (ed.) *Research in Community and Mental Health*, Vol. I. Greenwich, Connecticut: JAI Press, 1979, pp. 357–386.
13. Hollingshead, A.B. and Redlich, F.C. *Social Class and Mental Illness*. New York: John Wiley, 1958.
14. Jacobson, Shirley and Klerman, G.L. "Interpersonal dynamics of hospitalized depressed patients' home visits." *Journal of Marriage and the Family* 28 : 94–102, February 1966.
15. Jan, Lee-Jan. "Influence of relatives on the length of hospital stay." *Social Work* 22 : 60–61, January 1977.

16. Kaplan, Stanley M. and Curtis, George C. "Reactions of medical patients to discharge or threat of discharge from a psychosomatic unit of a general hospital." In: M. Greenblatt, D. Levinson and G. Klerman (eds.) *Mental Patients in Transition*. Springfield, Illinois: Charles C Thomas, pp. 7–15.
17. Levinson, Daniel and Gallagher, Eugene. *Patienthood in the Mental Hospital — An Analysis of Role, Personality, and Social Structure*. Boston: Houghton-Mifflin, 1964.
18. Liefer, Ronald. *In the Name of Mental Health*. New York: Random House, 1969.
19. Marx, Arnold J and Ludwig, Arnold M. "Resurrection of the family of the chronic schizophrenic: clinical and ethical dilemmas." *American Journal of Psychotherapy* 23 : 37–52, January 1969.
20. Myers, J.K. and Roberts, B.H. *Family and Class Dynamics in Mental Illness*, New York: John Wiley, 1964.
21. Myers, J.K. and Bean, L. *A Decade Later: A Follow-up of Social Class and Mental Illness*. New York: John Wiley, 1968.
22. Pokorny, A.D.; Thornby, J.; Kaplan, H.B.; and Ball, D. "Prediction of chronicity in psychiatric patients." *Archives of General Psychiatry* 33 : 932–937, August 1976.
23. Sall, Joan; Vosburgh, William W.; and Silverman, Abby. "Psychiatric patients and extended visit: a survey of research findings." *Journal of Health and Human Behavior* 7 : 20–28, March 1966.
24. Scheff, Thomas. "Legitimate, transitional, and illegitimate mental patients in a midwestern state." *American Journal of Psychiatry* 120 : 267–269, September 1963.
25. Simmons, O.G.; Davis, J.A.; and Spenser, K. "Interpersonal strains in release from a mental hospital." *Social Problems* 26 : 21–28, July 1956.
26. Steadman, Henry J. and Cocozza, Joseph J. "The criminally insane patient: who gets out?" *Social Psychiatry* 8 : 230–238, 1973.
27. Steadman, H.J. and Cocozza, J.J. *Careers of the Criminally Insane: Excessive Social Control of Deviance*. Lexington Books: Lexington, Massachusetts, 1974.
28. Vaughn, C.E. and Leff, J.P. "The influence of family and social factors on the course of psychiatric illness: a comparison of schizophrenic and depressed neurotic patients." *British Journal of Psychiatry* 129 : 125–137, 1976.
29. Weinstein, Louis. "Real and ideal discharge criteria." *Mental Hospitals* 15 : 680–683, 1964.
30. Weiss, Peter; Macaulay, Jacqueline; and Pincus, Allen. "Geographic factors and the release of patients from state mental hospitals." *American Journal of Psychiatry* 123 : 408–412, October 1966.
31. Yarrow, Marion; Schwartz, Charlotte; Murphy, Harriet; and Deasy, Leila. "The psychological meaning of mental illness in the family." *Journal of Social Issues* 11(4) : 12–24, 1955.

PART III

Special Topics

12

Alternate Views of "Schizophrenia" and Their Consequences for Therapy

JAY HALEY

Since Bleuler created the term "schizophrenia" in 1911 there have been revolutionary changes in the ways human beings are described. Criteria for classifying people into groups have changed, and so have explanations of human motivation. We no longer think that the shape of the skull or the physique of the body determine fixed character types, just as we have discarded the idea that masturbation causes insanity and illness is a sin. The classification "schizophrenia" has also been touched by change in this century. The communication and social theories of the 1950s, and the experiments with hospital milieus, led to new ways of defining and thinking about this diagnosis. Yet the result of these changes has not been more consensus about the definition of "schizophrenia." Instead, new ideas and descriptions have just been added to old ones.

It is a curious fact that any idea that was ever held about "schizophrenia" still exists in a group somewhere. New ways of thinking about the malady do not cause past ideas to be discarded. Since there is little or no scientific evidence to support *any* theory of "schizophrenia," people define the term in ways that fit their purposes and social situation. However, choosing one definition rather than another can have serious consequences because the fates of human beings are involved; it is not merely a matter of academic interest. Besides the effect on the person classified "schizophrenic," there are at least four areas of major consequences of different definitions: (1) the field of therapy, (2) the hospital milieu, (3) the family, and (4) the focus of research. Different premises about the malady and its consequences are outlined, and the set of premises most conducive to therapy is suggested.

SCHIZOPHRENIA IS A DISEASE

According to this view, "schizophrenia" is a clearly defined class and one can rigorously state whether a person belongs to it or not. Schizophrenic people can be differentiated from other people, and the malady is permanent because a person in that category can never become normal. If normality occurs, the person was misdiagnosed. The cause is assumed to be organic with a genetic base.

This is the extreme physiological definition of the category. Those who hold this view tend to consider the definition so obvious that it need not be questioned.

Therapy

No form of conversational or social therapy will influence the malady since "schizophrenia" is synonymous with "incurable." The person will never be self-supporting or fully functioning so therapists need not attempt rehabilitation. Drugs will modify the person's behavior if correctly prescribed and used in massive-enough doses. Neurological damage from medication must be accepted because drugging the person is all that can be done. An analogous condition is cancer where dangerous drugs are used because the problem is hopeless.

Hospitals

With this definition, the hospital can only offer a humane environment and keep the person from troubling the community and burdening his family. Hospitalization is not a form of treatment since the disease is incurable; it is more a haven and a retreat. If the patient makes difficulties in the hospital, severe forms of restraints are permitted, such as isolation rooms, shock, or even lobotomy in occasional cases since the person is not like other people and does not respond to ordinary restrictions.

Family

The family of the patient has not caused the malady by any action and is therefore innocent. They cannot be held responsible for transmitting a hereditary defect, although they might feel guilty about it. The family must suffer the consequences of having such a member (and also be concerned that another member might manifest the hereditary taint). The State should relieve the family by putting the troublesome person in custody at the family's request, and by giving disability payments. If other family members behave strangely or conflictually, it could be expected as the result of dealing with a "schizophrenic."

Research

By virtue of the definition of the disease, research must be confined to biological and hereditary variables. Because of the severity of the disease, more extreme forms of research are tolerated than would be allowed on other human beings. It is considered acceptable to completely change the person's blood, do deep brain probes, or experiment with powerful medications which have unknown long-term consequences.

SCHIZOPHRENIA IS A LATENT DISEASE

This theory is similar to the one above but allows more flexibility for contradictory data. In fact it is formulated in such a way that it cannot be disproved. The disease exists but might not ever be manifest since it must be "triggered" in some way by the environment. Therefore there are "schizophrenics" who have never had, and might never have, any observable manifestations of this hereditary disease. It can be intermittent in an individual when it does appear, so that stress and the social situation are a factor in the malady. The diagnosis is more difficult since the individual could be seen before or after the disease has appeared, and so not be diagnosed correctly. It is also possible to confuse other emotional states with the disease, such as hysterical states or behavior induced by drugs. When in remission, the person might appear normal, and so no one would know that he is really a "schizophrenic."

Therapy

The consequences for therapy are serious since this premise has controversial implications. The disease is incurable, but a therapist can be fooled into thinking that social therapy had some influence because stress was relieved and the disease temporarily subsided. Therapists who hope to achieve a basic change, or who show evidence of such changes, are naive. They think they might rehabilitate such a person, and in an exceptional case that might occur because of a stressless environment, but generally they will inevitably be disappointed in their efforts.

Hospitals

With this definition, the hospital must be made available during times of the manifestation of the disease, but not at other times. Determining the disease process can be difficult, since hospitalization might in itself cause the stress that brings out "schizophrenia," and which causes it to persist. Restraint and medication are used, and discharge is offered when the staff believes the person is "ready" to live outside with the disease. A protected environment is preferred, and permanent medication is recommended since future episodes might be prevented. Even at the risk of permanent neurological damage, it is best to maintain the victim on large doses of drugs.

Family

This theory is less attractive to families since it can be argued that the family was the stress that "triggered" the disease. However, it can also be argued that they did not really cause the illness because it is genetic, and they have only done what other families have done with their children. This particular child, however, suffered the underlying pathology which was triggered by the stress of normal living. Therefore the family did not cause the problem and must suffer the consequences of living with such a person.

Research

Biochemical research continues in pursuit of the elusive cause, but this theory also suggests that the social situation should be examined. Problems in child development are considered and family studies are conducted to determine the stress situations that might bring out the disease.

SCHIZOPHRENIA IS A PSYCHOLOGICAL PHENOMENON

With the shift to a psychological view, the organic and genetic factors are abandoned as causative. However, it is a courtesy to mention in the opening paragraph of any article expressing this view that there are possible organic and genetic causes yet to be found. According to this theory, schizophrenia is a distortion of thinking, perception, and affect which originated in infancy and childhood. At the point a psychotic episode took place, the "ego was overwhelmed by the Id." The decompensation occurred because the person faced a situation which put him or her under stress, and the ego structure disintegrated because of its fragility.

Therapy

Therapy is a possibility but success is doubtful because of the deep psychopathology involved. The therapy is expected to be so long-term and "deep" that only patients from wealthy families can spend the years that it takes to explore the roots of the problem in childhood. Since the problem is in the nature of the individual, the family is not involved in therapy. Isolation from the family in a private hospital has been considered the treatment of choice.

Hospitals

Hospitals cannot "cause" the problem but might exacerbate it if they are not humane environments. The main function of a hospital is to isolate the person from the community while long-term therapy is undertaken. Corrective emotional experiences and psychosocial development can also be achieved by ward groups and the hospital milieu. Medication is used for behavior control on the wards, but drugs are not considered therapeutic since insight into the psychological roots is of more importance. Staff members who hold this view but work for state hospitals wish they had the time to do long-term individual therapy with their patients to relieve the deep psychological problems.

Family

This theory is not attractive to families because it implies the family caused the problem. However, since the cause resides in infantile experience, the family cannot now be blamed. The problem for the family is that they must defend themselves against an ambiguous charge of causing the problem when no one knows what it was they might have done in that infancy and childhood period. Therefore, the family not only must suffer the consequences of living with a mad member, but must also suffer blame for causing in some mysterious and unknown way this deep psychological problem. Typically the mother is blamed because of her importance in the childhood period. The term "schizophrenogenic mother" was created in the late 1940s by a psychoanalyst when the psychological theory of causation became popular [2].

Research

Psychological testing is considered a valuable research endeavor.

SCHIZOPHRENIA IS A SOCIAL PHENOMENON

The social theory argues that the bizarre behavior of a "schizophrenic" is an adaptive response to his *current* social situation; theories of organic defects or early childhood traumas are abandoned as undemonstrated, if not unprovable.

According to this view, "schizophrenia" is a peculiar type of behavior which is adaptive to the peculiar type of social situation in which the person is embedded. That situation includes family, hospital staff, and the relations between family and the professional community. This view differs sharply from previous theories. With the social view, the problem is no longer defined as medical. Therefore medicating the patient is no more reasonable than drugging a delinquent or a criminal insofar as it is merely a device of social control. Calling the person "sick" and putting him in the care of doctors and nurses is a mystification contributing to the malady since there is nothing physically wrong with the person. The emphasis on the social situation makes everyone who is involved relevant to the problem, whether they are the intimates in the family living group or the collective society which appears to need a number of deviants in order to remain stable.

Therapy

This is the most hopeful view for therapy. It is possible to have the person return to normal if the social situation can be changed. Since the behavior is considered appropriate and adaptive to a social context, that context must be altered so that the person's responses can change. The social context includes the family and the professionals appointed by the community to deal with the person. One of the difficulties for the therapist with this view is that professional colleagues with a different hypothesis about "schizophrenia" are part of the problem. Insofar as the therapist is also part of the professional community and the social context, he or she is attempting to change a group while being a member of it. For example, to attempt to rescue a person from colleagues can replicate the group process within the person's family in which some members of the family attempt to rescue the person from the others.

Hospital

The hospital is part of the social situation called "schizophrenia" and therefore a brief hospitalization is recommended. Another alternative has been to involve family and hospital in a joint endeavor to change the problem person and in that process change both hospital and family. The usual treatment in the hospital cannot solve the problem since the problem resides in the community of which the hospital is only one part.

Family

This view is the least acceptable to families because they are defined as part of the problem. There are two views of family causation in the field.

1. The "schizophrenia" of an offspring is adaptive behavior to a family which has been abnormal and pathological over the years. The patient is only an expression of the bizarre thinking and perception and "double-binding" that has always permeated this family. In later years, typically at the age of leaving home, the young person manifests in an extreme way the family tensions and conflicts. The family uses hospitals and medication to restrain the young person while continuing to associate with him or her in deviant ways. This hypothesis is one

which families most oppose since they are not only blamed as a current cause of the problem but have also caused it from the beginning.

2. An alternative view is that "schizophrenia" is a response to a malfunctioning stage of family life and not to a type of family that has always been pathological. That is, a family might be as normal as any other until the stage when the young people in the family begin to leave home. At that point, the family becomes unstable, the community enters with agents of social control, and the outcome is one person diagnosed as "schizophrenic." Once that happens, one member starts a career as a mental patient and the family begins a career of struggle with, and caring for, a defective member. When a therapist enters this system to bring about change, the family—and the hospital staff—can react against the instability produced by the changes and so be viewed as people benefiting from the malady and therefore accused of causing it.

Research

Research involves the investigation of families, hospital milieus, and other social groups. Contrasting types of families are placed in experimental situations to see how each differs from another. This is still a new form of research. Problems of methodology, sampling, and dealing with different stages of family life have yet to be resolved. The ideal research would be longitudinal studies that used film recording of family behavior over the years. Then it would be possible to see what the behavior was like in families where "schizophrenia" later occurred, rather than use family members' unreliable reconstructions of history.

SCHIZOPHRENIA AS MANY TYPES

This view argues that there is not one "schizophrenia" but many different types. Some types could have an organic cause, others a social cause; some are "reactive" and some are "process."

Although this view sounds broad minded, it leads to confusion rather than clarity. It is extremely difficult to get a consensus among diagnosticians whether a person is schizophrenic, far less which of several types he or she might be. There are no specific criteria for hypothetical types and so no evidence that different kinds exist. This view is actually only an expression of the idea that "there is probably more than one kind" as a way of trying to explain away conflicting data. Essentially, such a view merely says the problem is complex, which indeed it is, without clarifying how to resolve the complexity. Even the issue of whether there is a "chronic" type and an "acute" type cannot be resolved without considering the obvious possibility that a "chronic" is an "acute" who has suffered a series of treatment failures and professional mishandling.

ATTEMPTS AT COMPROMISE

In the field of light, a particle theory and a wave theory can exist side by side. However, differing theories of "schizophrenia" are not so benign. A person's life depends upon people who have different theories and who also have power. It is not a matter of research theoreticians jousting for supremacy; severe consequences to families and professionals result from actions based upon the theories.

The professionals who debate the problem tend to be honestly puzzled by the extreme behavior of a person called "schizophrenic." It is argued that there *must* be something organically wrong with someone who behaves in such bizarre and extreme ways and does so year after year. The fact that no evidence of any biological cause of the disorder has ever held up on examination has been considered a frustrating aspect of the problem of research, and not a demonstration of the fact that there is nothing physically wrong with the person. It seems unbelievable that people could act with each other in ways that could "cause" a person to be so strange.

The two most extreme positions in the field are the most clear: those theoreticians with a social view argue that there is no physiological or genetic evidence for the cause of the behavior, and people can drive each other mad. Theoreticians with the organic view argue that people do not have such influence on each other and there must be an as yet undiscovered physiological cause. In between are the range of professionals who look for a theory which has a partial organic explanation and a partial social explanation. Yet it seems doubtful that a compromise position can be found when the issue is therapy, not research. If one is setting out to change people, a theory based on the premise that they are unchangeable cannot be accepted.

Even if a therapist accepts the idea that the problem might be organic but the person is still capable of therapeutic change, his or her therapy begins to founder by that compromise. If the idea of an organic abnormality is allowed, then the goal of normality for the person cannot be set. The therapist is automatically caught in a situation where he or she is attempting to achieve the goal of helping a person be partially handicapped. If the social function of the "schizophrenic" is to have the role of a failure in order to stabilize his or her social milieu—which is one theory of social causation—then encouraging the person to be socially handicapped is cooperating in stabilizing an abnormal situation. This is not therapy.

Should the social therapist accept a partial organic explanation, it means that he or she must approve of colleagues' handling of organic problems. This includes powerful medications, hospitalization, dangerous research procedures, and even psychosurgery in extreme cases. The therapist finds himself or herself collaborating in a therapy where medication is used that causes neurological damage in as many as 40 percent of the cases [1]. This is not therapy.

Conversely, if the organic theoreticians accept the idea that there is a social cause and the problem is not physiological, then they are agreeing that the issue is not medical. Nonmedical people should be in charge, and hospitals and doctors are inappropriate caretakers.

To summarize, if it was possible to compromise, then people with different theories could share a common approach and there might be a possibility of comprehensive treatment. The chance of a biological cause could be taken into account while the social situation was also emphasized. Past experience with such attempts at compromise show problems that cause such collaboration to fail. Self-fulfilling prophecies occur when a professional has the view that a problem is incurable. In such an instance, relapses are inevitable, and medications must be used even if in themselves they cause psychotic behavior and neurological damage. A therapist who has the goal of helping people become normal simply cannot collaborate with someone who holds the pessimistic view of the organic theoretician. If one tries to hold organic and social theories, the result is the view that there is an organic cause which is "triggered" by the social situation.

AN AWKWARD COMPROMISE FOR THERAPISTS

At the moment, professionals in the field of "schizophrenia" are collaborating whether they wish to or not. Quite diverse views meet one another in the hospital arena, and it is the clients and their families who take the consequences. The problem is how to manage cooperation among the professionals so that the obvious goals are achieved: the protection of the community, and help for the person in distress. To achieve such cooperation it would seem best to find consensus on an approach that does the most good and the least harm.

It would seem possible to arrange a general approach to the problem of "schizophrenics" which could operate in stages. The initial stages would emphasize the most benign and hopeful approach, and the later stages would adopt the more pessimistic views if the hopeful approaches have failed. A brief outline of such stages is offered here. In essence, they would be based upon the hypotheses about "schizophrenia" which were proposed earlier, but in the reverse order. The social theory is given the first priority since it has the most hope and apparently does least harm. Granted that mishandling a family in therapy during a crisis can cause harm, one must still accept the premise that professionals are competent to select an approach. That is, one should not necessarily oppose the use of drugs because of the incompetence of many practitioners who use drugs.

Stage 1

When a person who might be called "schizophrenic" is brought to community attention because of a threat to harm himself or others, the first step would be to immediately involve his family and other intimates in a meeting to plan what should be done. The first goal would be to keep the person in the community and not extrude him into custody. Competent crisis treatment has led to estimates that as many as 90 percent of those persons who behave strangely enough to cause trouble can be kept out of custody [4].

Therapists

To implement this stage there should be therapists who are competent to deal with crises. It also helps to have therapists who are tolerant of the range of behavior called "normal." (For example, when a working-class navy corpsman replaced psychiatric residents on an emergency service, the rate of admission dropped in half. The corpsman was more familiar with family arguments, drinking, and drugs than the residents whose experience with life had been medical school.)

Hospitals

Hospitalization would be avoided. If removal from the family was absolutely necessary, it would involve a stay in a relative's home, in a boarding house, in a motel, or in a general hospital where there would be no stigma of mental illness. A brief respite in a normal situation prevents the person being handicapped by losing his job or time in school. If medication is used, it should only be part of a bargain to persuade the family to keep the person out of the hospital and in the community and would be used briefly.

Family

The family would be advised that they were the best therapists for the person and also that the person was their responsibility. That is, the family would be told that they could not use the State to restrain the member but must do it themselves. They would be assured that they can do it themselves with competent professional help.

In cases of a threat of violence, the family would be asked to involve relatives and neighbors to help restrain the person. If suicide was threatened, the family would be asked to maintain a suicide watch to protect him or her. Families have successfully followed these procedures. Hospitalizing the person typically leads to the State assuming more and more responsibility and the family less and less, as the person sets out on a career as a mental patient.

To carry out this stage, it is necessary to train therapists to specialize in the therapy of families in crisis. They would need to be available 24 hours a day through the crisis period. It would also be necessary to involve the family in a period of therapy to resolve whatever instability in the family was precipitating these crises. The therapists would need to have the view that the problem person was perfectly capable of returning to normal behavior if the social situation was corrected. The expectation would be that the person return to school or work as quickly as possible on the assumption that doing normal things leads to normal behavior when the social situation is being changed, so that abnormal behavior is not necessary.

This general approach is applicable not only to people called "schizophrenic" but also to depressives, drug addicts, and other deviant people who are ordinarily placed in custody. A retarded person with occasional episodes of violence who is behaving under his abilities can also benefit from a family approach where behavior as near normal as possible is expected.

Stage 2

The operations of Stage 1 would be repeated. It is a common observation that often when a family meets a crisis and that crisis passes, there is one more crisis the family must handle before stability is achieved. For example, when a young person starts to leave home there is often an episode of bizarre behavior. As that problem passes and the young person starts to leave home again, another episode occurs in a less severe form. If the family is helped to survive the disengagement, the problem no longer continues. The family has gotten past a difficult stage of family life.

Stage 3

If social therapy has been attempted and the problem recurs a third time, the family is taking a step toward chronicity which requires a less hopeful approach. Possibly the therapists dealing with the problem failed to change the social situation. Possibly a more psychological or organic explanation should be sought. The first choice should always be the most hopeful one. In this case, the premise should be that the family was using outside experts as a way of stabilizing a problem cycle. Assuming that view, the two extreme approaches seem untenable: To refuse help is not possible since the community must be protected; to take the person away from the family is not helpful since the family continues to let the experts take charge of their problem person for still longer hospital stays.

There is a third approach. The person can be hospitalized, but the family is required to cooperate in the hospital program. The family must meet to decide about hospitalization, attend regular therapy interviews during the brief hospital stay, and have therapy interviews to plan discharge. That is, the family and the problem person are not allowed to separate. This is a practical approach which has been used [3]. Ideally, the family members should be asked to staff the hospital ward, run groups, do recreational therapy with all the patients, and generally participate in their offspring's custody program.

After discharge, the therapist who began with the family in the hospital should continue with them into outpatient care so that there is continuity. This approach minimizes taking the person out of the family into the hands of experts by mingling experts and family in a joint endeavor.

Stage 4

There are always cases that fail. At the point where previous competent therapy has failed again and again so that the problem person is back in custody, a revision of the hypothesis about that particular person would seem to be in order. It might be that therapists have not done a competent job, or that the State is paying the person to be disabled, or that everyone involved is caught in a cycle. Whatever the cause of the failure, the task is to provide the maximum help with the least harm. An expectation of the person living as a handicapped person will begin to develop among the people involved and must be considered. This could include a sheltered living situation, close supervision, and special care. Medication which risks physical damage should not be used. The hypothesis of possible organic damage does not give a professional the right to risk further damage with drugs.*

SUMMARY

This review of the different hypotheses in the treatment of "schizophrenia" suggests that markedly different views lead to extremely different consequences

---

* It seems evident that the anti-psychotic medications will be outlawed because of the damage they are causing. The problem for many psychiatrists when that day comes is that they will not be trained in how to do anything except medicate. The parallel between the defense of brain damage caused by anti-psychotic drugs and the defense of lobotomy was drawn by Cloe Madanes during a panel discussion protesting the use of damaging medications in the treatment of people defined as schizophrenic. The other panel members were Carol Anderson, Nancy Atwood, C. Christian Beels, William Carpenter, and Moderator William R. McFarlane. The meeting was called "Schizophrenia — New Approaches to the Family" and was sponsored by the College of Physicians and Surgeons of Columbia University on April 2 and 3, 1981.

for the person and his or her family. There is no solid research evidence to support any particular hypothesis about the cause of this malady. Therefore, the aim of professionals should be to choose hypotheses which lead to the most hope of change and to the least harm. The social theories of causation are the most hopeful; the organic and genetic theories are the most handicapping. Therefore, it seems logical to approach therapy in stages: the first stage should be a social approach, and only after all else has failed should the organic and genetic hypotheses be allowed to determine the destiny of individuals.

REFERENCES

1. Chouinard G.; Annabel, L.; Ross-Chouinard, A.; et al. "Factors related to tardive dyskinesia," *American Journal of Psychiatry* 136 : 79–83, 1979.
2. Fromm-Reichmann, F. *Principles of Intensive Psychotherapy.* Chicago: University of Chicago Press, 1953.
3. Harbin, H.T. "A family oriented psychiatric inpatient unit," *Family Process* 18 : 281–291, 1979.
4. Langsley, D. and Kaplan, D. *The Treatment of Families in Crises.* New York: Grune and Stratton, 1968.

13

The Family in the Hospital: Experiences in Other Countries

JOHN ELDERKIN BELL

This chapter aims to describe the first comprehensive study of a mode of hospitalization found in two-thirds of the world's countries. In these countries it is usual for relatives to accompany patients full-time during the course of hospitalization. It concludes with a description of some derivative applications of the principles and practices discovered in a broad survey of hospitals in developing countries.

The first part of this chapter presents findings and conclusions from an extensive NIMH study of family participation in hospitals in Africa and Asia, conducted by the author and Elisabeth A. Bell, child psychologist. The study includes detailed descriptions of many hospitals and other medical and psychiatric facilities. The full report is presented in Bell [1].

Commonly, mental hospitals work toward two almost mutually exclusive ends: the rehabilitation of the patient, which is the desired goal; and his or her adaptation and integration within the hospital community, which too often results in the tragic concomitant of institutionalization. While institutionalization has been avoided for many patients in our most progressive mental hospitals and in the community programs that emphasize alternatives to hospitalization, there continue to be patients who have become isolated from home, work, and community, so that they are unable to live effectively outside an institutional setting.

In general and specialized hospitals for the treatment of "physical" illnesses, the relations of patients, families, and medical staffs cannot be simply characterized. At one extreme are hospitals or programs within hospitals where the patient is regarded as the only consumer and the strengths that are in families are ignored, so family members are virtually eliminated from partnership in the care of the patient. At the other extreme are those hospitals that welcome families as primary and full participants in the total care of the patient. In general, it may be said that the attitude toward the family as colleagues with patients and staffs has become increasingly positive in the past 20 years in the United States. Nevertheless, there is still enough dissatisfaction among families to create public relations problems for hospitals, even to the point of initiating malpractice suits.

My own involvement with hospital-family relations began about 1960 in efforts to develop family group therapy with hospitalized mental patients and their families. The family treatment approaches that were proving so effective in outpatient practice were not generally succeeding with patients in mental hospitals, especially among those hospitalized for more than a very brief period. Even rehabilitation of discharged patients in their homes was not generally succeeding if the duration of hospitalization exceeded about three months [10].

AN INTERNATIONAL STUDY

At my initiative, in February 1963, the National Institute of Mental Health began a formal program oriented toward several major goals:

1. To deepen understanding of the nature of family-hospital relations;
2. To learn the principles and practices that appear to facilitate and impede family participation in the hospital community;
3. To evaluate the effects of deliberate professional interventions into family-patient-hospital interactions;
4. To improve family-hospital articulation toward increased family solidarity through application of scientific findings to demonstrations; and
5. To devise and develop group alternatives to families for hospitalized patients whose family ties are or must be irrevocably broken.

The study began with an exhaustive search of the literature on the family and the hospital, and a decision to investigate a few hospitals in Africa and India where it was reported that some of the family accompanied each patient and stayed with him or her during hospitalization. This practice was occasionally referred to in reports about hospitals there, and the intention to study it arose particularly from ready an article by Kohlmeyer and Fernandes [8]. A decision was made to study in considerable depth not more than half a dozen hospitals where it would be determined in advance that excellent representations of family-hospital articulation could be found.

Twelve possible sites for study were identified through extensive international correspondence with informed persons. However, efforts to arrange the fieldwork met with discouraging consequences. Problems of overworked staff in the hospitals, lack of housing for visitors, language barriers, potential difficulties of "noncontributors" in staff interrelationships, and the length of time required for gaining orientation to the hospital, the wider community, and the culture were cited as impediments; these were confirmed by consultants. Accordingly, the study plan was revised to a pattern of brief visits to a large number of carefully selected facilities (153) in 27 countries of Africa, the Middle East, and Asia. I was assisted by my wife, Elisabeth A. Bell, child psychologist, who gave special attention to the provisions for child patients [5].

In each hospital we first held an interview with the medical officer in charge, usually the hospital director, and other top staff. The parts of the hospital that would be likely to provide observational data for us were identified and a tour was made in each. If more extensive onsite observation was needed, arrangements were made to return to a ward, a clinic, an area where a particular staff person would be at work, or where there seemed to be a potential opportunity to extend our knowledge.

For the most part the information available was organized around the following questions:

- Who comes to the hospital with the patient?
- What do relatives do in the hospital?
- What impact does family participation have on the hospital and how does it organize to take care of it?
- What prevents or deters family attendance?
- What are the benefits and disadvantages in family-hospital articulation?
- What steps may be taken to reduce the isolation of patients in our country?

The first issue to which we gave our attention was the kinship of those who came with the patient. From culture to culture, hospital to hospital, and ward to ward, great variability in the makeup of the family was observed. Attendance of relatives not only represents aspects of kinship and economic roles, but such diverse roles demanded by the ability to perform tasks of a very specific nature, such as:

- Waiting in line in place of the patient.
- Supporting the patient during the waiting period.
- Reducing the patient's resistance by persuasion, cajoling, or humor.
- Learning about the patient's illness.
- Learning about the hospital.
- Making or participating in decisions relative to hospital entrance, surgery, other forms of treatment, and correlative decisions about family matters—who will remain with the patient, who will go home, how affairs will be managed at home.

- Simply waiting outside in response to patient or staff request.
- Finally, and most importantly, feeding patients. This homely activity is accomplished in many ways—by cooking, by purchasing food, by securing it from diet kitchens or a canteen, or by transport from home.

Including the family in admission activities and permitting them to undertake helpful functions enabled them to bridge the gap between home and hospital. Admission and the first few days of hospitalization were identified as among the most critical periods in determining whether family relationships would be preserved. Some, in fact, argued that this period was more important than the stage when it becomes evident that hospitalization will be a long-term process.

THE FAMILY AND PHYSICAL CARE

The functions most commonly expected of family members when they stay with the patient in the hositals come under the category of physical care: feeding the patient, clothing him or her, making the bed, bathing and exercising, watching and protecting.

Feeding included securing, storing, preparing, cooking, and serving food and the related activities such as gathering, purchasing and transporting fuel, making fires, and washing pots, pans, and dishes. Also, family members brought water, juices, or soft drinks, sometimes to assist in the forcing of liquids. When the food came from home, it meant symbolically that the patient was eating from the same table as his relatives. When food was not brought every day, it was common for the family to bring it on Sundays or holidays. Patients who could afford it might prefer the hospital diet as a sign of status.

Watching the relatives we would observe them sorting out their belongings; bargaining with a woman who had brought in a load of fresh maize; returning from the markets with bananas, firewood, beans, shop packages, gourds full of milk, baskets of greens, or bags of peanuts; toting baskets of wood on their heads; positioning three stones together to form the support for the cooking pans, and kindling the three sticks pushed between; laughing, making jokes with, and teasing their neighbors; rushing to the ward with a bowl of food, making sure that the food was hot when the patient received it. Providing clean clothes, diaper service, and bed linen; bathing and exercising the patients; barbering and hairdressing; escorting patients into almost all areas except those maintaining sterile conditions; toileting the patient; functioning as orderlies or janitors; protecting the patient and monitoring the patient's condition; these illustrated the use of family members for highly personalized care by familiar methods and standards.

Insofar as treatment activities were concerned, great variability from hospital to hospital was observed. In the majority of hospitals, relatives joined with staff in performing various kinds of treatment services under staff supervision which seemed often to be remote, implicit, or nominal rather than direct and active. Each hospital had defined those nursing activities which relatives were prohibited from doing. Permission to conduct simple evaluative tests, to monitor patient status, to administer drugs and some physical treatments were withheld in some hospitals and granted in others; there was extensive variability in practice.

COMMUNICATION PATTERNS IN FAMILY-HOSPITAL ARTICULATION

It became obvious that the family in the hospital is a source of important information to the institution and to the community. It is also a means of transmission of information and a significant part of the hospital's total patient-oriented communication system. This is not usually an abstract, intellectualized activity, but a highly motivated, personalized function concerned with the patients, engaged in by family who love them, and enlisting staff who have publicly announced their desire to help. The communication is evident through actions as well as expressions.

In the simplest terms the network includes the following component parts: patient; staff; nonstaff within the hospital, including relatives and other patients; family at home; and the patient's home community. Since most of these units consist of many individuals, the system is complex indeed. From the hospital's point of view, however, the situation is even more complicated, for the basic network for one patient overlaps with similar ones for each of the other hospital patients.

When relatives stay in the hospital and become a direct part of the communication network, the changes affect communication patterns between the relatives and the hospital more than in other dimensions, for much which was invisible and inaudible becomes seen and heard.

Of course there is some communication with relatives when they do not come, but it is indirect, that is, through intermediaries, and consequently subject to distortion. If staff wish to send messages, many methods may be available to them, but the messages as sent may be garbled in transition or misapprehended under circumstances where how they are received is difficult to evaluate. Likewise, messages from family to staff may be misunderstood and evaluated inaccurately, leading staff to erroneous assumptions about the family and inappropriate actions toward them or the patient.

As in our country, in admission the family serve as informants for staff. During the course of hospitalization the family continue this role. This shows up in the amount and nature of what they tell about the ongoing course of the patient's illness or of the process of treatment. When the family has the opportunity to observe the patient continuously over each 24-hour period, in a majority of cases they provide more information needed by the physician than any staff member can. They may not monitor some processes as effectively as staff or electronic devices, but in general the consistency of their relationship with the patient offers a distinct advantage for securing evaluations of his or her status and information to answer medical questions. They know better than others the usual ways a patient acts and can more readily detect signs of improvement or deterioration. There is a more developed baseline of information against which to judge the extent of change.

Also, opportunities are sometimes available to family for securing information about the patient's condition that others may not have. Some patients may tell the family more easily than a doctor or nurse about feelings, pains, and problems. This would not always apply, however. In general, the family would be able to comprehend better than staff what the patient is saying in efforts to communicate. Some patients are so shy, so frightened, so suspicious, so reserved, so inarticulate that only almost indecipherable cues about their condition transmitted by nonverbal signs may be available to staff or family. The family probably has more skill in reading the meaning of these messages.

The family also communicate to the staff how they expect the patient to be treated. The primary message is contained in the family's own handling of him or her, which suggests attitudes that staff might adopt. If the family is tender, affectionate, considerate, and gentle, most staff will tend to follow suit in the presence of the family, even though this may be somewhat foreign to their usual manner. If the family seems not to care or to be impatient or angry, staff may then initiate them, or seek by example to modify family attitude.

Staff are able to use the opportunity in family attendance to reassure; to counsel; to solicit help; and to convey and correct conceptions, attitudes, and action patterns. The hospital setting offers an environment in which receptivity and readiness for response to staff may be heightened. The family of the mentally ill person, whose illness has made him or her unbearable at home, see staff channeling behavior in new and more constructive directions and from them pick up insights and techniques to be used in the hospital and at home. They learn also about the use of drugs in behavior amelioration and become part of the process of control through medicaiton. If the patient is ambulatory and has the ability, he or she may secure prescribed drugs and assume responsibility for taking them, watching for side effects, and bringing him or herself back for evaluation and control of the drug regimen. When a patient cannot manage this by themselves, his or her own family may provide the most immediate helping resource.

In addition to communication in reference to illness and treatment, the families are in active communication with the patient on their own behalf.

Checking on the patient's care at the hospital, testing out whether suspicions about mishandling have a factual basis, and reassuring themselves are natural expressions of their concern and anxiety. Relatives can use feeding and caring for the patient as opportunities for sizing up the situation, perhaps without even needing to talk about a matter that would disturb the patient, his or her relations with the staff, and confidence in and benefits from the treatments. Families do not generally conspire to be silent, but may find sufficient communication with the patient in other ways to lessen their own anxieties.

Further, family and patient together seek understanding of the illness and its consequences. For the most part this was felt to be good—they learn from one another. They explore their perplexities, sharpening the questions they want to ask staff, and they develop more ability to respond to staff. But there are difficulties, too, for their communication with one another may restrict their need to extent their contacts, and may limit sources of answers to their questions and restrict the potential fund of information available from others.

The communication of the relatives of one patient with those of others also serves many purposes. A primary one is to exchange operational information. Much of the orientation to the hospital community is accomplished by oral transmission of rules, regulations, expectations, adaptive methods, dangers, taboos, staff characteristics, authority, and physical layout of the hospital. This speeds the adaptation of the relatives, who meet one another in corridors, at the kitchen, waiting outside examination rooms or surgery, in the wards, or on the grounds. Naturally this adjustment is easy in hospitals that are simple in design and operation, but the same type of adjustment appears to have been achieved in complex urban medical centers. It creates problems, too, if more than accommodation to the current ways of doing things is sought. Since the communication is informal and outside the staff's relations with families, it can perpetuate undesirable as well as desirable customs.

In the few instances of active family participation in mental hospitals on a full-time basis, the families provided controls over bizarre behavior and reduced the extent to which any patient would be allowed to conduct himself or herself outside ordinary social limits. This extended beyond what one family might be able to accomplish with a patient, for the family effectively set the tone and brought community standards into the hospital.

When families are together in a ward or hostel they gradually assume cooperative arrangements to assist one another unless there are contraindications in customs about relations with others. A mother will watch her neighbor's child while his or her mother is marketing or cooking; the family next door will feed a patient for a day or two while the family goes home to look after the crops, to check on the children there, or to interview an employer.

Perhaps the greatest help that comes from the interchange among families is in reduction of their sense of isolation. One could often see groups of relatives chatting with one another. In a sense they lighten the mood of the hospital especially when they are able to socialize comfortably with one another away from the patients' beds. One staff physician said, "The relatives bring fun into the hospital." The families also reassure one another.

The staff use communications with relatives for their own purposes, such as, to accomplish treatment objectives and to speak on their behalf to the patient. Or course one of the most important uses of staff relations with the family is for education. When the family know from staff about the nature of the illness, the meaning of symptoms, the reasons for treatment, and the expectations about the course of the hospitalization, they become capable of supplying answers at the moment of questioning and of reassurance at the point of anxiety.

The final area of communication deals with the link between the patient and his or her home community, especially with those family members who remain at home. It also deals with the link between the patient's family in the hospital and their home community. Formal methods, such as writing, telephoning, and sending telegrams are sometimes resorted to. We were told that in many places where electronic transmission was unavailable, the "grapevine" or "bush telegraph" was singularly rapid and effective; and sometimes even where mechanical devices could be used, the native methods are speedier and more reliable.

SOCIAL AND PSYCHOLOGICAL SUPPORT

In those hospitals where the family has ready access, psychosocial support from a family to a patient is provided by the relatives whether they visit periodically or stay with the patient. The nature, pertinence, intensity, and duration of the support will relate to the length of time the family is with the patient, but not exclusively. The extent of the patient's need, his receptivity, the roles imposed on the family by the community, and their religious attitudes affect the way the family members behave with the patient. The quality of the support they give seems to differ when it is given consciously from when it is given secondarily during routine action toward the patient.

In those hospitals where family members are there throughout their patient's stay, to speak of the family's offering social and psychological support as though it were a separate action would misrepresent what happens. Such support is mainly an indirect consequence of the actions of the family in the hospital. On the other hand it should not be inferred that there is no conscious effort to give such support to the patient through his illness and hospitalization, even though the family attention may be centered on domestic functions or on active participation in treatment. As the families bring their own life into the hospital and carry it on there, they also provide mutual support to one another.

There are many hospitals abroad, however, of the pattern usual in the United States, where the family members do not stay, are not allowed to bring food, where staff handle all patient care, and where the relatives are only there to visit. Visits of relatives are then plainly for social and psychological support.

PHYSICAL ARRANGEMENTS FOR FAMILY PARTICIPATION

To permit families to come into the hospital it is necessary to allow them to use existing facilities or to provide specially organized space and equipment. In the majority of hospitals visited the provisions for the relatives were unplanned. Families were expected to supply what they needed for their own care and comfort, and already constructed buildings or furnishings were adapted by the families to their own uses. However, in some places hospitals had given special thought to how the relatives could live and work in the hospital and had made some arrangements for their activities. Even in the most highly developed arrangements, the accommodations were not elaborate, although they permitted many functions.

Certain space and equipment might be regarded as the minimum required for family residence and participation. This would include facilities for shelter, sleeping, a source of food (canteen, cafe, or market) if they do not bring food from home, sanitation and bathing, refuse disposal, laundering, storage, waiting, and visiting. Other facilities, beyond the bare minimum, would include space and equipment for recreation, worship, education, employment, and privacy; these were found infrequently on our visits.

Provisions and services in the environs of the hospitals often supplemented those found in the hospitals, and on occasion operated in their place. Transportation, communication services, markets, restaurants, shrines, and living accommodations were found in various forms. In some instances whole villages, apartments, or residences were constructed in the nearby community by the hospital or independent proprietors for use by the families.

Certain principles that should apply in the development of facilities for relatives stand out:

1. Space is required for family members, the functions they are to perform, and the activities the hospital will initiate with them.

2. The hospital's facilities should promote family identity and solidarity by allowing the family to have the most direct and continuous relations possible with the patient.

3. Facilities for the relatives plus the patient should be organized around single families; those for relatives alone may be planned for joint use by a number of separate families simultaneously or sequentially.

4. The environment in the hospital should approach the home environment as much as possible and permit easy assumption of customary functions in the new setting. Humbleness of facilities does not necessarily

represent lack of medical vigilance. It may show more real concern for the relatives by reducing the problems of transition from home to hospital and back.

5. Equipment should be simple. As Dr. During of the Children's Hospital in Freetown, Sierra Leone, said: "If relatives can use it, fine; if not, then it should be usable by untrained staff; if not, then by overworked and underpaid nurses who can't waste time on complexities; if beyond this, then only if highly trained manpower is available and can be spared."

6. Facilities must allow possibility of open communication (visual, auditory, verbal) with other patients, relatives, and staff. Interfamily actions must be allowed for educational, social, cathartic, and mutual support purposes.

7. Appropriate attention must be given to sanitation and safety. Every environment compromises with absolute sanitation and safety, so the compromises might as well be ordered in part by concerns for human and social well-being. Space must show clear differentiation of those activities from which family are restricted.

8. Relatives must have easy access into and out of the hospital and the patient's room. Physical and human (e.g., staff) barriers promote patient institutionalization. Entrance of the family must be welcomed and be as easy as or easier than admission for a patient.

9. Though facilitation of family participation with the acutely ill is critical, hospitalization of the chronically ill creates special burdens in continuing family participation and requires particular facilitation, for example, space for moving in familiar objects, means for providing familiar and preferred foods, socialization with family and others from the community, privacy when with the family, reduction in dependence on hospital staff and surroundings, retention of ties with home, inclusion of work, recreation, and other pursuits (religious, education, etc.) in the hospital.

10. Too much regularity in the spatial and color arrangements of facilities, in furnishings, in sizes of space, and in relation of interior to exterior deters relatives from participation and promotes patient isolation and dehumanization.

11. Areas should be provided to fill the relatives' need to get away from patients at times for the welfare of the patient and for their own privacy, rest, or socialization.

12. There must be a free flow of the community into the hospital in human traffic, delivery, and symbols of the community (sights, sounds, objects).

13. Space must be flexible to permit adaptations to various family-patient configurations and to changing community and cultural conditions, that is, there should be immediate and long-range flexibility.

14. Patients should be exposed more to normal healthy people than to other patients in the artificial environment of the hospital.

15. Transportation from home to hospital and back must be rapid, easy, inexpensive, and accessible.

INSTRUCTION OF THE RELATIVES

Staff of many hospitals we visited saw the full range of their associations with relatives as a chance to educate them and thereby reduce their tensions, to improve their attitudes and health, and to increase their usefulness to patients. Staff took moments to teach at the time of admission; in clinics; on the wards during rounds or treatment procedures; during care activities such as cooking, bathing, feeding; when preparing for the patient's rehabilitation; and in follow-up care. These informal opportunities in individual relations were often supplemented by formal classes. In general, education was voluntary for the family, but the effort was made to take advantage of quickened motivation, to meet demands for knowledge at the times of readiness to learn, and to organize and pace lessons to provide them in assimilable doses. Hospitalization was even extended in some instances for the purposes of education, and transportation was arranged to bring family members back to the hospital for follow-up sessions.

The most significant and general area of teaching in the hospitals related to the patient's illness. The instruction of the family at the patient's bedside, and the direct answering of their questions was probably the most frequently used method. This was complemented by the example of how the doctor or nurse handled the patient, although language barriers sometimes reduced understanding of what was happening. Participation of relatives in programs on the wards also is a means of instruction. Some nurses were extremely skillful at involving the relatives. Some treated the families as concerned and competent helpers; some as though they were children with whom the nurse would waste her time if she tried to teach them or use them to help.

ORGANIZING THE HOSPITAL FOR FAMILY PARTICIPATION

To organize a hospital to include the relatives, a number of steps were suggested by hospital administrators. First, it was pointed out that an *overall policy to incorporate the relatives* needs to be stated, followed in practice, and enforced with the authority of those in charge. Second, it was suggested that much attention must be given to organizing *the authority* within the hospital to take families into account and to provide examples of their acceptance. The doctor at the head of the hospital sets the tone that is reflected by staff. Typically, the medical officer in the hospital promoted family participation by the way he or she handled internal procedures in the hospital and particularly with the staff. Here the prevailing policies about families were expressed, promoted, elaborated, and refined.

A third step in organizing for family participation consists in *setting forth procedures* that allow relatives to function optimally within determined practices. A variety of methods was encountered from hospital to hospital.

Access to the Hospital

Records and statistics of family attendance. No hospital visited had a record system built around the family as the unit. All records were oriented to a primary patient, with variable practices in regard to inclusion of more than identifying information about some family members.

Controlled availability of staff. Normally a balance has to be obtained between what families and staff desire in regard to the intensity of their relations. If families are not satisfied, pressure on staff for more time and help mounts. Previously effective efforts at control over the families often breaks down at that point. To a degree the family's convenience, as well as that of the staff has to be served.

Staff supervision of families. Some methods for supervising the family when it comes to the hospital have to be in operation.

Joint conference with families. When families are around the hospital, there are always ways of learning about their conditions, expectations, hopes, anxieties, irritations, suggestions, and evaluations. Some hospitals have established conferences with families by invitation and by staff assignment. Sometimes these have included contacts with several families simultaneously. There is a problem in making the families feel free enough to express themselves, especially in the beginning when they have stereotyped ideas about the hospital, its life, and its staff. Many of these ideas have to be unlearned in order to secure open communication. A climate for communication has to be developed, but even under optimal conditions there will be areas of reservation where the communication can be only nonverbal. Equally important for openness is revising the stereotypes that staff accumulate about families. Staff ideas that begin "all families. . . ." should be suspect, just as similar ideas about "all patients" should be challenged. Such generalizations mean that the approach to the families has become institutionalized when, to the greatest extent possible, it should be individualized.

Staff conferences about families. Occasionally these were encountered.

Procedures for resolving difficulties with families. Conferences with families and staff are both effective methods for preventing problems that could be created in the hospital by family members and for achieving solutions to those that have arisen. Sometimes, but rarely as a first choice, discipline through the assertion of authority is required. Not infrequently, families will negotiate with one another and work out improved ways to handle awkward situations. Firmness about agreed-upon rules, such as those that control space, reduces tension.

Staff privacy. Almost every hospital, when asked where family members could not go, had some closed areas to describe. The restricting of some areas which were open elsewhere seemed in part to be tied to the availability of personnel to supervise and to a general climate of impersonality. Especially for the mental patients it was stressed that there are advantages in reducing the mysteries about the environment and the procedures that occur in it. But even in the most open mental hospitals there were some areas off-limits to patients and relatives, at least for some times during day or night.

Procedures for discharge. When hospitals are open for families to come in, they are open for departure, too. Not only may family members leave, but over and over we heard about patients being taken out when permission to leave had not been sought and would not have been granted. The procedures for control of discharge, for adequate preparation for convalescence and rehabilitation, and for follow up were found to need support by education of relatives as well as patients, even though hospitals recognized that there were advantages in the eagerness of patients and families to return home.

Defining staff and family roles. The final step necessary to organizing for family participation was defining the roles for family and staff. The roles for the family were expressed in general terms as well as specifics. The definitions were by fiat and from everyday practice. They led to agreed-upon activities, mostly by operational consensus which resulted in the support of staff and family— whether enthusiastic, implicit, grudging, or tentative.

In general, the family roles were established on the base of those brought from home and community. But they were extended or modified according to the demands of a patient's illness, expectations of staff, and limitations and requirements of the physical and social environment. Since these variables were potent in their influence, we saw, as has been described earlier, many different tasks being taken on by relatives. For instance, hospitals reported having advised relatives to come; having told them that their participation was important; having instructed them that they were to help; having conveyed their expectations of cooperation; having specified activities and how and where they could be done; having sought to individualize activities to the particular patient and family, and in many other ways having structured the families' roles and functions.

Families were not passive in following hospital direction, however. In many hospitals they proved largely intractable as far as staff were concerned, with staff finding that their own roles were strongly patterned by what relatives would permit. Perhaps this could not have happened unless it served some purposes of which staff were unaware, but it led some staff to feel "put upon." Families often seemed to act as though the hospital were part of their own community which they could shape to their own liking. This facilitated their continued and effective participation.

Specialized staff for families. Although there was some theoretical discussion of this possibility with staffs, no instance was discovered in the 153 medical settings.

FRIENDS AND CRITICS OF FAMILY PARTICIPATION

Most of the professional people with whom we talked had mixed feelings about family participation within their hospitals, no matter what its extent. A statement that the family can always do things for the patient better than staff would be patently ridiculous, but the idea that staff can always function better than the family is also ridiculous. Some tasks can always be done better by the family, such as some forms of communication; some can always be done better by staff, for example, the many operations that require specialized skills. Some things are exclusively the functions of one or the other; activities growing out of family roles naturally require relatives, while surgery and X-ray technology, for example, require staff. But in many respects there is overlap in capabilities; then choice about who is to do what is made on the basis of factors other than qualifications, as, for example, by authority, custom, or deference. It must be remembered, also, that either the family or the staff may hurt patients. These human relations are not always benign. The family member who says something caustic each time he or she approaches the patient may not be more hostile or destructive than the nurse who bumps into the patient's bed every time she gets near it. Family ties and professional training may provide channels through which either love or hate may flow.

One of the advantages often mentioned was that the presence of the family reduces hospital costs. The most important economic benefit is in the reduction of the staffing budget, especially for staff providing nursing services. The extent of the reduction depends on the division of labor between family and nurses, a matter which is sometimes decided at the bedside, sometimes by hospital policy, sometimes by government directive, and sometimes by labor unions. We found most typically that separation is made between basic care and professional nursing services, with the former being assigned to the family and the latter to the staff. But from hospital to hospital there is great variation.

The advantages in quality of care are sufficient to give them independent importance in the list of benefits of family participation in hospitals. We were told that the nurses are more responsive to patients when the family is present.

Their work is demanded by the family as well as the patient—and the family is not helpless, as some patients are, so they are better able to say what they want and to evaluate the nurses' performances. Several nurses and doctors who had previously worked in hospitals where it is not customary for relatives to be present reported to us that the relatives who visit the hospital are more likely to panic needlessly and to make unreasonable or untimely demands on staff than do those who stay with the patient.

Of further importance in respect to quality of care is the attitude toward patients that develops when families are present. The doctors and nurses are said to adopt the family's positive attitudes toward the patient. This is not deliberate—it just grows—and since relatives are usually eager to serve the patient well, the staff is also. This counteracts tendencies to impersonalization and callousness in working with patients. Of course, not all families set good examples for the staff, but in those instances professional training leads staff members to attempt to counteract the detrimental effects of harsh attitudes and thoughtless actions on the part of family members.

A third area of advantage is the psychological condition of the patient and his or her family. We were told that the patient is much calmer when the family is present continuously; less is demanded from him or her by way of social adjustment; there is more continuity with the past and the future; there is more protection from anxiety-provoking circumstances; customary methods relieve the patient from disturbances; and he or she is spared the distress of separation, or the fear of it.

Some of the people, living conditions, and routines to which the patient is accustomed are carried right into the hospital with him or her. What a comfort there is in the familiar, especially when anyone is weakened by illness. Commonplaces are valued for themselves, and they carry symbolic virtue by speaking reassuringly of the ordinary run of things. While they may foster some nostalgia, preoccupation with what is absent is overcome by the nearness of those who are closest to one.

We were told that the relatives as well as the patients benefit psychologically. The relatives do not wish separation from the patient, especially when this might be interpreted as neglect in their home community. Also, they profit from the volume of anxiety-relieving information that becomes available when they are present.

Actual medical benefits followed from the presence of the relatives. The most apparent were observed among the children where the calmness was regarded as healing. Children were quietly moving about when mother was there. They were active up to the level of their capabilities and desires, and never frantically mobile nor overrestrained.

With adult patients the same ease in achieving optimal levels of activity appeared. The physical environment that made access and egress free for the relatives offered the same facility to patients. They came and went in a natural way that did not enforce inappropriate passivity, but allowed complete rest if indicated.

In some types of treatment the family's help accomplished what no staff, no matter how accessible, could do. A pertinent instance related to the postsurgical disorientation so common after eye surgery and the way family members were able, simply by their presence, to hold the patient to reality. A similar advantage was reported in the reduction, although not elimination, of confusion in the period immediately following electroconvulsive shock for mental patients.

On the negative side, relatives introduced many "unknowns" to the wards. There were repeated comments about distressing interference with treatment while the patient was in the hospital, ostensibly because the relatives knew no better. A number of times instances were described when foreign substances, deleterious in their effects, were given to patients. Perhaps even more important was the continuation of a poor diet, perpetuating or accentuating malnutrition, that was at the root of many illnesses and associated as a factor in many others. Against such practices, a few hospital administrators seized the educational opportunity to train patients and families, and brought their investment of staff time in direct clinical service to patients into balance with their efforts to prevent future illness.

We found a division of opinion about the advantages to staff in being able to use the relatives for certain chores. In general, the relatives relieved staff of menial and nontechnical work, permitting trained personnel to concentrate their effort on higher level work. Not all staff see this as an advantage, and it would not be in all cases.

Those hospitals that supported the idea of inclusion of family members saw this as good public relations. They had found that the relatives who knew at first hand what happened to patients were even better at publicizing the hospital than those patients who had been treated successfully.

The full-time presence of family members appeared to prevent artificiality in their relations with their patients and to modify the content of their communication. Many of the topics of conversation to be expected during a brief visit were no longer relevant. To ask the patient how he or she is today is unecessary. To inquire about sleeping, eating, pain, symptoms, medical treatment, doctor's evaluation, wishes, needs, and so on, would be redundant, since the information has been provided already in the continuous relations. The patient is not now a host entertaining guests and putting relatives into this unnatural position. The focus of the relatives' attention on the practical functions of feeding, bathing, toileting, laundering, fostering comfort, and taking care of maintains customary relations even though the balance of the relationships in the family is upset by the illness and removal from the home into a foreign setting. The psychological supports expected in the visit during visiting hours in a Western hospital were tendered without self-consciousness, because they derived from the activity of the relatives through the basic language of action.

Family participation may help many but not all; it may be possible in particular wards in many hospitals, none in others, and throughout the hospital in still others. It may be advantageous, if used with discrimination and with the support of scientific justification, but the risks may offset the values in some instances, in some settings, and with some patients.

Following the study phase of the total project, attention turned to educating professional persons and applying the ideas and principles that emerged from the study. This developmental phase began in 1965 and might still be said to be in progress. It has been and continues to be represented in widespread educational efforts, in lectures and workshops, intensive courses in health-related academic settings, targeted efforts to implement principles and practices in hospital and community programs, and continuing conceptualization of the actual and potential family-related practices that will link families with medical and psychiatric programs. Within programs seeking to support the best of current and potential institutional practices, partnerships between families and hospitals and other medical programs, family-centered programs are being advanced, albeit slowly.

Study of the hospitals abroad stimulated many ideas for revising hospital and other medical programs in the immediate settings where I had direct or indirect entrée. Even prior to publication of the book that set forth the full report on the study, educational efforts in the form of lectures, seminars, and workshops were initiated [1]. These seemed to stimulate some changes in services.

Perhaps the earliest direct application of the findings of the study involved a week-long workshop during which I described and showed pictures of the transformation of a former nurses' residence at Harari Childrens Hospital in Salisbury, Zimbabwe, into a hostel where mothers or fathers could live when a child has been hospitalized. This added direction to ongoing efforts to adapt a vacant nurses' residence at another children's hospital for some useful purpose other than temporary housing for students or staff. The residence was redesigned into quarters for temporary family living during hospitalization of a child. The hostel was eventually remodeled and is now known as the Ronald McDonald House.

Another early attempt at application of the findings proved unsuccessful. It concerned a problem encountered by many Mexican-American patients in a local mental hospital. They missed the beans, chili, tortillas, and tacos that are staples of their regular diets. The problem was particularly severe for persons hospitalized for long periods. An effort to arrange for a modification of the diet in this hospital failed when the superintendent with whom I was consulting quoted a State regulation which he claimed, as it turned out inaccurately, forbade the bringing in of food.

In contrast, but much later, in the Palo Alto Veterans Administration Hospital a program was gradually instituted in a service for long-term patients. In this program family members were permitted to purchase meals on major holidays when the canteen was closed; thus they celebrated the "feast" days with family members who could not leave the hospital. A critical factor was the development of support by top staff in administration, finance, dietetics, nursing, and building management. Recognition of the readiness of families had to be developed so as to plan and carry out the arrangements. That it took the planning staff three years to achieve success may surprise some, but that represents the reality of the resistances encountered and the extent of negotiation required to overcome them.

Another early but important application of findings was developed in 1969 as the Family Focus program. This was an intensive project concerned with the introduction of family content into the curriculum for students in the Division of Physical Therapy at the Stanford University Medical School. A federally funded training program was developed and run within a prefabricated home built on the campus to function as temporary living quarters and a training center.

In this seven-year project, now being continued and represented in content throughout the curriculum of the Division and in derivative practice, projects, and programs, newly handicapped patients spend the last three days of hospitalization in the home. The patient was transferred from a hospital ward into the home and lived there with his or her family. Responsibility was shifted from staff to the family, and medical support was given in much the same manner as services might be provided in a home by community services. The family and the patient all learned to adapt to the conditions and relations occasioned by the new disabilities. Follow up in the home after discharge from the hospital strengthened the family impact of the program and facilitated adjustments to changes occurring during continuing rehabilitation. The dramatic impact of direct association with families under stress served to redirect many components of the total professional training program, and deeply implanted family orientation to the provision of services.

These early applications, begun more than a decade ago, have been followed by many other projects and new ideas which can only be referred to briefly here. Central was the emerging definitions of the process of importing ideas and making them work in this country, a model which has reference as well to taking ideas from setting to setting in this country. The model as developed involved the following principles:

1. Know, at least in general, what you are looking for—a target—sometimes to be thought of as a problem to be solved.

2. Learn where to observe.

3. Direct your observations purposefully, that is, keep your own role clear and intentional.

4. Be receptive to: the seeming universals—what is everywhere potentially visible; the exceptions or novel alternatives.

5. Store the information; keep thorough records.

6. Document findings.

7. Reflect on what has been learned.

8. Perhaps the most important step, abstract the principles implicit in observation. While direct transfer of models from elsewhere does occur and may be most productive, the more general relevance of observations comes from attempts to formulate the underlying concepts that can then free the mind for devising applications that are relevant to the new site.

9. Devise the action steps and test out the program methodologies in direct operations, with sensitive fine adjustments to meet the ongoing and emerging demands in the setting.

The efforts following this conception have been quiet but progressive for the settings within which they have been applied. They have made impacts at various program levels from overall hospital policy to activities conceived and initiated in response to single families. Primary has been the sensitizing, educating, and mobilizing of staff, for families commonly have more readiness to participate in patient care than is usually acknowledged. At the same time, the changed circumstances for families associated with long-term care, and especially in reference to older patients, result in modifications in family patterns which must be supported by staff and facilitated where they benefit the patient and the associated family members.

Examples of the further program activities include:

1. A home-based rehabilitation program for patients without families to care for them. This program was based on a rehabilitation village in Thailand where two chronic schizophrenics and a leper lived together and made a success of noninstitutional living, both in daily care and in establishment of a modest business. The leper had severe physical limitations but intellectual competence; the schizophrenics were floridly psychotic but retained the strength to do physical tasks under the leper's direction. None of the individuals could manage alone in the community, but together they achieved self-support, and freedom from institution living.

In the community project that applied the principles behind this successful household, a group of patients from the Palo Alto Veterans Administration Hospital, none of whom had family, were transferred to a home in the community. The patients were matched in advance on the principle of complementing the separate limitations in each patient by strengths in another member of the group. Thereby, a home for five seemingly nonrehabilitative patients was set up and operated without live-in staff—not, it must be admitted, without ups and downs, an occasional severe crisis, and eventual termination. Nevertheless the project had a long enough duration to demonstrate the potentials of such programming [7].

2. A targeted program to facilitate the process of integration of families into the Intermediate Care Service providing treatment and care for patients who need continued hospitalization in the two hospitals under single administration that form the Palo Alto Veteran's Administration Hospital. Branches of this Service are found in each hospital. In both, committees of staff were organized in 1973 to promote family affairs. These interdisciplinary committees have been at the center of efforts to analyze what is occurring to families in relation to each unit, and of developing new activities beneficial to both families and the medical program.

In addition to the food program mentioned above, the activities have brought about modifications in ward programs, redirection of volunteers toward serving as surrogate family for patients who have no relatives, development of socializing activities through use of family members as volunteers, education of families about specific medical conditions common among the patients and the needed treatments and follow up; problem solving through conferences that involve groups of family members and staff, delegations of functions formerly performed by staff to families, development of the participation of family members in patient-centered social and recreational events, improving the sensitivity of staff to family problems, concerns, ideas, and resources for taking part in patient care, and even such mundane problems as assuring the availability of some parking spaces close to the hospital for relatives who through age or other problems are themselves somewhat limited in capacity.

The general model has not been based on psychotherapy or family therapy. Deliberately the focus has been placed on modifying the factors that impact on the welfare of the family. The process has been given introductory formulation in a developing model titled Family Context Therapy [4]. The basic intent is "to change environmental conditions that cause or accentuate family difficulties, and to construct contexts that promote family well-being" [2].

Set forth in the model are a series of possible action interventions:

1. Assess, plan and initiate modifications of family-hospital relations.
2. Delegate responsibilities to families in accord with staff consensus.
3. Analyze courses and outcomes of patients' hospitalizations to determine and encourage modes of family relations specific to each program.
4. Abstract constructs regarding hospital-family relations.

Such constructs might concern variables such as:

- time periods in hospitalization;
- the direction of activities within hospital-family relations—whether initiated by staff toward families, or by families toward staff;
- the spaces where relations take place;
- the criteria specified by the hospital governing its relations with families;
- the changes in the institution over time that affect families; and
- the place of the hospital among all the social institutions that are impinging on the families.

Derived from these constructs, program modifications have been designed and can be improved so that the process of modification of hospital-family interactions can move from random toward orderly programming.

SUMMARY

A project initiated in 1963 to study family relations with hospitals in developing countries where families often take a vital role in patient care has followed an organic growth process from that time. Findings from the foreign study were applied directly in hospitals and professional training to provide models of activities and services for families. Adaptations were also devised and applied in selected health settings. Out of this 15-year program the method called Family Context Therapy was devised [4]. The continuing conceptualization and application of the method gives promise of improving relations between families and medical institutions, and in broader application, between families and many of the social institutions throughout communities.

REFERENCES

1. Bell, J.E. *The Family in the Hospital: Lessons from Developing Countries.* Washington, D.C.: Government Printing Office, 1969.
2. Bell, J.E. "La familia en los hospitales en paises en desarrollo." *Neurologia—Neurocirugia—Psiquiatria (Mexico)* 14 : 69–78, 1973 (In Spanish).
3. Bell, J.E. "Family in medical and psychiatric treatment: selected clinical approaches." *Journal of Operational Psychiatry* 8 : 57–65, 1977.
4. Bell, J.E. "Family context therapy: a model for family change." *Journal of Marriage and Family Counseling* 4 : 111–126, 1978.
5. Bell, J.E. and Bell, E.A. "Family participation in hospital care for children." *Children* 17 : 154–157, 1970.
6. B.S. Brown and E.D. Torrey (eds.) *International Collaboration in Mental Health.* Rockville, M.D.: National Institute of Mental Health, 1973.

7. Bell, J.E.; McDonough, J.M., and Toepfer, H. "Achieving community living by preplanned interdependence." *Psychosocial Rehabilitation Journal* 1 : 7–18, 1976.
8. Kohlmeyer, W.A. and Fernandes, X. Psychiatry in India: family approach in the treatment of mental disorders. *American Journal of Psychiatry* 119 : 1033–1037, 1963.
9. Sasano, E.M.; Shepard, K.F.; Bell, J.E.; Davies, N.H.; Hansen, E.M.; and Sanford, T.L. "The family in physical therapy." *Physical Therapy* 57(2) : 153–159, 1977.
10. Schwartz, C.G. "Perspectives on deviance: wives' definitions of their husbands' mental illness." *Psychiatry* 20 : 275–291, 1957.

14

Family-Organizational Linkages

MARVIN B. SUSSMAN

INTRODUCTION

Family units as primary groups are increasingly becoming assertive and evaluative in their relationships with bureaucracies such as human service organizations and agencies because of: (1) increasing maturity of family members in relation to rights, entitlements, and available service options; (2) alleged or actual mismanagement of available resources by bureaucratic functionaries; (3) sky-rocketing costs of formal institutional services; (4) the beginning desire of some human service establishments to develop a complementarity with families in caring, treating, controlling, or educating its members; and (5) the increased voicing of ideological and moral positions on returning to a family form that is adaptive, intact, and controlling of its members.

A related issue is the family's desire for autonomy and independence in the face of growing dependence on large-scale organizations, not only for services but for economic maintenance, jobs, shelter, food, and pleasure. Have society's organizational systems reached their absorptive capacity to handle subordinate and dependent families? Are our institutions and organizations so overburdened and mired in dependency that they cease to be creative or productive in relation to their original missions and seek, if not salvation, at least peace and perpetuity in boundless rules and regulations?

The fact is that although families are making noises about the accountability and responsibility of bureaucracies and the need to take care of themselves now and in the future, families and bureuacracies need one another. Complex societies such as ours cannot continue over time and provide its members with some quality of life if families and bureuacracies did not develop a complementarity of essential functions. Such understanding and appreciation of one another's activities and functions provides bases for more equitable and dignified family-bureaucratic organization linkages and relationships. It also furnishes space for families to take charge of their own lives, to exercise available options, and to express their own individual cultural ways transmitted over generations.

This chapter is primarily conceptual and theoretical. It presents a linkage model of families and bureaucracies which, like all models, contains assumptions, definitions, processes, and variables. Its usefulness lies in its ability to explain observable behavior. The model, for example, can be used as a diagnostic tool, enabling the observer to pinpoint: (1) probable causes, correlations, and points at which therapeutic interventions are most appropriate, and (2) reasons for successful and unsuccessful outcomes as a consequence of interventions, events, and situations.

What follows is a definition of terms and concepts; descriptions of the unique functions and activities of families, kinship groups, and bureaucracies; assumptions and analysis of linkage between family structures and organizations; and proposed linkage models.

DEFINITIONS

Family and Kinship

Family is defined in a variety of ways depending on the values of the observer; the intended use of the definition in any given situation; the structural properties of the unit i.e. the actors—the single parent, nuclear, or three-generation household family; or the dynamics of interaction and functions being performed. One of my colleagues, expressing momentary frustration, defined the family as a group of individuals—usually parents and children—formed by the acts of marriage and procreation, linked together in some system of exchange and role reciprocities and ruled by its sickest member. A therapist who holds to this view is supported by many good arguments.

Individuals are members of several types of family structures concurrently, and some of these memberships change over the life course as transitions from one stage to another occur. A primary group—the family—is created by the act of marriage. The unit referred to as the "nuclear family of procreation" consists of husband and wife living together with children obtained by procreation or adoption. In American society, this family usually resides in a household apart from either set of parents. Until World War II, the dominant role assignment was for the male to be gainfully employed in the labor force, and thus the predominant economic provider, while the female was the homemaker and had the major responsibility for rearing children. This nuclear unit was and remains the legally sanctioned family form and is responsible for the torts of its members.

Adult members of this nuclear family of procreation are also members of the nuclear family of orientation which is the unit in which they were reared, consisting of sibs and parents. The family of gerontation is composed of three generations consisting of grandparents and relatives. In addition, the in-law family is another form in which the individual has membership as a consequence of marriage. Cultural prescriptions and social norms guide allowable relationships and exchanges between self and mother-in-law, father-in-law, sibs-in-law, and other collaterals which make up this in-law family.

There are numerous structures under the rubric of family which obligate its members through voluntary or compulsory means. Only two important types are presented here: the classical extended family, and the modified extended family [5,6,20,23,24]. The classical extended family is a series of nuclear families living in close proximity and bound together in a series of exchanges and reciprocities. Similar occupations of its providers or involvement in a corporate family economic enterprise are the elasticities of this form. This structure establishes a hierarchical authority structure for governance and the nuclear units subordinate their individual goals and behaviors to the normative demands of the larger groups. Such classical extended families are still found in rural areas of the United States and among ethnic minorities.

The modified extended family also consists of nuclear family units which are not necessarily propinquitous and who develop voluntarily with one another a series of exchanges and reciprocities involving economic, service, and personal support. The stress is on voluntary relationships and exchanges. There is no strong cultural prescription, legal mandate, or rule of descent to enforce promises or relationships.

Our culture recognizes a multilineal descent system. That is, the individual can claim descent from four lines beginning with grandparents; eight with great grandparents; 16 lines, four generations removed; 32 lines, five generations removed, and so on. The number of lines doubles with each subsequent generation. Therefore, no descent line, as is the case in a primogeniture system, has any particular claim on the individual's abilities, assets, or person. Our inheritance system and attendant obligatory behaviors are limited to the life span of the nuclear family. Claims which parents may have on their children are largely gone when these children marry. Hence, familial status cannot demand claims obligations. Personal voluntary relationships among family members are the basis for the existence and functioning of the modified extended family.

Finally, there is one other family form which has manifested and is growing in incidence because of radial changes in the demographic pyramid caused by lowered fertility and increased survival of persons over retirement age. It is the "everyday family," consisting usually of persons who are not related by blood or marriage, are of different ages, live in the same neighborhood, and treat one another as if "they are family" [22]. The structural forms vary; some function as large nuclear units while living in separate households, and others as classical or modified extended families [16].

These structures provide both similar and complementary functions with varying degrees of frequency and intensity. It is critical to visualize these units as flesh and blood systems which influence the perceptions, feelings, attitudes, decisions, and behavior of its members in matters of everyday living and those involving life-course transitions.

Bureaucracy

A bureaucracy, on the other hand, is a complex structure with roles and responsibilities rigidly defined. Persons hold positions in a hierarchy that is usually shaped as a pyramid. Increasing responsibility and authority is correlated with a higher niche in the pyramid.

The principles of span of control and time; specificity and integration of function; and mass production with interchangeability of parts and activities are fundamental to the workings of a bureaucratic organization. The control and time notion is based on the assumption that the time one person has to supervise adequately a large number of persons is limited; to effectively supervise (control) requires a few persons reporting to the supervisor. Hence the hierarchical ordering of positions. Also, jobs in a bureaucracy are highly specialized, each job has a specific function and set of activities. The product or outcome is the result of the integration of all functions. According to organizational theory, mass production—capitalizing on the interchangable part or behavior—should result in a product or service at the lowest possible cost. Workers are trained to do these specialized jobs and they are replaceable. Merit is the norm for reward in the organization. Families and bureaucratic organizations do different things for its members and these differences are endemic to their basic structures.

SPECIFIC PROPERTIES OF FAMILY STRUCTURES AND ORGANIZATIONS

The basic assumption is that all human societies require linkages and appropriate behaviors in relation to functions which are complementary to institutions and families [5,6,7,9,10,11,8,12,2,22]. Prior to describing the dynamics and processes of these linkages, the properties and special characteristics of families and organizations are presented. The objective is to demonstrate the difficulty of and necessity to develop a balanced complementarity between two systems which vary extensively in their functions and in what they provide for their members.

Families as primary groups are best suited to care for their members because their structure is the most competent to handle unusual events and idiosyncratic behaviors. They can provide space for the family to function as an emotional system.

More formal organizations, such as hospitals and long-term care establishments, are more suited to handle standardized and recurring events. They use technical knowledge and workers in such organizations and make judgments on the basis of merit. Members' careers and futures depend upon their proven job experience and success.

Adult members are not thrown out of the family because they cannot function effectively, although inability to perform roles successfully may be a contributing factor to the increasing incidence of divorce. But the breakup of a marriage is "dissolving the company," and is not the same as job termination. Individuals have a right to fight the intended separation, and many do. Also, children, especially young ones, cannot be "discharged" for not performing all of their tasks competently or not living up to expectations.

The parent who is a poor provider or caretaker is not going to be thrown out of the family even if he or she violates some standard or law, for example, commits child abuse. Even in such dire circumstances, the child may be taken away from the family, but the family persists.

Families tend to excuse the torts of their members, correcting behaviors which may become deviant, and attempt to live as best they can with the oddball behaviors of various members. Families do not operate on the principle of merit.

If negative or inappropriate behavior occurred in a more formal structure such as a business or service institution, e.g., a psychiatric hospital, the merit criterion would be applied. If it was demonstrated that technical competence was inadequate, some corrective action would be taken, such as shifting the individual to a new position or effecting a discharge.

Formal organizations are more competent in handling the activities of a large number of people who are of diverse backgrounds and sustaining and integrating the work of specialists. In contrast, family members undertake the multiple tasks of running a household. The usually establish a division of labor in which one or more members share the performance of the same tasks and may take on one another's tasks under certain conditions and situations. In contrast, institutions, such as nursing homes, use experts to perform "family" activities such as cooking, chauffeuring, cleaning, purchasing, and repairing.

The family is structured favorably to provide an emotional environment which allows for the development of intimacy, love, and solidarity. Formal organizations by their structure and objectives, unless they are treatment institutions such as small private psychiatric hospitals, cannot do this with any consistency or profit. Emphasis on providing a safe and loving haven for workers and clients may mean not getting the job done.

In organizations such as psychiatric hospitals, medical schools, or homes for the aged, secretaries are supposed to type and correspond; nurses are supposed to care for the ill; physicians are supposed to diagnose and treat; educators are supposed to teach and train; researchers are supposed to investigate; maintenance people are supposed to clean and polish; and all these specialists are coordinated into a model intended to achieve the institutional objectives. It is not primarily an emotional system as is the family, although individuals working in such formal structures may convey and achieve for themselves some level of emotional gratification and acceptance.

If human service systems do respond with warmth, good feelings, real concern, honesty, love, and intimacy to their clients, achieving their specific objectives may be enhanced. Emotional well-being in a formal organization may enhance productivity. However, it is not a primary objective of formal structures, and emotional gratification is more likely to be obtained in small primary groups such as families. Another assumption of the linkage conceptualization is that although human beings need meaningful primary group relationships and emotional and social support from others for their mental and physical health, it is also essential for their survival that they relate successfully to organizations. Factors which enter into such family-organizational linkages are the predictability of the event, contingencies, economies of primary group activities, and frequency of the event. The following examples illustrate these points.

An aged person with some form of chronic brain disorder who is living alone may become ill and be unable to function, even to the point of not being able to call someone for help. No one can predict the onset of illness, and even if one could, the professional who might do some good may never get there. Also, there is no way to insure that the expert in this kind of situation, whether a policeman, social worker, emergency ambulance attendant, or physician, would be able to help such a person. Such unpredictable events occur constantly in the lives of individuals, and unless there are people available, such as family members or friends, the person is unlikely to obtain help in critical situations.

Situations where there are many contingencies are likely to be more effectively handled by primary groups, rather than by formal human service systems. Some years ago, in connection with a study of the natural history of diabetes, I assumed the role of patient/anthropologist at a large metropolitan hospital. Over a period of nine months, I spent approximately 200 hours as a "patient" observing the diabetes clinic of this particular teaching hospital. Efforts were made to have all patients with diabetes adhere to a strict diet. Exercise and insulin completed the triage for survival of the diabetic patient. A therapy program involves a number of professionals: nutritionists, nurses, physicians, and counselors. It was a costly program in which formal instruction was given. I discovered that the program was eminently unsuccessful.

Diabetic patients, especially those who came from the ghetto areas and were near retirement age or elderly, told me that what they were getting from the nutritional professionals was "bullshit." Although the information was rational and based upon the best knowledge derived from scientific experiments at that time, these patients were reacting to what appeared to them to be the total ignorance of the professionals about how indigenous people live and manage their households. The experts did not know how the poor purchase food, their dependence on credit, the lack of selection of items and the high mark-up in neighborhood stores, food preferences, and the inability to do comparison shopping and go to stores other than those closest to one's household.

The professionals were interested in helping the diabetic patient; in this instance, mostly the poor and aged. However, either because of their ignorance or insensitivity to the problems of such patients—fear of being mugged in the streets and the physical limitations of their diabetic condition, both of which did not permit them to venture too far from home; and the costs of such foods—their response was "bullshit." Reflecting on this experience which occurred over 20 years ago, it is obvious that in a situation in which there are so many contingencies, it would have been best to involve the biological or "everyday" family (informal support network) of these patients, and provide them with the information and necessary resources to achieve a balance of diet, insulin, and exercise. Such primary group members, with vast experience to handle problems of this kind, might have been able to do a better job in maintaining quality diets for diabetic patients than were achieved by the professionals.

The major rationale for having large-scale organizations is to cut costs. The greater the number of services provided, the lower the price. However, there are situations in which organizational activities may be counterproductive, i.e., it may cost more in overhead to provide the particular service. The availability of science and technology to families and other primary support systems may result in their being able to handle situations at a lower cost than a large-scale organization. For example, picture a situation in which an elderly person with a history of mental illness lives in the household of a member unit of the extended family, or lives in the same neighborhood or community of this household, or in a community where there is a viable support system. The elderly person—through communication with network and family members via visitation, phone, or use of a home computer—would be able to monitor his or her health effectively thus prevent a more serious illness or disability as a consequence of neglect. Techniques for monitoring diseases such as diabetes or high blood pressure are becoming increasingly available. As a consequence, medical experts have time and energy to treat the more critical cases and emergencies.

The family has a greater capacity than organizations to handle infrequently occurring events and contingencies. Such crisis-type happenings require members of families or other primary groups to act immediately. Experts of service systems may either not be available, or bringing them into the situation may not make a difference or be the best use of their expertise. Also, it is likely to be very costly. Even if one wanted an expert, in an infrequent occurring situation, he or she may not be available. For instance, grandfather has wandered away from the house. He has done this before; in fact, he does it on a fairly regular basis. Does one immediately call the police or go out to look for grandfather?

An aging mother is prone to migraines that seem to occur just prior to the time she is to get her social security check. She worries because she has heard about the theft of such checks and how hustlers and muggers stay around the mailboxes or visit on the day the checks arrive. Do you call the doctor to treat this condition, or do you give assurance and suggest that she take a few aspirin or other medication that the physician has prescribed?

You are at a family gathering and your uncle, age 81, complains of feeling ill. His heart appears to have stopped. Your immediate reaction is to ask someone to call the emergency squad while you try mouth-to-mouth resuscitation, raise him to a sitting position, and do appropriate techniques which you have learned in your Red Cross class.

These illustrations demonstrate that formal organizations, especially those which provide human services, can be effectively utilized for their expertise when called upon to handle situations and events which are beyond the capacities of families. It also suggests that families can function in situations using science and technology to provide economies of a small scale in situations where experts cannot be trained or coordinated, and in those areas where no expertise has been developed and professionalized.

THE FAMILY AND BUREAUCRACY IN COMPLEX SOCIETIES: THEORETICAL BASES FOR LINKAGE

Complex societies consist of bureaucratic organizations and primary groups interrelated by a coincidence of interdependence and conflict. Each organization has specialized functions, an ethos, norms, and values which command the loyalty and identification of its members. Students of bureaucracy have extensively developed the theme of the incompatibility between the bureaucratic organization and the primary group as exemplified by the family (Litwak and Meyer, [10]). In line with Max Weber's classic theory of the nature of bureaucracy, it has been repeatedly stressed that the primary group, because of its particular structural properties, goals, and functions, is antithetical to the purposes, needs, and functions of the bureaucratic organization. For this reason, social distance between these two organizational forms has appeared to be a prerequisite for their mutual survival in a society.

The high level of differentiation of function in industrial society places extraordinary pressure on the nuclear family and collateral members of the various kinship networks to capitulate to the normative demands of bureaucratic organizations. The more extensive, permanent, and powerful system (the bureaucracy) may logically be expected to dominate the lesser and weaker one (the family) if there are necessary changes in relationship which require role modifications. Yet, some families develop a modus operandi for handling the demands of bureaucratic organizations while maintaining their own internal structure and function, and under certain conditions and situations, may surpass the bureaucratic organization in the extent of their influence.

The structural characteristics of these two types of institutions have been cited to lend support to the presumed position of family subordination. The bureaucratic organization is based on an ideology of efficiency and rationality and functions instrumentally and in a scientific and objective manner to achieve its goal, an orientation which is necessary for the continued survival of complex societies. The family, on the other hand, is an effective structure in which behavior is a response to emotional feelings and sentiments with little regard for objective analysis. As the social sphere of bureaucratic institutions has extended, their greater power presumably has allowed them to preempt the more important adaptive functions once performed by the family. The latter structure has been left with only such tasks as socialization into generalized roles and identities, and tension management of family members, chores which more rationally ordered organizational systems cannot perform or find acceptable because these objectives lack specificity.

Accommodation is an alternative concept to preemption through which to view primary group-bureaucratic relations and to analyze the structural basis of the division of labor which exists between family and organization. Note that certain purposes and goals are vital to the persistence of the society itself and all of its institutions. For example, family and bureaucracy both share the valued goal of survival and support it with available means and resources. The functions of a family and a bureaucratic organization are complementary in this respect, a complementarity which has been achieved by means of accommodating behavior on the part of each of the participating structures. This is possible principally because these interaction systems have developed expertise in performing their functions and, therefore, need each other.

Although accommodation is a better concept to invoke in this context, contest is also involved. Both structures jockey for position which aims to reinforce or maintain discreteness in established spheres. A give-and-take process is implied in which the hostilities of each party are mitigated and the structures become linked. A contemporary efficiency model which is based on differentiation of functions supports the argument that primary groups and bureaucratic organizations accept each other's expertise. Each has its own specialists who socialize novices into the performance of specific and diffuse roles; effectiveness determines which of these structures will be paramount in a particular area. In addition to this toleration of role expertise, structural interdependence enhances the need for the entire network to sustain each link so that it may perform its unique function, since structures and functions are interrelated.

The purposive rationality of the bureaucratic setting—which is best actualized in the professional expert—serves to complement and support the affective and expressive functions of the family—in which roles of another character predominate. Although its sphere and membership may be considerably less extensive than that of the bureaucratic organization, the family has intrinsic features which are invaluable in affording sustenance and personal identity to its members. It is an institution that has long experience in handling affective matters and responding to them in an intuitive fashion. Because of its limited range, ample opportunity is provided for individual emotional expression and gratification, and the individual enjoys a sustained orientation toward group belongingness that may support him even in the face of the most shattering crises.

Litwak and Meyer [11] identify three categories of tasks in which primary group members are most efficient and effective: (1) those which require sufficiently simple knowledge, permitting nearly anyone to perform them or to instruct others in their performance; (2) those which raise problems that neither the family nor experts have enough knowledge or consensus to analyze and solve; and (3) those related to idiosyncratic events.

Tasks of the first category would include taking care of one's own or another's physical needs, such as those associated with rising, bathing, eating, dressing appropriately, keeping personal schedules, shopping, and leisure activities. Instruction in these chores is well left to socialization agents such as parents or siblings.

Although expert advice would help the performance of the tasks of the second category, they remain in the primary-group sphere because experts are not prepared to deal with them. Many important individual and social matters must be decided by untrained persons. These include such questions as: What is the "best practice" in child rearing? What does one have to do to attain marital happiness? What is the best way to help an aged parent who has been independent all his life and now should be assisted? What criteria should one employ in selecting a mate? The contribution of an expert is of limited value in deciding such issues and problems; their resolution relies heavily on the experience and folk wisdom of persons in primary or reference groups.

Category three includes those infrequent happenings, such as floods, fires, or earthquakes, for which special preparation would be wasteful. These events are unique, and responses to them cannot be predicted or patterned; their anticipation must be limited to considerations of community survival. Preparing individuals for definite roles in connection with events of unusual character would constitute a squandering of talent. Furthermore, observation and experience reveal that individuals involved in disasters turn nearly exclusively to family members to provide succor and comfort. Survivors of disasters are generally unable to function effectively in rescue-and-help roles until they are apprised of the fates of family members. Rescue or service agencies are not sought out at such times to satisfy emotional needs, even when they are prepared to extend this type of help.

These functional adaptations among structurally different organizations are viewed as illustrations of the manner in which two parties, having identified areas of common concern, might mitigate their hostilities and accommodate their differences. This should not be permitted to overshadow awareness that both cooperation and contest are operative and perceptible. Areas in which bureaucratic-familial relations are mutually supportive coexist with others in which relations are not so well adjusted. This fact concerns us here because conditions of widespread social change are likely to affect the direction of interinstitutional relations; new points of conflict and cooperation will emerge.

THE LINKAGE, LIFE SECTOR, AND OPTION CONCEPTS

Linkage

Despite these bases for the structural efficiency and functionality of family-bureaucratic organizational relationships, a division of labor and complementarity of functions does not exist universally in the real world, where structures have disparate goals, procedures, and roles. Actually, there are overlapping areas of ambiguity in the functions and activities of the family and bureaucracies, and competition often borders on conflict over control of interactions.

One important reason for the persistence of the family in modern society is its role in the linkage process; it counteracts domination by bureaucratic organizations through using interstitial groups and socializing its members for competence in linking roles. Consequently, it is appropriate to analyze the socio-psychological bases of linkage for the family.

The linkage phenomenon is based on a number of assumptions. First, it is both a process and a condition interrelating groups, organizations, and individuals. The particular pattern is the linkage condition; how it is formed is the process. A second assumption is that in any linkage, especially between structures, it is possible for one participant to be or become subordinate or superordinate to the other, even after institutionalization of the relationship has occurred. Consequently, in any relationship, the family can be in a superordinate position wielding influence and affecting the policy, structure, and activities of bureaucratic organizations. Or it can be subordinate, accommodating the normative demands of the formal structures.

Another assumption is that the family can optimize its possibilities of survival, enjoy some quality of life, and sustain intact its interactional system and territory if members develop handling, manipulating, and mediating skills in linkage activity. Competence in interpersonal relationships, use of options, and problem solving are prerequisite and appropriate activities of a family socialization system [3,18,27]. Still another assumption is that linkage operates within some system of reciprocity based on bargaining. Specific exchanges are of unequal value; reciprocity is maintained when each bargaining part receives sufficient payoff to maintain the relationship, rather than accept the alternative of breaking off [4,13,17,19].

Life Sectors

In highly complex industrial societies diverse services are performed by rapidly expanding bureaucratic organizations with elaborate administrative mechanisms. Individuals in primary groups are thrust into a bewildering maze of interrelationships. An individual in contemporary society has so many options that it has become analytically useful to create the concept of life-sector categories of major activities. A life sector is an area of activity usually occurring in a defined territory and which can be observed to have a beginning, duration, and an end in time. Life-sector categories include economic, governmental, health, leisure, residential, and family activities. It is presumed that individuals and groups function within these areas to meet their needs and achieve their objectives.

Options

Options are opportunities available to a family member or a family for role participation in different life sectors. The availability, knowledge, use, and successful outcome of an option sequence depend upon cultural, structural, experiential, situational, and personality factors [21,25].

The option sequence begins with availability and optimally ends with a successful outcome. Steps after option availability include: awareness of all possible options; knowledge of routes to option use; selection of one or more options; training or socialization into role behavior requisite for appropriate utilization of the option; and option outcome, the goal of the option sequence.

One linkage point is the family's initial contact with bureaucratic organizations concerned with medical treatment and rehabilitation in the health life sector. The availability of medical care and rehabilitation options depends on: the financial position of family; knowledge, awareness, and motivation of family members including the patient; and location of kin, friends, and peer group members.

Awareness of options may come from a number of sources, including linkage groups and bureaucratic organizations. At this stage of the option sequence, the personal resources, motivation, needs, and objectives of family members are determinants of the type and extent of the linking role to be performed in behalf of the family. In addition to the information on health care options provided by linkage groups and bureaucratic organizations; kin, peers, friends, and work colleagues may be sources of knowledge. Also, knowledge of health care may be obtained from the mass media and other communication and education sources.

Commencing with awareness of the routes to achieve the option, family members and representatives of linkage groups activate linkage roles until an option outcome is achieved. Here is a strategic point in the linkage sequence. Awareness of options and awareness of routes to option achievement are two distinctively different phenomena. Option awareness implies knowledge of theoretical possibilities of adequate treatment and rehabilitation for the family member, while awareness of routes involves a realistic appraisal of available health care facilities given the variety of constraints already enumerated.

A decision regarding the selection of one or more options depends initially upon an appraisal of realistic possibilities of achieving the option outcome. It is at this stage of the option sequence that a particular service is selected. If options for health care are restricted because of discrimination, a special interest group or voluntary association may be sought to assist in increasing options in this area. In some instances, the family may become the target of selection for betterment because a particular community action group feels that increasing options in health care for the mentally and physically ill is in the best interests of the larger society.

If options in health care are restricted because of limited funds and high costs of services, there may be a joining with linking institutions which are part of the marketing system. A credit union, consumer's organization, mutual benefit society, or kinship group may be able to assist with information, money, and other services connected with the care of the ill member. This selection process does not preclude the joining or a linkage group for more general reasons, e.g., to promote harmonious relationships, effective communication, or improve living conditions.

All members of families take on linking roles at some time during the family life cycle and their own life course. Some of these roles are initiated by the family and others by outside groups and organizations. Circumstances, situations, age and sex of members, family needs and objectives, the presence or absence of linking groups, and policies and programs of bureaucratic organizations regarding linkage are among the factors that determine whether the individual family member takes the iniative in linking with bureaucratic organizations. These factors also determine if the family representative uses an interstitial mediating group to effect linkages. The extent to which a member will take on linking roles on behalf of the family depends upon the skill of the particular individual, level of need, motivation for achieving specific family objectives, and interaction patterns within the family.

This illustration indicates that family members are not passively acted upon by the needs or demands of bureaucratic organizations. Linking activities are endemic to the family. Taking on linking roles provides opportunities for changing one's status and power position within the family. Linking roles are essentially socializing ones. The family representative or linker develops skills and knowledge for handling bureaucratic organizations and uses these to meet family needs and objectives in a particular life sector. He may teach other family members or hide his expertise in an assumed aura of ignorance in order to maintain position within the family. A more sanguine view is that the linker acts in the family's best interest and socializes other members for competence sufficiently for them to function in behalf of the family without necessarily jeopardizing his or her status as an expert in this particular linking role.

Although some family members are expert linkers, possess generalized competencies, and can initiate linking activities in a variety of life sectors, they tend to work in particular sectors with a set number of linkage groups and bureaucratic organizations. In consonance with our conceptualization of differentiation into the life sectors of contemporary urban life, a single family member is not likely to be *the* linker for the entire family. In traditional or transitional societies in early stages of development, one family member may link the family to organizations in all life sectors. Rural immigrants to urban areas may also have one family member function as the linker until other members become acculturated and socialized into modern roles which involve linkage activity.

LINKAGE-RECIPROCITY MODEL

Linkage involves a system of exchanges of unequal value within expectations of reciprocity and continuous bargaining by representatives of groups and organizations for a preferred advantage in the linking relationship. Real or perceived payoffs must occur in order to sustain linkages.

Bargaining is encountered more frequently where linkages are based on choice rather than compulsion. There is voluntary entrance and egress from the linkage compact and there is the possibility of leaving the linkage if the payoff is deemed inadequate. Even where cultural prescription, legal edict, or tradition bind a family to a linkage group or bureaucratic organization, bargaining of a different order ensues. Techniques ranging from "putting on" to "putting down" a form of confrontation are used. An up-to-date variant of confrontation is "Gheraos," used most successfully in India in labor-management linkages and in Japan in student-university nexuses [14,1]. It is an organized physical act of holding an authority figure, performed by a group of individuals, students, workers, irate ADC mothers, and so forth, who do not want the "blood" of the organizational functionary but are willing to hold the official without food until he gives in to their demands. There are similar bargaining tactics in total care institutions where individuals organize to change their position in a system they cannot voluntarily leave.

Exchange, reciprocity, bargaining and the specific tactics used in gaining an advantage in any relationship are characteristic of all combinations of linkages. If linkage groups such as the Ombudsman-type do not provide payoffs for the family; the family will try to join one which does, or work to change the leadership, or decide to deal directly with the bureaucratic organization. Linkage groups, especially those which work so that they become quasi-bureaucratic in structure, may over time institutionalize norms, policies, and procedures. They thereby lose the flexibility which enabled them to perform adequate integration activities between the family and the bureaucratic organization and to meet the particular needs of primary groups.

In presenting a word diagram of a reciprocity-linkage model it should be emphasized that reciprocity does not automatically mean harmonious exchanges based on a rational approach to human interaction. Group life has to accommodate a number of contradictory processes, goals, and norms. Conflict is endemic to all human interaction, but so is accommodation. Achievement of individual, group, or organizational goals is counterbalanced by situations requiring cooperation among structures; *other-* rather than *self-oriented* activities in order to achieve desirable goals which command total resources. Goals are superordinate, that is, they are not the sole property of a single structure and require reciprocal action with commonly shared expectations.

Given the available theoretical postures, ours recognizes that if a structure or group provides what individuals need and desire, then it has functionality for these participants. Systems of relationships are woven into a matrix of reciprocity—exchanges of unequal amounts and of different types received by interacting individuals or groups. Structures are maintained and have functionality, or they go out of business, or become dysfunctional according to the effectiveness of reciprocity networks.

For the purposes of illustrating this model (see Figure 14-1) I have selected the family and the school. Each structure has goals; a set of identities; a role system to handle internal and external interaction; a commonly shared set of expectations; an ideology which defines relationships; and a conceptual posture

Figure 14-1   Reciprocity-Linkage Word Model

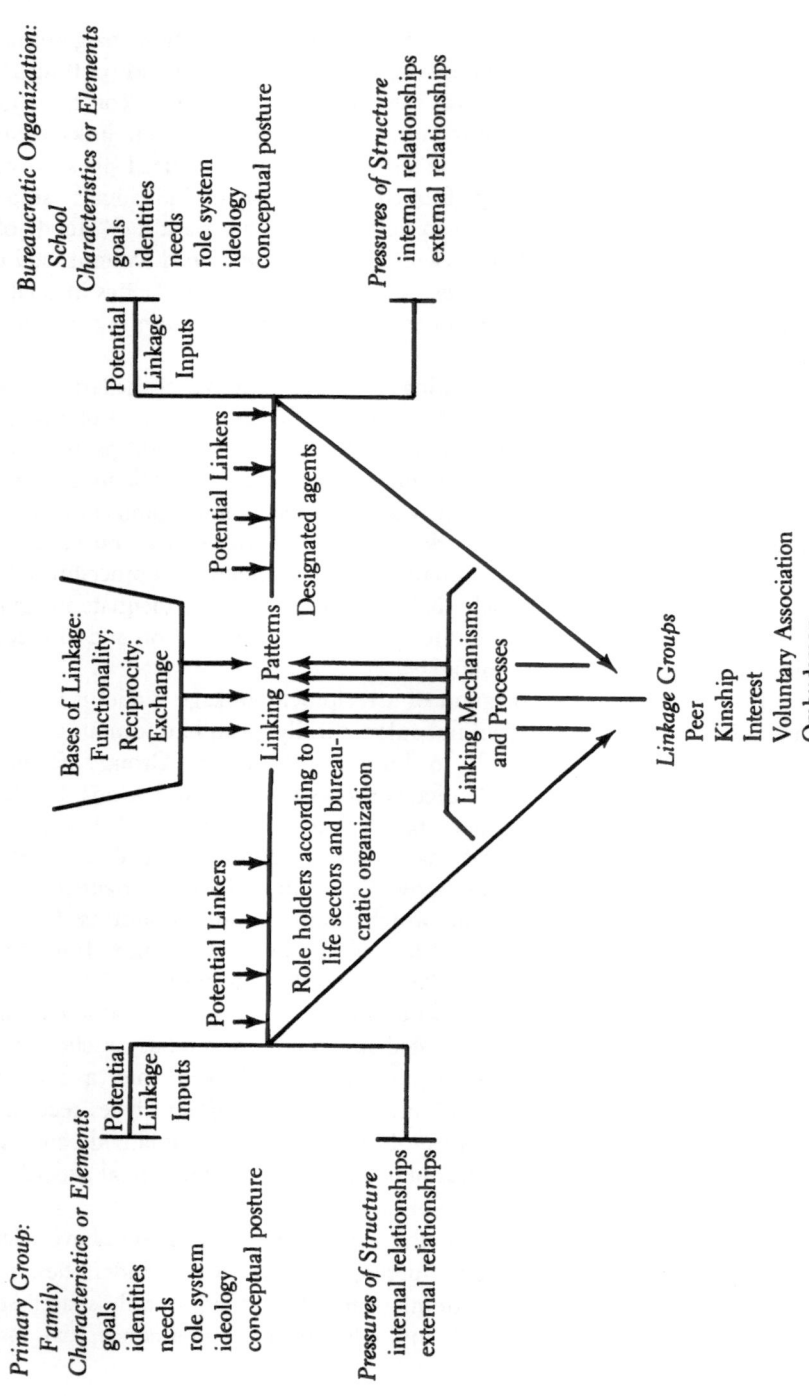

for viewing, interpreting, and reacting to ideas, situations, interactions, and so forth. Virtually all characteristics and elements of structure can be listed as linkage inputs since they may either facilitate or constrain interaction between the family, linkage group, and bureaucratic organization.

The internal structure pressures of any system are directed toward two problems: (1) internal relationships, and (2) external relationships. These are considered to be potential linkage inputs. The constant pressure within the structure is to modify the existing arrangements of superordination-subordination (status), power, socialization of novices, decision-making processes, and patterns of influence and cooperation. External structures provide "options" as well as pressures for individuals to use in readjusting roles, identities, goals, conceptual apparatus, and so forth—both within the family and in extrafamilial relationships.

In this illustration the external structure, the school, is seeking to educate family members for the purpose of assuming so-called modern identities and roles. Family members, mostly children in this situation, are school agents in carrying inputs back to the family and thus introducing additional pressure on the internal structure of the family. The reciprocal of this school family process is also operating. The family school process creates forces to change input demands of schools varying according to level of modernism, existence and activities of linking associations, location and origins of educational system, and other factors.

Any member of the family can be a potential family linker and the emergence of a particular one is dependent upon which life sector and bureaucratic organization are involved, as well as internal family relationships. For the bureaucratic organization, on the other hand, the linkers are likely to be designated and assigned to these roles. Actual linking functions may be carried out by nonassigned persons through the informal network of the bureaucratic organization.

Peer, kinship, interest, voluntary association, or Ombudsman linkage groups—"third party" structures—may be referred to and used by both the family and the school. The approach and extent of use of these linkage groups in mediating and advocating activities depend on whose "farm club" is the linkage group. Does it "belong" to the family or the bureaucratic organization?

Linking-bases provide the rationale for the linking process, and "payoff" is its most important product. Linkage mechanisms involve communication between structures and interactional relationships of "linkers" such as child, parent, or teacher within and between both structures. The processes are reciprocal acts and imposed self-constraints. Reduction of the differences in cognitive styles is also a critical process. Conflict between the two structures is limited (effecting cooperation) through the development of mutual aid patterns and the delimitation of the pressure for dominance of structural inputs in relationships with other structures. A rapprochement involving shared responsibilities and competition without annihilation is a necessary condition of interstructure relationships. The linkage mechanisms and processes operate within a two-way funnel system between structures.

SUMMARY

In this chapter I have defined terms and variables and analyzed the structures and functions of bureaucracies and various family forms. I viewed linkage from within the family and surveyed how families form connections with groups and organizations in various life sectors, initiate the linking process, try to develop the competence of its members in linking roles in order to handle and manipulate bureaucratic organizations, and create and use linking groups. This analysis of linkage has been largely ignored in conceptualizing primary group—bureaucratic organizational relationships.

On the conceptual level, a paradigm of the linkage process involving primary structures, interstitial groups, and bureaucratic organizations was suggested; the relationship between the linkage process and the option sequence was proposed; and the theoretical bases for a linkage network, whether it has volunteer or conscripted participants, was presented.

Much of sociological inquiry has been concerned with the problem of ordering this interaction at the primary group level, and a number of theoretical models have been developed to account for both internal and external sociobehavioral characteristics of such groups. Linkage theory is a conceptual framework which explains the interface between primary groups and institutions. Three major positions have been taken concerning this relationship. According to Max Weber, the norms, objectives, practices, and ideologies of families and institutions are so contradictory that conflict between the two is inevitable [27]. Talcott Parsons, while acknowledging the presence of conflict, reemphasizes the diametric opposition and perpetual conflict posited by Weber. Conflicting norms, goals, and means do exist, but both family and institution can function smoothly if they are isolated from each other [15].

Litwak and Meyer have developed a synthesis of these theoretical postures suggesting a "balance theory of coordination between bureaucracy and primary groups" [10]. Again, conflict is an acknowledged component of the relationship, but the suggested posture is more moderate than that of either Parsons or Weber. These is a way to develop balance between primary groups and more formal organizations since each system has different purposes and structure and hence performs different functions. Formal organizations operate on principles of logic, rational thought, merit, mobility, specialization, and differentiation and are best suited to achieve standardized outcomes. Primary groups, such as families, are best suited to handle more idiosyncratic and less repetitive events and behaviors.

A human service organization—a formal organization—can provide clients with a monthly check, pay Medicaid fees, and provide homemaker services. The family—a primary group—neutralizes severe crises and stress with expressions of love, intimacy, solidarity, and care.

The needs of individuals are best satisfied by the functions performed by both of these two diverse systems, the bureaucracy and the primary group: "Coordination between the primary group and bureaucracy is requisite for survival and harmonious relationships, and such coordination is effected when groups and institutions are close enough but not too close" (Sussman, 1977b). If the bureaucratic institution and the family are too far apart or too near, the results are fear, suspicion, and a lack of cooperation.

Although the family is often thought of as being subordinate to the bureaucracy; in any relationship the family can be in a superordinate position, wielding influence and affecting the policy, structure, and activities of bureaucratic organizations. It is precisely this superordinate position of the family which is of interest here, since theoretically the family can bring to bear a significant amount of power and control in a given situation. In order to do so, however, the family members must have knowledge, solidarity, and cohesion equal to the task. In the 1980s families will be on the move in relation to bureaucracies: organizing, making representations, and using linkage groups to develop a satisfactory complementarity with large-scale organizations.

REFERENCES

1. Aoi, K. and Morioka, J. Personal communication on these tactics used in Japan in the 1960s, 1970.
2. Dobrof, R. and Litwak, E. *Maintenance of Family Ties of Long Term Care Patients: Theory and Guide to Practice*. U.S. Department of Health, Education and Welfare Publication, ADM 77-400, 1977.
3. Foote, N. and Cottrell, L.S., Jr. *Identity and Interpersonal Competence*, Chicago: University of Chicago Press, 1955.
4. Levi-Strauss, C. "The principle of reciprocity," In: Lewis A. Coser & Bernard Rosenberg (eds.) *Sociological Theory* New York: MacMillan, 1957, pp. 204–294.
5. Litwak, E. "Extended kin relations in an industrial democratic society." In: Ethel Shanas & Gordon F. Streib (eds.) *Social Structure and the Family: Generational Relations*. Englewood Cliffs, NJ: Prentice-Hall, 1965, pp. 290–323.
6. Litwak, E. Occupational mobility and extended family cohesion." *American Sociological Review* 25 : 9–21, February 1960a.
7. Litwak, E. "Geographic mobility and extended family cohesion." *American Sociological Review* 25 : 385–394 June 1960b.
8. Litwak, E. and Figueria, J. "Technical innovation and theoretical functions of primary groups and bureaucratic structures." *American Journal of Sociology* 73 : 468–81, 1968.
9. Litwak, E. and Meyer, H.J *School Family and Neighborhood: The Theory and Practice of School-Community Relations*. New York, 1974.

10. Litwak, E. and Meyer, H.J. "A balanced theory of coordination between bureaucratic organizations and community primary groups." *Administrative Science Quarterly* 11 : 31–58, June 1966.
11. Litwak, E. and Meyer, H.J. Administrative styles and community linkages of public schools: some theoretical considerations. In: A. Reiss (ed.) *Schools in a Changing Society*. New York: The Free Press, 1965.
12. Litwak, E.; Meyer, H.; and Hollister, D. "Theories of linkage between bureaucracies and community primary groups—education, health and political action as empirical cases in point." Paper presented at the *Annual Meeting of the American Sociological Association*, Montreal, Canada, 1974.
13. Mauss, M. *The Gift, Forms and Functions of Exchange in Archaic Societies*, translated by Ian Gunnison, London: Cohen & West Ltd., 1954.
14. *(The) New York Times. Dispatch from New Delhi, India*, August 10, 1969.
15. Parsons, T. and Bales, R.F. *Family Socialization and Interaction Process*, Glencoe, IL.: The Free Press, 1960.
16. Ross, H.R. *How to Develop a Neighborhood Family, An Action Manual*. Miami, FL.: Northside Neighborhood Family Services, Inc., 1978.
17. Schelling R. *The Strategy of Conflict*. Cambridge, MA.: Harvard University Press, 1960.
18. Smith, M.B. "Competence and socialization." In: John A. Clausen, (ed.) *Socialization and Society*. Boston: Little, Brown, 1968.
19. Thibault, J.W. and Kelly, H.H. *The Social Psychology of Groups*. New York: Wiley & Sons, 1959.
20. Sussman, M.B. "The family today: is it an endangered species?" *Children Today* 48 : 32–37, March–April 1978.
21. Sussman, M.B. "Family, bureaucracy and the elderly individual: an organization/linkage perspective." In: Ethel Shanas and Marvin B. Sussman (eds.) *Family, Bureaucracy and the Elderly*. Durham, NC.: Duke University Press, 1977, pp. 2–20.
22. Sussman, M.B. "Adaptive, directive and integrative behavior of today's family." *Family Process* 7 : 239–250, September 1968.
23. Sussman, M.B. "Relationships of adult children with their parents in the United States." In: Ethel Shanas and Gordon Steib, (eds.) *Social Structure and the Family: Generational Relations*. Englewood Cliffs, NJ: Prentice-Hall 1965, pp. 62–92.
24. Sussman, M.B. and Burchinal, L.G. "Kin family network: unheralded structure in current conceptualizations of family functioning." *Marriage and Family Living* 24 : 231–240. 1962a.
25. Sussman, M.B. and Burchinal, L.G. "Parental aid to married children: implications for family functioning." *Marriage and Family Living* 24 : 320–332, 1962b.
26. Sussman, M.B. and Brooks, M. "Comparative family research: a nine nation study." In: H.Y. Tien and F.D. Bean (eds.) *Comparative Family and Fertility Research*. Leiden, Holland: E.J. Brill, 1975, pp. 73–89.
27. Weber, M. *The Theory of Social and Economic Organizations*. Translated by A.M. Henderson and Talcott. Glencoe, IL: Free Press, 1947.
28. White, R. "Motivation reconsidered: the concept of competence." *Psychological Review* 66 : 297–333, September 1959.

15

The Family of the Chronic Mentally Ill Patient: Ally or Adversary?

STANLEY E. WEINSTEIN

The past 25 years have been a period of growth for mental health movements that have had great impact on the care of the chronic mentally ill patient. Foremost developments were the introduction of the tranquilizer and psychoactive drugs and an emphasis on deinstitutionalization. The community mental health movement, highlighted by the 1963 Community Mental Health Act, provided the impetus for a shift that has taken thousands of patients from state hospitals back to their communities. According to the U.S. Bureau of Census, persons in mental institutions represented the highest percentage of persons institutionalized in 1950 and 1960. This number one rating was relinquished in 1970 [32]. Institutions caring for the aged and dependent are now responsible for the largest percentage of institutionalized persons. Although care has shifted away from mental institutions, the number of new patients being diagnosed as schizophrenic continues to increase beyond the overall percentage increase anticipated in the general population in this country. The reason for this increase is that although there is a decrease in the population growth rate, there is an increase in the population between the ages of 15–44—the ages in which schizophrenia has the highest incidence rate [32]. Attention to schizophrenics is important because, excluding alcoholics, schizophrenics comprise the largest population of chronic mentally ill patients. There were approximately 1,111,389 schizophrenics under care in1977–78 [31]. Chronic mentally ill patients are those in whom the disability is present for a long period of time and involves continuity of hospitalization and/or a number of hospitalizations [31].

These past 25 years have also seen the development of two significant movements having direct involvement with the chronic mentally ill: the self-help movement and the widespread use of family therapy as a treatment modality. Since the family constitutes the primary natural support system, one would assume that these movements would develop side by side. Such is not the case, and this chapter examines how they have developed and the obstacles to the involvement of families as allies with mental health professionals in the treatment of chronic mentally ill patients.

SELF-HELP GROUPS FOR THE MENTALLY ILL

The development of self-help groups can be viewed, according to Levy, as a political and sociological phenomenon as well as a psychological one. These groups are often perceived as a response to the failure of society to meet the needs of its members [26]. Alcoholics Anonymous (1935) and Recovery, Inc. (1937) were the start of the self-help movement for individuals with problems that were not being successfully treated or cured by professional mental health groups. Since then, numerous self-help groups have developed, such as: Schizophrenics Anonymous (1962), Terrap (1964), Neurotics Anonymous (1964), The American Schizophrenic Association (1969), Emotions Anonymous (1971), Families Anonymous (1971), Phobia Self-Help Groups (1972), The Samaritans (1974), Manic-Depressive Association (1975), National Anorexic Aid Society (1977), Depressive Anonymous (1978), and Survivors of Suicide Victims (1978) [14]. This list is far from complete but it indicates the rapid rise in such groups during the 1960s and 1970s. Katz and Bender [22] suggest that people join self-help groups for two major reasons: (1) many individuals feel rejected and frustrated by the larger society and its institutions and feel powerless over decisions made affecting them, and (2) many of these people feel manipulated, categorized, and depersonalized.

Levy [27] lists five conditions for a self-help group:

1. The primary purpose is to ". . . help and support its members in dealing with their problems and in improving their psychological functioning and effectiveness."

2. The origin and sanction of the group rests with the members themselves.

3. "It relies upon its own member's efforts, skills, knowledge, and concerns as its primary source of help, with the structure of the relationship between its members being one of peers, so far as help-giving and support are concerned."

4. It is composed of members sharing a "common core of life experience and problems."

5. Members control the group's structure and operation.

Katz and Bender [22] provide the following definition of self-help groups:

Self-help groups are voluntary, small group structures for mutual aid and the accomplishment of a special purpose. They are usually formed by peers who have come together for mutual assistance in satisfying a common need, overcoming a common handicap or life-disrupting problem, and bringing about desired social and/or personal change. The initiators and members of such groups perceive that their needs are not, or cannot, be met by or through existing social institutions. Self-help groups emphasize face-to-face social interactions and the assumption of personal responsibility by members. They often provide material assistance, as well as emotional support; they are frequently 'cause' oriented, and promulgate an ideology or values through which members may attain an enhanced sense of personal identity.

There are many reasons why self-help groups have developed so rapidly and are involved in so many areas. Gardner and Riessman suggest that it is partly because of the "do-it-yourself ethos in the society" and fiscal constraints [13]. After studying different kinds of self-help groups, Levy reported that the groups are ". . . not only trying to help their members deal with their identified problems, but they are also serving to meet their members' most fundamental human needs—needs for empathic understanding, for enhanced self-esteem, for meaning, and for an opportunity to express their feelings and share their experiences with another."

Although self-help groups have typically been composed of, and provided for, individual patients, other organizations have developed to serve the family. Groups for families include those with a member who has autism, mental retardation, and more recently, schizophrenia. Some of these groups include: Alliance for the Mentally Ill (Wisconsin), California Association, Families of the Mentally Disabled, Family and Friends of the Mentally Ill (Mississippi and South Carolina), Parents of Adult Mentally Ill (Georgia), Schizophrenia Support Group (Washington), and Threshold (Maryland) [26]. Hatfield reports how a new relative and consumer movement in support of individuals with major mental illness has developed in the late 1970s and how in 1979 100 of these groups came together and formed the National Alliance for the Mentally Ill [18]. The objectives of this organization are:

- Coordination of activities of state and local advocacy groups
- Serving as an information collection and dissemination center
- Monitoring existing health care facilities, staff, and programming for adequacy and accountability
- Promotion of new and remedial legislation
- Fostering public education
- Promotion of community support programs, including appropriate living arrangements linked with supportive social and vocational rehabilitation, and employment programs

- Providing for family support
- Promotion of research (preventive, treatment, rehabilitation and cure)
- Delineation and enforcement of patient and family rights
- Liaison with other national and international mental health organizations
- Promotion of alternative treatment modalities

There have been a few studies on self-help groups for relatives of schizophrenic patients. Levy studied the National Schizophrenic Fellowship—a self-help group whose members consist mainly of parents of schizophrenics in England [25]. This organization has 140 branches and 3,300 families. Few individuals with schizophrenia are members, even though they could join. Levy found, as did Hatfield, who studied the Schizophrenic Association of Greater Washington, that most members were parents, female, and middle class [19,21].

SCHIZOPHRENIA AND CHRONIC MENTAL ILLNESS

There has been some confusion as to whether all individuals diagnosed as schizophrenic are chronically mentally ill. Often the two are perceived as synonymous by clinicians, families, and statisticians. In recent years there has been some awareness of the difference in diagnosis and treatment of the patient with an acute psychotic episode and that of the patient who is psychotic and chronically mentally ill. This results from the idea that duration of symptomatology is a major variable in treatment, prognosis, and, now, diagnosis.

The American Psychiatric Association defines "Schizophrenic Disorders" as those containing psychotic features, including delusions, hallucinations, or certain thought disturbances. The onset occurs before age 45 and has a duration of at least six months [2]. This is differentiated from the new diagnostic category, the "Schizophreniform Disorder" which is of less than six months duration. Other aspects of the schizophrenic disorder include an anticipated recurrence and deterioration of both social and occupational functioning: "The prognosis is especially poor when the prodromal phase has taken an insidious downhill course over many years" [2].

Diagnostic criteria have been described, but what about etiology? A recent editorial in the *Journal of Nervous and Mental Disease* addressed the reality and frustration of the limited knowledge concerning mental illness and possibly, in particular, knowledge of chronic mental illness. Dr. David Mechanic wrote: "The disturbing fact is that explanations of mental illness are so numerous because we know so little. In a scientific vacuum anything goes, and there has been no shortage of people willing to expand their favorite theories" [30].

A disease has been categorized and diagnosed; the cause is unknown; now the question of treatment arises. May comments:

Given the level of care that is now available and the treatment methods that are commonly used, about one-third of all schizophrenic patients will do relatively well and return to a reasonable level of functioning. One third will become hard core failures, continually more or less severely disabled and spending a great part of their lives in hospitals and under equivalent protection and support. The remainder, the partial treatment failures, will occupy an intermediate status. [29].

The one-third that will do relatively well are probably those now considered suffering not from schizophrenia, but from a schizophreniform disorder. This conclusion was reached based on the American Psychiatric Association statement on the treatment of schizophrenia: "A complete return to premorbid functioning is unusual, so rare in fact, that some clinicians would question the diagnosis" [2].

FAMILY THERAPY AND SCHIZOPHRENIA

The development of family therapy as a treatment modality and the use of family dynamics as an explanation for the etiology of symptomatic behavior occurred in large part over the last 25 years. Although Nathan Ackerman has been considered the founding father of family therapy, there were a number of events that contributed to this development [9]. The first was the child guidance movement in which not only the child patient, but a parent (usually the mother) was brought into treatment. The second contributing event was the numerous research projects investigating schizophrenia following World War II. Sullivan looked at relationships [34], Fromm-Reichmann wrote on the "schizophrenogenic mother" [11], and other researchers studied schizophrenics and their families [7,38,29]. Much of the early literature on family therapy centered on the family with a schizophrenic member, usually an adolescent or young adult. In 1956, Bateson, Jackson, Haley, and Weakland published a paper titled, "Toward a Theory of Schizophrenia" which described how the "double bind" pattern of communication found within a family can lead to schizophrenic symptoms and how relationships within the family lead to this situation [6]. Haley also described in one of his earlier books how to treat families with a schizophrenic member [17]. Bowen studied families with a schizophrenic member and wrote that schizophrenia was a generalized family problem ("the family as the unit of illness") and that family psychotherapy was the treatment of choice [7]. In the past few years, however, Bowen has modified his previous enthusiasm and indicated that it is extremely difficult to change the fundamental structure of the family with a schizophrenic member [8]. Ackerman indicated that family therapy can be useful in the treatment of psychosis [1]. This inference, made primarily from research attempts to understand the process of schizophrenia and characteristics of families in which there was a schizophrenic member, led to recommendations for treatment. Whether fully intended or not, family therapy was being presented as the treatment of choice for schizophrenia. The literature did not, however, usually differentiate between acute schizophrenia (now the schizophreniform disorder) and a chronic schizophrenic patient. The literature has also published very few outcome studies of family therapy with such families. Rubinstein reviewed the literature on the use of family therapy for schizophrenia and concluded that the family of the schizophrenic is a "complex system," and that schizophrenic behavior is not easily modified [33]. At this time there is no evidence that family therapy or any other known psychotherapy or somatic treatment will *cure* a chronic mentally ill patient. This does not mean that mental health professionals cannot help these patients and their families lead more productive lives with more options for them as individuals and as a family.

In the past decade there has been a renewed emphasis on the psychosocial aspects of the chronic patient; and this has led to the development of a number of model programs [4]. Some of these programs have shown successful ways in which a chronic mentally ill individual can be helped with independent living, employment, and social relations. However, there are views that differ in regard to whether to include the family. One view is that the family is antitherapeutic and creates an environment which perpetuates or exacerbates the disability [36]. Those who support this position often want to exclude the family and focus completely on the individual and his capabilities. The opposing view is that the families have been burdened by the mentally ill relative and need help in coping with the situation [23]. Obviously, there is a grey area in between in which therapists may be ambivalent regarding the involvement of the family but welcome the support that they can provide for the patient and the treatment program. This support is frequently different than the expectation for participation they have from other patients and families. The literature on family therapy has not adequately addressed the treatment of the chronic mentally ill and their families. Recently, a small number of family therapists began to confront this problem and there are reports of referrals being made from state hospitals to family therapy clinics for the treatment of chronic mentally ill patients.

Besides differentiating between the schizophreniform patient and the chronic mentally ill patient, therapists need to begin exploring the differences between the chronic mentally ill who have been hospitalized and/or institutionalized, and those chronic mentally ill who have never been hospitalized. Since the recent emphasis on deinstitutionalization, a new population of chronic patients have come for treatment and many will not be hospitalized. Acute and chronic schizophrenic patients have too often been perceived by family therapists as a homogeneous group when it comes to treatment approaches. However, the goals, skills and attitudes of therapists working with chronic patients are different than those required for traditional family therapy; these differences need to be reflected in the treatment program.

SELF-HELP GROUP FAMILIES AND FAMILY THERAPY

In the past, most university programs and community mental health centers have given low priority to the chronic mentally ill. Some reasons for this are: the lack of satisfaction for the clinician; the multiple problems presented by many patients, including lack of basic living skills; the social distance between many therapists and schizophrenic patients; and the lack of resources of both the patient and the community mental health system to address these problems: "Chronic populations are frequently classified as 'hopeless' by the mental health profession . . ." [31]. Often a diagnosis of schizophrenia is to a mental health professional what the diagnosis of cancer is to a general practitioner of medicine. One means the death of the body and the other means the death of the functioning mind. "Hope" has been a significant variable in all forms of psychotherapy [10], but unfortunately, mental health professionals have often given up hope for these patients and see life in a state hospital as the inevitable outcome. Talbott reported on a recent survey in a professional newsletter in which every member of the American Psychiatric Association, as well as each council committee and district branch, were asked for their opinion on the problems "engendered and encountered by chronic mental patients" [35]. Only 156 responses were received from a membership of 25,000, giving some indication of the interest in this problem as shown by much of the professional community.

With the recent emphasis on deinstitutionalization, most of these patients are being discharged to their families [19,31]. Many mental health professionals and community programs have not attempted to provide mental health programs for these patients and their families. In this connection, Talbott recently wrote: "All segments of society should be aware of the fact that we are dealing with care, not cure . . .," when referring to the chronic mentally ill [35]. This is not intended to mean that they cannot be significantly helped. Even though *cure* is seldom a realistic goal for many diagnosed mental illnesses the improbability of cure is often taken as evidence that nothing can be done. Earlier theories of schizophrenia and this absence of hope are perceived by families as abandonment by the mental health profession, as punishment for producing a chronic mentally ill relative. Appleton reports:

In spite of theories of double-bind, schizophrenogenic mother, and infantile trauma, we have no evidence that the mothers of schizophrenics caused their children's illness. In many cases they have been taking care of youngsters who do not socialize, rarely smile back, are awkward, cannot learn and have temper outbursts, often without reason. Such mothers (and their husbands) should be given help and treated with respect rather than with subtle contempt.

The families of chronic mentally ill patients have organized and recently have begun telling the professionals what they want: "Families must assert their right to a life of their own. They have been maligned, and professionals have failed to see the suffering they endure" [21]. In line with this direction, Kanter finds: "Most relatives of schizophrenics are extremely sensitive to any suggestion whether implicit or explicit, that they are the cause of their relative's distress. They feel guilty and blamed by both client and community, yet somehow sense . . . that they are not solely responsible for their relative's disturbance" [23]. In Gardner's and Reissman's study of the self-help movement, they state: "Implicit in the self-help thrust is a profound critique of professionalism" [13]. Hatfield found that the majority of families found friends (84 percent) to be more helpful as a resource than therapy (55 percent). Persons with a mentally ill relative want to talk to others who have known the same experiences. They are sensitive to blame and believe that "Being a relative of a mentally ill person is devastating enough" [20]. Barter noted that "Families often feel depressed and guilty at their failure to be of more help to the patient . . ." [5]. Thus blame is a major issue between families and therapists; and in particular, family therapy—the use of which seems to imply that families are responsible. Psychoanalytically oriented psychotherapies have not only blamed parents but also have blocked family members' attempts to participate in the treatment. Even family therapies that indicate that the current life situation is responsible for the development of the symptoms may not adequately alleviate their burdens. The bind for many family members is that even though they may dislike the professionals, they are dependent on them for medication and hospitalization. Levy found that the attitude of family members toward professionals was "ambivalent" [25]. A conspiracy of mutual distrust often develops between the therapist and the family, and often the patient is in the middle.

FAMILY AND THERAPIST INCONGRUITIES

The concern over being blamed by mental health professionals is not unique to the families of the chronic mentally ill, but is often a concern by many families whenever psychiatric treatment is sought. The professional response should not be to "blame" but to hold families "responsible" for working with the therapist and the patient when they agree to be part of family therapy. The difference in the definition of these two words is crucial, because it determines the attitude that both families and mental health professionals bring to this cooperative therapeutic effort. According to Webster's New World Dictionary, the definition of *blame* is: "1. to accuse of being at fault; condemn (for something); censure 2. to find fault with (for something) 3. to put the responsibility of, as an error, fault, etc. (on someone or something)." The definition of *responsible* is: "1. expected or obliged to account (for something, to someone); answerable; accountable 2. involving accountability, obligation, or duties (a responsible position) . . ." [37].

Although therapists and families enter into treatment contracts with expectations that all parties be responsible, this does not necessarily have to develop into disapproval of the family; which constitutes blame. The lack of congruence between families and family therapists may be over the issue of "intentionality" which is not addressed by the definition of blame. Families do not intentionally make a relative schizophrenic, even if future research would indicate clearly that family functioning may be a contributing factor. Tentative data, derived from theorizing and unproven research, have unfortunately shaped the views of many mental health professionals. Most family therapists treat families as if they have not intended to make a mistake and therefore are not to be blamed. However, by indicating that the family needs to do something differently, the clinician is implying that something is not being done correctly or as well as possible. While many families reject the need for family therapy, they do indicate that they need help coping with a chronic mentally ill relative [19]. Family therapists can agree that families have been burdened; the dilemma is about the etiology of the problem, namely, is it linear or circular causality? Does the pathology originate in the individual or the family, or is it the interaction between the two? If a clinician believes the family has intentionally or unintentionally caused the pathology, he is apt to see their need to cope as a defense against the guilt that is inevitable in such a situation. In subtle ways, the therapist can blame the family. All data are tentative so perhaps it would be best to say that, at this stage: (1) there is no proof that families cause schizophrenia; (2) families need help in coping; (3) families can and should be responsible members of a treatment program to help chronic mentally ill relatives; and (4) future research should be supported to further explore these issues.

Another aspect of the incongruities between the families of chronic mentally ill patients and family therapists is shown in conflict over the definition of treatment problems. Therapists have frequently looked for cure or expect "normality," while families look for management and an absence of blame [16]. A family therapist might view hospitalization as a means of stabilizing the problem and keeping the family member dysfunctional [15]. The family, on the other hand, may see hospitalization as a respite for them and an opportunity for their relative to stop decompensating. The very statement that there is hope the patient may achieve normality can be disruptive to a family that has learned to cope by giving up hope.

SUMMARY

Self-help groups are less threatening than professional treatment and usually combine friendship and helping [24]. One unique feature of self-help groups is that both needy member and helper receive benefits [12]. Self-help groups are support systems by and for people with a shared experience and often a shared view of professionals. When one considers the lack of knowledge, the inability to cure, the theories that blame, and the lack of attention by the most skilled and experienced clinicians, it is not difficult to understand the plight of these families. Deinstitutionalization, while certainly more humane and appropriate than the alternative, has often placed the responsibility for the care of chronic mentally ill patients back on families.

This does not mean that families should determine treatment. However, many families have experienced a series of therapists and therapies without any positive results and they can easily question why they should continue in the process when there is little benefit for them or their relative. When the professional has not brought about any change in the functioning of the patient and recommends what the family perceives as unrealistic demands, he loses his credibility. Family therapists can and often do recognize the plight of families and also know that helping the family to change will lead to significant change and sometimes cure in a patient with psychotic symptoms. These patients have been capable of independent functioning and go on to live normal lives. However, those patients typically seen as chronically mentally ill may not respond, and it is not appropriate to consider "normality" as a realistic expectation. This is the dilemma: When does one shift one's expectations and goals from helping someone be normal and capable of independent living to helping a family live with and manage the behavior of a relative and offer him opportunities for a productive life? Is the cutting point the six months necessary to diagnose someone as schizophrenic? It is not possible to pick such a specific time due to our lack of knowledge and the range of capabilities and strengths available to families and individuals. A more realistic suggestion would be three to five years in which attempts to change the individual are initiated by a competent therapist. Family therapy can still be the treatment of choice because of its inherent supports and the investment families can make to help their relative. A major factor is the attitude of the therapist. However, after many attempts have failed, ". . . such families need advice concerning appropriate expectations for patients, specific techniques for managing disturbing behavior and the availability of community resources" [21].

How does a family therapist reconcile this need for hope and the expectation for normality with a family who needs help in managing an individual for whom "normality" is unrealistic? The answer might be to consider elements from both areas in cases in which normality has not been achieved in a reasonable period (more than six months). The family therapist must support the family while ascertaining the steps necessary to move the individual closer to appropriate developmental functioning. The goal is for a flexible model in which all available resources are utilized for optimal psychosocial and vocational functioning. The expectation of the therapist should be that the individual can achieve the next developmental step and that the family should be involved to achieve this step. As in all family therapy, congruence is needed between the family, the individual, and the therapist. Normality is to be considered a potentiality in these cases, but the day-to-day work is on the achievement of realistic tasks and goals for the chronic mentally ill patient. It is this congruence that often determines whether the family of the chronic mentally ill patient will be an ally or adversary.

REFERENCES

1. Ackerman, Nathan. "Family therapy." In: S. Arieti (ed.) *American Handbook of Psychiatry*, Vol. 3. New York : Basic Books, Inc., 1959.
2. American Psychiatric Association. *Diagnostic and Statistical Manual*, Third Edition. Washington D.C., 1980.
3. Appleton, William S. "Mistreatment of patients' families by psychiatrists." *American Journal of Psychiatry* 131 (6) June 1974.
4. Bachrach, Leona L. "Overview: model program for chronic mental patients." *American Journal of Psychiatry* 137 (9) September 1980.
5. Barter, James T. "Successful community programming for the chronic mental patient: principles and practices. In: John A. Talbott (ed.) *The Chronic Mental Patient*. Washington, D.C. : The American Psychiatric Association, 1978.
6. Bateson, Gregory; Jackson, Don D.; Haley, Jay; and Weakland, John. "Toward a theory of schizophrenia." *Behavioral Science* 1 (4) October 1956.
7. Bowen, Murray. "Family psychotherapy." *The American Journal of Orthopsychiatry* 31 (1) January 1961.
8. Bowen, Murray. *Family Therapy in Clinical Practice.* New York : Jason Aronson, 1977.
9. Brodkin, Adele M. "Family therapy: the making of a mental health movement." *American Journal of Orthopsychiatry* 50 (1) January 1980.
10. Frank, Jerome D. "Therapeutic components of psychotherapy." *Journal of Nervous & Mental Disease* 159 (5), 1974.
11. Fromm-Reichmann, F. "Notes on the development of treatment of schizophrenics by psychoanalytic psychotherapy." *Psychiatry* 11, 1948.
12. Gardner, Alan and Riessman, Frank. *Self-Help in the Human Services.* San Francisco : Jossey-Bass, 1977.

13. Gardner, Alan and Riessman, Frank. "Self-help models and consumer intensive health practice." *American Journal of Public Health* 66 (8), 1976.
14. Gardner, Alan and Riessman, Frank. *Help: A Working Guide to Self-Help Groups.* New York New Viewpoints, 1980.
15. Haley, Jay. *Leaving Home.* New York : McGraw-Hill, 1980.
16. Haley, Jay. *Problem Solving Therapy.* New York: Jossey-Bass, 1976.
17. Haley, Jay. *Strategies of Psychotherapy.* New York: Grune & Stratton, 1963.
18. Hatfield, Agnes. "Alliance for the mentally ill: a challenge to mental health delivery. Unpublished report, 1980.
19. Hatfield, Agnes B. "Help-seeking behavior in families of schizophrenics. *American Journal of Community Psychology* 7 (5), 1979.
20. Hatfield, Agnes and Howe, Carol. "Mutual help groups for families of the mentally ill. Unpublished report, September 1979.
21. Hatfield, Agnes B. "Psychological costs of schizophrenia to the family," *Social Work* 23 (5), September 1978.
22. Katz, Alfred H. and Bender, Eugene I. *The Strength of Us.* New York: New Viewpoints, 1976.
23. Kanter, Joel and Lin, Anchen. "Facilitating a therapeutic milieu in the families of schizophrenics." *Psychiatry* 43, May 1980.
24. Knight, Bob; Wollert, Richard W.; Levy, Leon H.; Frame, Cynthia L.; and Padgett, Valerie P. "Self-help groups: the member's perspectives." *American Journal of Community Psychology*, 1980.
25. Levy, Leo. "The national schizophrenia fellowship: an english self-help group." *Social Psychiatry*, in press.
26. Levy, Leon H. "Processes and activities in groups." In: M.A. Lieberman, L.D. Borman et al. *Self-Help Groups for Coping with Crisis.* San Francisco: Jossey-Bass, 1980, pp. 234–271.
27. Levy, Leon H. "Self-help groups viewed by mental health professionals: a survey and comments." *American Journal of Community Psychology* 6 (4), 1978.
28. Lidz, Theodore; Fleck, Stephen; Alanen, Yrjo; and Cornelison, Alice. "Schizophrenic patients and their siblings." *Psychiatric Journal for the Study of Interpersonal Process* 26 (1) February 1963.
29. May, Philip R.A., "Schizophrenia: overview of treatment methods." In: Alfred M. Freedman, Harold I. Kaplan, and Benjamin J. Sadock (eds.) *Comprehensive Textbook of Psychiatry* Vol. II Second Edition, Baltimore, MD : Williams & Wilkins 1975.
30. Mechanic, David. "Editorial: explanation of mental illness." *Journal of Nervous and Mental Disability* 166 (6), June 1978.
31. Minkoff, Kenneth. "A map of chronic mental patients." In: John A. Talbott (ed.) *The Chronic Mental Patient.* Washington, D.C.: The American Psychiatric Association, 1978.
32. National Institute of Mental Health. *Psychiatric Service and the Changing Institutional Scene,* 1950–1958. DHEW Publication No. (ADM) 77–433, Superintendent of Documents, U.S. Govt. Printing Office, Washington, D.C., 1977.
33. Rubinstein, David. "Family therapy of schizophrenia —where to? —what next? *Psychotherapy and Psychosomatics* 25, 1975.
34. Sullivan, Harry. *Interpersonal Theory of Psychiatry.* New York: W.W. Norton, 1953.
35. Talbott, John A. "What are the problems of the chronic mental patient—a report of a survey of psychiatrists' concerns." In: John A. Talbott (ed.) *The Chronic Mental Patient.* Washington, D.C.: The American Psychiatric Association, 1978.
36. Test, Mary and Stein, Leonard I. (eds.) *Alternative to Mental Hospital Treatment.* New york: Plenum Publishing Corp., 1978.
37. *Webster's New World Dictionary,* 2nd Edition, Guralnick, David B. (ed.) Cleveland OH and NY : William Collins & World Publishing Co., Inc., 1970.
38. Wynne, Lyman C. and Singer, Margaret T. "Thought disorders and family relations of schizophrenics." *Archives of General Psychiatry* 9, September 1963.

16

Family Therapy Supervision on a Psychiatric Inpatient Unit: Implications of an Ecological Epistemology

JOAN M. SCRATTON AND PATTI M. SEMAN

It has been observed that "the family therapy field is more sophisticated developmentally in its therapeutic methodologies than in the areas of training and supervision" [33]. A review of the literature lends support to that position and confirms the lack of any formalized body of theory about family therapy training and supervision. Kniskern and Gurman likewise note a paucity of research investigating family therapy training. This parallels the state of research on training in individual psychotherapy, a modality with a much longer history and acceptance within the psychiatric establishment [31]. Training in family therapy in both formal academic and free-standing institutes has by and large taken place under the auspices and influence of charismatic leaders in the family therapy field (e.g., Ackerman, Whitaker, Satir, Bowen, Nagy, Haley, Minuchin, and Palazzoli) whose theoretical assumptions have dictated the training and supervisory model. Notably missing from the literature is any specific reference to family therapy supervision in a psychiatric hospital—the subject of this chapter.

What follows is a description of family therapy supervision of psychiatric residents on an inpatient psychiatric unit of a university hospital. Implications for the application of an ecosystemic epistemology to a traditional psychodynamically oriented academic institution are addressed. Basic

There is no senior author of this paper which is a shared collaborative effort.

For the sake of literary clarity, the personal pronoun "he" has been adopted throughout this text except when specific reference is made to the primary family therapy supervisors on the inpatient unit, each of whom is female.

assumptions affecting choice of supervisory model and training goals and tasks are delineated. Significant aspects of the supervisory relationship and supervisory modality are examined from a systemic perspective.

TOWARD AN ECOLOGICAL EPISTEMOLOGY

The past two decades have witnessed a radical theoretical shift from predominantly psychodynamic and deterministic explanations of individual behavior toward an ecological paradigm. The ecosystemic perspective refocuses the unit of observation to the boundaries of living systems and their transactions. It is concerned with "the relations among living entities and between entities and other aspects of their environment" [21].

The significance of this perspective for clinical practice is that it offers an adaptive view of the individual in continuous mutual interpersonal transactions with the environment. This shift expands the meaning and function of human behavior beyond the essentially pessimistic constraints of psychic and biologic determinism to an organizational notion of human transactions. The conceptual underpinnings for this new world view of the human condition [13,32] derive from multiple sources, for example, general systems [10] and cybernetic [49] theories, structuralism [39] and the hypotheses advanced by the information [42] and communication theorists [8,45].

In contrast, the "interdisciplinary" model has relied on the efficacy of the therapeutic milieu and the contributions of discrete disciplines for the treatment of psychiatric and behavioral disorders. Increasingly, the "interdisciplinary" paradigm has been subjected to critical evaluation vis-à-vis an ecological systems approach. This unifying holistic model transcends disciplinary boundaries offering both a new way of thinking and an operational format.

The application of this paradigm to an inpatient psychiatric setting presents a formidable challenge so long as the linear (cause→effect) thinking characteristic of the classic medical model prevails. The dangers of superficial or simplistic misapplication of general systems terminology notwithstanding [9,20] the authors are persuaded by Auerwald's argument that "the ecological systems model, by clarifying and emphasizing the interfaces between systems allows for the use of a variety of theoretical models which have to do with interactional processes and information exchange. These models form bridges between the conceptual systems of single disciplines [6]."

It would be misleading to suggest that the family therapy psychiatric inpatient training program about to be described was the result of a carefully formulated program design based on an ecosystemic perspective. Instead, the theoretical assumptions and philosophy represented in this paper reflect an epistemological shift evolving discontinuously over time from an interdisciplinary to an ecosystemic paradigm. This radically affects one's perception of human transactional systems and challenges established theories of change. The gap between epistemology and clinical implementation is acknowledged as we struggle with the task of transcending linear formulations in the translation of theory to training and practice. It is assumed that such a shift cannot be imposed upon an academic system from without, and, that a process of internalization is a necessary prerequisite to lasting systemic change.

The need for academic disciplines to be at the forefront in the evolution and implementation of the ecosystemic paradigm, and for the incorporation of an ecological philosophy into core curricula has been recognized [7,16,21,43]. Yet, although every clinical discipline has more or less independently come to acknowledge the dramatic effects of context on the human psyche and on human behavior, to date, each has failed adequately to translate this knowledge to clinical practice.

At the practice level, considerations relating to the preservation of professional "turf" and the economic dictates of a bureaucratized society have essentially determined the nature and constraints imposed upon mental health care delivery systems. This has tended to preclude extension of conceptual knowledge beyond disciplinary boundaries. Perhaps it is no accident that the family therapy movement, which has by and large evolved without respect to professional disciplines, is in the vanguard in this respect. It represents one area of clinical training and practice which has seriously attempted the operationalization of an ecosystemic paradigm even as it struggles to identify and remedy evidence of regression to linear thinking within family therapy, theory, and practice.

This chapter highlights the crucial nature of the inpatient family therapy supervisor's role at the interfaces between the conceptual frameworks of the various disciplines involved in the treatment of the hospitalized psychiatric patient and the various systemic levels—biologic, psychologic, social, and individual—within which symptomatology is manifested. Subtle shifts in operational style and conceptualization of supervisory goals and tasks are still in a process of evolution and development as we gain in practice wisdom and experience. Meanwhile, the fact remains that in an endeavor where leaders in the family field have predicted failure [19,23], a viable systemic family therapy training model has been successfully established within an academic psychiatric institution firmly rooted in the psychodynamic tradition.

PROGRAM DESCRIPTION

Introduction

The authors advisedly limited this chapter to a description of family therapy supervision of psychiatric residents on an adult inpatient unit. Family therapy supervision is also provided to some psychiatric nursing staff and to those graduate social work students assigned to the unit. In addition, junior medical students in the psychiatric clerkship are invited to observe family sessions behind the one-way mirror and, in those instances where the student has been assigned the role of "primary therapist" to the hospitalized patient, to participate in the resident's supervision.

The decision to focus this chapter solely on resident supervision was in part based on the centrality given to the training of psychiatric residents on the inpatient service and the hierarchical issues and challenges this raises in a multidisciplinary training program. It had been assumed that the psychiatric resident would be more likely to have difficulty in accepting supervision from faculty of another discipline than, say, the staff nurse and/or the social work student. This is, however, debatable, particularly in the case of the psychiatric nurse trained within a hierarchical medical model wherein the physician is expected and required to establish his authority and accept responsibility for the outcome of therapeutic interventions. Issues related to case assignment and power struggles inherent in complementary resident/student or resident/nurse co-therapy relationships could be the subject of another paper. It is postulated that systemic issues raised in relation to the family therapy supervision of psychiatric residents on an inpatient service will have relevance to the supervision of nursing staff and social work students who also form a part of the therapeutic community within which the training is taking place.

Historical Context

Prior to 1974, when a four-year mandatory training in family therapy was built into the core curriculum of the psychiatric residency program at the University of Maryland Department of Psychiatry, family therapy on the adult inpatient service had traditionally been provided by psychiatric social workers with an occasional interested resident participating as co-therapist.

The historic moment to which the genesis of mandatory family therapy supervision within the residency program can be ascribed occurred in 1973 at a clinical services committee meeting. Casual reference was made to the coincidence of a married couple being simultaneously hospitalized in the University of Maryland Hospital. In the course of discussion, the following facts emerged:

1. Husband and wife had been assigned to different wards, each with a separate resident designated as primary therapist.
2. Within the course of diagnostic assessment and treatment, marital problems inevitably surfaced.

3. The two resident therapists (each of whom had been assigned an individual psychotherapy supervisor) decided to meet with the couple in a brave attempt at marital co-therapy.

4. Unsupervised, and without training or experience in a complex therapeutic modality, predictably, their interventions proved counterproductive.

The vehement protestations of one of the authors as to the "irresponsibility" of allowing the uninitiated to intervene in the marriage and family life of disturbed hospitalized individuals, without benefit of direct supervision (in a setting where individual psychotherapy supervision was mandatory), led to an invitation to provide supervisors and family cases for those residents requesting family therapy training. In an early climate of resistance and lack of institutional support, a small outpatient family clinic was established, with the director also assuming responsibility for coordinating family therapy training in the residency program. The mandatory four-year training requirement came into effect during the following year. From these inauspicious beginnings, family therapy training has gained momentum to a point where it has become accepted as an integral and viable part of the psychiatric residency program.

Several factors undoubtedly contributed to the changing level of acceptance, recognition, and support which has taken place over time: (1) the paradigm shift in the social and behavioral sciences toward a unifying holistic model based on an ecological epistemology challenging the linear assumptions of traditional medicine [6,7,16,43]; (2) the recognition that training in individual psychotherapy alone is not sufficient for the education of the psychiatric generalist and the need to include marital and family therapy in the core curriculum of a psychiatric residency program [34]; (3) the timely emergence of a psychiatrist role model, who, in his position as ward attending, set about transforming one of the three inpatient psychiatric wards into a model for a family-focused short-term inpatient facility*; (With some idiosyncratic differences, all three wards have for several years had a firmly established family treatment program.) (4) the existence of a faculty nucleus of trained family therapy supervisors, predominantly social workers, whose skills had been underutilized; (5) the appointment of two recognized leaders in the family therapy field to the part-time faculty of the Department of Psychiatry (Jay Haley and Cloe Madanes). Since 1976 they have provided a one-year (one day a week) elective training program in family therapy to post-graduate fourth year residents and child fellows.

---

*For a more detailed description of a family-focused inpatient psychiatric ward model emphasizing nursing staff participation, see Harbin, Henry T. A family oriented psychiatric inpatient unit. *Family Process* 18 : 281–292, 1979 [27].

The Setting

The most intensive exposure to family therapy typically occurs during the second post-graduate year of the psychiatric residency. This takes place on the adult inpatient service of the Institute of Psychiatry and Human Behavior, where the resident may have up to five patient families in therapy at any one time. An average of 82% of patient families have been engaged in family therapy over the past three years. In addition, family intake interviews and family group meetings are conducted on a weekly basis by nursing staff. This is an acute-care facility for male and female patients, ranging in age from adolescence to old age, covering a broad spectrum of diagnostic categories and socioeconomic statuses.

Family therapy supervision is provided by full-time psychiatric social work faculty assigned to each of the three wards, with backup supervision from one of the authors and a former ward attending psychiatrist who was an early graduate of the family therapy training program (Henry T. Harbin, M.D.). More recent graduates of the residency training program have since been recruited to provide psychiatric role models and to augment the inpatient family therapy supervision already provided. The training typically involves from two to three hours of formal family therapy supervision per week for each resident, including a minimum of one hour of live supervision using a one-way mirror and telephone. It should be noted that all of the inpatient family therapy supervisors are sophisticated in ego psychology and psychoanalytic concepts and are graduates of the Family Therapy Institute of Washington, D.C. (co-directors: Haley and Madanes).

Inpatient Family Therapy Training

The residents assigned to the inpatient unit of the Institute of Psychiatry and Human Behavior are, for the most part, family therapy neophytes who are required to begin working with patient families as soon as they join the unit. In addition to direct supervision, a basic weekly seminar is therefore offered during the first two months on the service, with an introduction to techniques of interviewing, identifying sequences of behavior and structure, giving directives designed to bring about change within dysfunctional family systems, and the acceptance of responsibility for outcome. The seminar is geared specifically to problems related to the treatment of families of hospitalized patients in an acute-care facility with emphasis on family participation in decision making with respect both to treatment and discharge planning. The therapeutic use of the weekend leave of absence, or "therapeutic furlough" is also highlighted. The resident is sensitized to hierarchical issues within the ward system which, if ignored, may prove deleterious to good patient care and is taught to recognize his own role as a member of that system.

At this early stage of training, the emphasis is on learning by doing the supplemented with selective use of video tapes and with minimal reference to literature. At the beginning of the second semester when the trainee is presumed to know what he needs to know, the same instructors (Henry T. Harbin, M. D. and Joan M. Scratton, M. S. W.) offer a weekly eight-session basic concepts seminar in family theory. This consists of an introduction to general systems [7] and communication theories [45], including the original double bind hypothesis [8] and later revisions [1,26,47]. A brief comparative study is made of strategic [24], structural [35], and "Bowen" [11] system theories and their influence on the family therapy field. Finally, selected publications on outcome research in family therapy are critically evaluated for validity and reliability.

TRAINING GOALS AND TASKS

In this early phase of the resident's training in family therapy, specific goals and tasks are identified as germane to an inpatient psychiatric setting:

1. To introduce the psychiatric resident, not to a body of theory, but to a new orientation to the human dilemma transcending linear explanations of behavior [6,25]. This, in turn, will suggest a variety of therapeutic options rather than any one method of treatment applicable to every situation.

2. To teach the trainee how to formulate an ecosystemic diagnosis and to devise a treatment strategy for each problem situation. Observed repetitive dysfunctional sequelae of interactional behavior within the family system, together with the family's response to the therapist's directives, will form the bases for a hypothesis concerning the function that individual symptomatology serves for the family as a whole.

3. To discover and nurture in each individual trainee those unique qualities of intellect, personality, "style," and aptitude which can be utilized creatively and empathically in interpersonal transactions.

4. To identify and accommodate to individual learning patterns and pace, utilizing paradoxical techniques in handling initial resistance, e.g., encouraging the resident to maintain a "healthy skepticism," while approaching new ideas and practices with an "open mind."

5. To enable the trainee to develop the ability to observe ambiguous and seemingly contradictory bits of behavior and translate them to their underlying metaphorical meaning. In other words, to metacommunicate in supervision and, selectively in family sessions, about observed family communication patterns.

6. To teach the trainee the potential for growth and transformation within a crisis situation threatening to family homeostasis and to recognize crisis as providing optimal motivation for change. The resident will also be taught techniques for inducing crisis in a rigid family system in order to bring about change.

7. To provide a developmental framework for the observation of human behavior. A psychiatric problem is defined as an adaptive attempt to resolve a transitional developmental crisis within the life cycle of the family, requiring total family commitment and participation for its resolution.

8. To teach that behavior is multidetermined, recognizing the role that deviance plays in supporting the social order [17], and relabelling deviant aspects of behavior for what they represent on an interactional level, i.e., an adaptive, often protective, response to system dysfunction [4,46] This avoids the twin pitfalls of relieving the individual of all responsibility for his behavior while resorting to reductionistic linear explanations often amounting to little more than a sophisticated game of shifting blame between parents, society, and individual biochemistry, depending on one's conceptual point of reference.

9. To provide the trainee with basic perceptual (observation), conceptual (translate observation into meaningful language), and executive skills (therapeutic intervention) [15].

Basic Assumptions

The implementation of family therapy supervision on an inpatient unit was undertaken with prior awareness of systemic problems inherent in such an enterprise. The following assumptions influenced the process:

1. The model of family therapy and theoretical orientation will, by and large, dictate the model of supervision. Specifically, the adoption of a directive, task-oriented, noninterpretive approach to family treatment based on a systemic view of family structure will be reflected in the supervisory paradigm.

2. The introduction of family therapy training within a psychiatric residency program rooted in the classical psychodynamic tradition will be met with covert or overt opposition, disparagement, and skepticism [23].

3. Given the linear, rational science base of medicine and prevailing psychoanalytic belief system, conversion to an ecosystemic epistemology will represent a major challenge for the psychiatric resident and initial resistance will be inevitable.

4. The training of the psychiatric resident in an ecosystemic approach to family therapy will threaten and be resisted by both ward staff and the administration unless ways are found actively to involve them in the process.

5. Endorsement of such a program will require active support from psychiatric role models who have status and visibility.

6. The family therapy supervisor will need to respect the hierarchical structure of the milieu (e.g., the resident's authority as primary therapist) while establishing authority of expertise in the supervisory relationship.

7. The traditional trust and authority vested in the physician is a powerful tool in a strategic approach to systemic change where the therapist's need to take charge is axiomatic.

8. The resident who demonstrates clinical competence in one modality is likely to be clinically effective in most treatment situations requiring psychological-mindedness, dynamic understanding of metaphorical levels of communication, empathy, flexibility, and openness to new learning experiences.

9. It has been observed that the patient's behavior cannot be considered apart from the social context within which it occurs [14,44]. Not only does the therapist's behavior become part of that context and significant for change, but the supervisor also forms part of the therapeutic system influencing and being influenced by the contextual course of events.

10. Psychiatric problems are seen as developing within the total biopsychosocial life context of the patient. This includes not only the individual, his family, and the community, but also the therapeutic subsystems (e.g., the ward milieu) within which deviant behaviors are observed.

11. Because the family therapist views abnormal behavior as an adaptive response to an abnormal situation, it is presumed the individual cannot change unless his situation (including the therapeutic milieu created by the hospital system) changes.

These are some of the challenges and problems inherent in the introduction of family therapy training and supervision on an inpatient psychiatric facility. In the opinion of the authors, these issues are much less critical in an outpatient setting where the therapist, supervisor, and family operate with more autonomy free from the powerful constraints of a highly structured ward setting with all the self-regulative and adaptive accommodations of a microcommunity.

Therapeutic Modality

A strategic task-oriented model of family therapy and supervision based on a structural analysis of the family hierarchical system has been adopted advisedly as the treatment method of choice for patients with severe problems in impulse control and/or the everyday management of their lives. Such a model provides needed external structure and direction. Experiential growth models and the exploratory, insight-oriented approach to family treatment were rejected because of limited usefulness for a patient population hospitalized in an acute-care facility and diagnosed with major affective, organic, schizophrenic, or conduct disorders. The model was selected for its pragmatism, lending itself to crisis-oriented, time-limited treatment with built-in provision for continuing family therapy on discharge from the hospital (e.g., the outpatient family clinic of the Institute of Psychiatry and Human Behavior).

The model was considered basically congruent with the shift within the mental health service delivery system toward brief hospitalization and emphasis on community-based treatment of psychiatric disorders. A therapeutic assumption was that long-term hospitalization becomes increasingly counter-productive for most psychiatric patients. It is noted that premature discharge may also occur where another two or three weeks in the hospital would have been necessary to solidify gains and prepare the family for resumption of responsibility on discharge.

Implications for Supervision

Given this treatment model, there are several implications for supervision. The supervisor will be teaching a time-limited, directive, problem-solving approach which requires specificity, creativity, and flexibility on the part of both supervisor and trainee. Hierarchical boundaries will be respected within the supervisory relationship. Supervisory responsibility for outcome will be acknowledged and accepted, allowing for appropriate risk taking and, where necessary, heroic interventions in response to seemingly desperate situations. The supervisory model will be more family- than supervisee-focused, and oriented toward the present rather than the past. Learning will take place within a positive context of support and respect for the resident's attempts at transformation of a dysfunctional system. Reliance will be placed more on observed therapist/family interaction than on therapist self-report. Supervision will be characterized by the immediacy of here-and-now directives and intervention. Finally, analogies between therapist/family interactional system and that of the supervisor/therapist dyadic system will emerge. For example, supervisory strategies often mirror those of the therapist actively engaged in giving directives designed to provide families with options, opportunity, and alternative routes to the creative realization of their goals.

Supervisory Model   Ideological differences apart, there is consensus in the literature on the primacy of supervision in family therapy training and the fact that the supervisory model will tend to reflect philosophical, theoretical, and therapeutic orientation to the family and the human condition [31,33].

The supervisory model of choice in this instance is "live" supervision, wherein the supervisor guides the therapist, using direct observation and intervention during the actual family session [36]. The live supervision model is perceived as most congruent with training and treatment tasks and goals on a short-term psychiatric hospital unit. It was quickly realized, however, that live supervision utilizing a one-way mirror and telephone intercommunication was logistically impossible for every family case, both because of the number of family therapy cases each resident was expected to carry and limitations on accessibility to one-way mirrors and videotape equipment, also widely utilized by other clinical faculty within the Department of Psychiatry.

Self-Report Supervision

In these circumstances, the selective use of the more traditional models of self-report supervision (the issue of reliability notwithstanding) [24,36] and co-therapy were adopted as necessary and, at times, useful adjuncts to live supervision. The advantages and limitations of both these models of family therapy supervision have been addressed in the literature [24,36,41,48]. Those programs emphasizing personal growth models of supervision (i.e., therapist-oriented training models) favor both co-therapy and self-report, while family-focused cognitive models tend to favor direct supervision emphasizing the acquisition of therapeutic skills and competence.

The self-report model is utilized pragmatically to provide the supervisor with an updated overview of the current interactional status of every family case both with respect to treatment and after-care planning (a necessary component of short-term hospitalization). An additional bonus is that it provides the resident trainee with more time for reflection, assimilation, and careful consideration of strategic options than live supervision generally affords, particularly when the designing of more complex directives (e.g., paradoxical injunctions) is involved.

Co-therapy Training Model

A case for co-therapy training has been made [41,48], including the advantage of providing the resident with a family therapy role model. Questions arise when the family therapy supervisor is not of the same professional discipline as the resident, or where identification with the supervisor (of whatever discipline) may actually inhibit the creative use of self. The neophyte family therapy trainee whose anxiety level is such that he "freezes" in live supervision may benefit initially from the "show-me-how-to-do-it" aspect of co-therapy on a strictly time-limited basis. There is a problem of complementarity inherent in the co-therapy training model which has not been sufficiently addressed, in that the supervisor assumes and is clearly designated the one-up position of "expert" in the eyes of the family, with the resident trainee relegated to a more or less passive "one-down" position at variance with his authority status as primary therapist to the hospitalized patient. Co-therapy is clearly contraindicated when live supervision is utilized, since it requires one-to-one direct telephone communication between supervisor and therapist during the therapy sessions.

Live Supervision

In a classic paper on live supervision (1973), Montalvo formulated direct innovative supervisory techniques analogous to the structural (Minuchin) family therapist's attempts to "create a sense of competence in family members by reshaping and reframing reality through the creation of therapeutic events" [33]. Montalvo's model is based on the assumption that "any family can absorb and orient the therapist and direct him away from his function as a change agent; that any therapist can be caught behaving with the family in ways that will reinforce the very patterns that brought them to therapy" [36]. He also assumes a significant gap between the therapist's self-report and what is actually observed to happen within a family therapy session.

One of the more useful and pertinent aspects of the Montalvo article is the section on "learning from mistakes," i.e., the "inevitable" and "natural" mistakes on the part of the therapist, mistakes which reveal the permeability of boundaries between a person's own perspective and his interpersonal and physical environment [36]. Montalvo quotes Ortega ". . . reality happens to be, like a landscape, possessed of an infinite number of perspectives, all equally veracious and authentic" [37].

The live supervision model affords the supervisor three possible alternatives: telephoning the therapist, convening a brief strategy conference outside the training interview, or entering the training interview. Brief teaching and planning sessions are arranged before and after the family sessions [40]. It has been the authors' experience that these sessions sometimes tend to be too brief and perfunctory to serve a useful training purpose. (The broader issue of the vast expenditure of professional time, skills, and hardware in an optimal family therapy training program utilizing this model has not been addressed.)

Rickert and Turner list among the advantages of the live supervision model versus the traditional consultation/self-report model: less opportunity for collusion against the family and for distortion of self-report sessions; less time wasted giving diagnostic information so that more time can be devoted to the trainee's effect on the family system [40]. Montalvo adds the all-important variable of timely opportunity for correction of therapy mistakes [36].

The issue of timing of supervisory intervention in the therapeutic process is considered crucial [24,36,40]. For instance, the supervisor transmitting his own sense of urgency to the supervisee can serve to throw him out of step with the family pace. On the other hand, supervisor reluctance to intervene, whether based on ambivalence regarding the use of the supervisory model, sensitivity to the trainee's feelings, or mirroring trainee reluctance to interrupt family members, can result in loss of the optimal moment for therapeutic intervention and change, ending in therapeutic stalemate.

In order for the supervisor's telephone interventions to facilitate learning and at the same time ensure that the family will be enabled to move beyond a repetitive sequential impasse toward problem resolution, the supervisor must be able to assess the trainee's level of knowledge, skill, learning style, and pace. This is essential if the supervisor's interventions are not to be experienced as intrusive, infantalizing, or disruptive to the therapeutic process on the one hand, or, at the other extreme, as oracular pronouncements defying critical questioning or metacommunication. The latter situation is more likely to occur when the supervisor has an established reputation in the field and where the style of supervision is impersonal and problem focused.

For the clinician-supervisor utilizing the live supervision paradigm, an alternative model suggests itself whereby supervisor and trainee are in a sense co-partners working in close unison to achieve agreed upon therapeutic goals contracted with the family. An analogy might be the orchestral conductor and soloist performer transaction, whereby the finely tuned interplay of conductor/performer is as much the artistic creation of the one as of the other, and the ultimate performance becomes a shared responsibility and achievement: "Both student and trainer can draw on their respective creativity, allowing for the nurture of their capacity to grow together" [3]. For such a model to work, the level of understanding between supervisor and trainee must be optimal. The team approach of Palazzoli and colleagues is interesting in this respect combining as it does the oracular power of a modern day Greek chorus with the direct interventive supervisory tactics of the structural school of family therapists [38].

Concern has been expressed in the literature regarding the efficacy of the live supervision model for family therapy training. Whitaker, for instance is convinced that ". . . observation and technical indoctrination by the supervisor tends to make the supervisee less confident of himself and more dependent on a technical method" [48]. Therapist dependency on supervisory interventions, disruption of the therapeutic process, and interference with the therapist's evolvement of his own style are common criticisms and reservations advanced about this training model [33]. One might add to these reservations trainee apprehension of criticism, fear of exposure, and the pain of learning publicly [30]. In this regard, informing trainees that they can expect to frequently fail may provide a liberating experience from the constraints of overpreoccupation with how they will measure up in the supervisor's eyes [40]. In group supervision, Haley establishes the rule that no one may criticize the work of anyone else unless he can offer a positive alternative [24]. Montalvo has the last word in this controversy: "Live supervision is, after all, only one more arrangement for guiding the therapeutic process. Its main asset, its capacity for getting closer to empirical happenings rather than self-reports about them does not make it more foolproof than any other arrangement involving humans [36]."

The Supervisory Relationship

Central to any model of supervision is the supervisor/supervisee relationship. It has been hypothesized that the nature of this relationship will be dictated as much by theoretical persuasion and training model as by supervisor personality and style: "Experientally oriented and psychodynamically oriented programs tend to emphasize the personal growth aspects of training and the affective lives of the trainees, whereas programs operating from structural, behavioral and strategic perspectives are more family-focused than therapist-focused" [18].

Within the hierarchical model of live supervision the supervisor accepts ultimate responsibility both for the successful treatment of the family and for the development of a competent therapist. Of necessity, supervision will be quite directive, particularly in the early stages of training. Such a model of supervision engenders an intense working relationship between supervisor and trainee, in which issues of authority, power, and control sometimes assume paramount importance. Haley states unequivocally that "one cannot *not* have a hierarchical trainer-trainee relationship" [24]. The hierarchical nature of the relationship is, however, controversial. Ackerman takes the diametrically opposite view that "whatever the method of supervision, the relations of the trainee to instructor are egalitarian, not hierarchical" [2]. Within Bowen's family therapy training program, the concept of family therapist as "coach" also applies to the supervisory relationship [11]. Fogarty, (a Bowenite) stresses a personal self-disclosing relationship with the trainee, congruent with the experiental teaching paradigm he has adopted [22].

Whatever the model of supervision, a relationship of mutual trust and respect is essential in order for learning to take place. This can best be achieved by the supervisor first establishing his competence to teach the trainee perceptive, cognitive, and executive skills, and second, by establishing early with the trainee a clearly defined contract of mutual expectation and goals. For example, with the use of live supervision, the supervisor would be wise to follow Haley's "call with reluctance" agreement, so long as it is made perfectly clear at the outset that when the supervisor calls with a direct instruction that *must* be obeyed, the trainee therapist will follow through on that instruction without argument or dissent so as to avoid possible harm to a family or a family member. Both Montalvo [36] and Haley [24] have established "ground rules" to meet the various exigencies which might arise in the course of live supervision.

Montalvo notes the capacity within the supervisory relationship for elusive relationship shifts that can occur without necessarily involving either person's awareness. (Within an analytic paradigm these shifts would be labelled transferential.) By whatever name, Montalvo graphically presents all-too-familiar ways "in which a supervisee can take what a supervisor thinks to be a crucial suggestion and make it into an incidental and powerless operation" [36]. Similarly, he pinpoints subtle problems in the timing of the supervisor's interventions—just too early—just too late—which result in disruption of the supervisee's performance [36].

Within the live supervision model both supervisor and supervisee risk themselves within a professional self-disclosing relationship—which has nothing to do with sharing observations about one's own unresolved personality conflicts, values, or personal life style—that is focused directly on the shared task of bringing about therapeutic change within a dysfunctional family system. "Structural theory states that problems in families develop when the interpersonal or hierarchical boundaries between relationships are transgressed. Similarly, supervisors working from this therapeutic perspective believe that when the hierarchical nature of the relationship is consistently violated the efficacy of both trainer and trainee is diminished" [33].

The authors agree with the necessity to establish early on the supervisor's authority and expertise within a complementary supervisor/supervisee relationship. In practice, however, they have experienced the relationship as a sequential, developmental process with a gradual shift from an hierarchical toward a more collegial relationship as the resident trainee gains in experience, knowledge, and skills, assuming more and more direct responsibility for the therapeutic outcome [5,28]. Thus, the shift is from a structuralist perspective during the early stages of training toward a more egalitarian posture whenever the resident's training is developing along expectable lines during the course of the training year.

Parenthetically, in the third and fourth post-graduate years of the family therapy training in the residency program described, the developmental learning process is expected to accelerate, with the trainee ultimately taking maximal responsibility for his own learning. This process demands optimal expertise, flexibility, and accommodation on the part of the supervisor. At this level, a neo-collegial arrangement is possible without loss of supervisor status and authority. This affords potential advantage to the graduating resident who will require a capacity for independent judgement in the clinical situation [12].

The identity problem of the psychiatrist/psychotherapist has been addressed in the literature. Brody proposes a return to the traditional family physician role. He also stresses the need for the psychiatric resident to have an in-depth exposure to those relevant aspects of (his) field available to nonphysician psychotherapists [12]. Martin stresses the need for professional role models in the training of a psychiatrist [34]. In this instance, it happens that all of the faculty supervisors with primary responsibility for family therapy supervision on the inpatient service are clinical social workers. They combine the dual functions of clinical teaching and direct patient care, particularly in the area of aftercare planning. As stated earlier in this text, "secondary" or backup supervision is presently provided by family therapy supervisors, including psychiatrists, who, in most instances, are not directly involved in the ward milieu and its decision-making processes. This presents a systemic dilemma in that the secondary supervisor may at times find himself at odds with, and relatively powerless to affect, decisions made by ward staff at variance with the family treatment plan. The centrality of the ward social worker's position as family therapy supervisor cannot be overemphasized in this regard, providing as it does both opportunity and challenge for systemic change from within. (For an elaboration of this issue, see the section entitled "Discussion," in this chapter).

In any academic institution with a multidisciplinary faculty, concern with such issues as professional identity, hierarchical status, and role diffusion will never be far from the surface. No single professional discipline is exempt from such preoccupation which ultimately proves counterproductive and frequently prophetically self-fulfilling.

Insistence on the need for role models of the same discipline may reflect psychiatry's preoccupation with its own identity vis-à-vis other medical specialities and the need to establish what is unique to psychiatry at a time when "psychotherapists" from a diversity of disciplines and persuasions are proliferating [34]. The reality is that family therapy is a field where no one discipline is preeminent and no one method is applicable to all situations. It is suggested that the issue of role models for family therapy training may have been overstated and that the espousal of a truly ecosystemic epistemology would transcend such interdisciplinary concerns by clarifying interfaces between the conceptual systems of respective disciplines while capitalizing upon the richness and breadth of scientific knowledge and humanistic philosophy contained in such diversity. Meanwhile, Kaslow notes a greater willingness on the part of the psychiatric residents to accept supervision and instruction from "sister" disciplines [29]. In the last analysis, however, the major issue is supervisor competence.

SYSTEMIC ISSUES AND DILEMMAS

Once an ecosystemic view of the world is accepted, it is no longer possible to remain myopic and confined to the knowledge of traditional disciplines. Given that any therapeutic context is determined by converging systems, the family therapy supervisor on an inpatient psychiatric unit is at a major nodal point where the task is to select relevant data and to determine their clinical application. At the same time, the supervisor is a member of a therapeutic system which is engaged in powerful, contradictory pulls toward homeostasis or change. A case in point might be a conflict both for the faculty supervisor and resident trainee between training requirements and perceived family need (e.g., the requirement that the resident treat a number of long-term individual patients on the inpatient service). The family therapy supervisor at the boundaries of interlocking subsystems is paradoxically vulnerable yet strategically positioned for the introduction of change.

Data Selection and Family Misuse of Medical Information

On the University of Maryland Baltimore Campus, the therapeutic system includes a number of professional schools and the faculty and staff of a major teaching hospital. This provides the context for the family therapist's interventions while adding to the complexity of the decision-making process.

"Patient care," or "psychiatric treatment," including a repertoire of treatment modalities, is influenced by: (1) departmental philosophy (in this case, psychodynamic, with increasing neuropsychological emphasis): (2) the hospital milieu composed of multidisciplines, each highlighting its particular orientation and treatment philosophy and, (3) a number of medical subspecialities other than psychiatry contributing to the diagnosis and treatment of "the patient." All of these networks impact on trainee understanding of the problem as well as creating reciprocal relationships between these systems and the family, influencing what should be done about it and how the family should be treated.

The family therapy supervisor in this situation needs to be an expert in systemic process both at institutional and family levels. Knowledge of family process will alert him to the possible misuse by family members of seemingly "objective" data in the service of homeostatic maintenance. The supervisor's task is to instruct the trainee in communicating these data to the family in such a way as to produce constructive change. The issues of data selection and the dysfunctional family's use of medical information in order to resist change are demonstrated in the following clinical example of family therapy failure.

Mr. and Mrs. C, a highly intelligent, sophisticated, middle-class couple brought their 14-year-old son, Tony, to the University Hospital, a center with an established reputation for expertise in neuropsychiatry. Because of the "abrupt onset," the parents were convinced that Tony's presenting problems of school refusal and temper tantrums at home when he did not get his way were neurologically based.

The parents came requesting the full battery of major neuropsychological tests. Initially, family therapy supervisor and resident made the decision to align with the family and to join their resistance to dealing with obvious family problems by recommending the tests. Psychiatric examination had revealed minor "soft sign" neurological findings only, insufficient to explain the presenting problems. When test results raised some neurological questions (while stressing that the basic issues were psychological), the family called in expert neurologists to debate the findings. Expectably, the experts rose to the academic challenge, and, as the sophistication and sophistry of debate increased, attention was successfully diverted further away from the familial conflict that was maintaining the problem. The ultimate paradox was that, test results notwithstanding, the need for the parents to pull together in order to respond effectively to Tony's behavior would remain.

Utilizing the multidisciplinary hospital system the parents succeeded in rigidly locking themselves into a position where the conflict was with the neurologists and, therefore, no solution was available to them as parents. The strategy at that point was to negotiate discharge, with outpatient family therapy, hoping that as the problems re-emerged at home, the parents might be more willing to work directly on Tony's behavioral problems.

Instead, after an explosive two weeks, the family reapplied for admission, this time to a prestigious out-of-state hospital where the whole process began again, only to have the original findings confirmed. This institution recommended, however, long-term psychiatric hospitalization which reportedly "stabilized" the family. In this instance, family therapy supervisor (a nonphysician) and resident were in complete agreement that family therapy was the treatment method of choice, but were defeated by parental need to prove the local experts wrong and find support for their linear explanation of Tony's problems.

Defining Hospitalization as a Family Crisis

The concept of introducing instability into a dysfunctional system in order to bring about change is at variance with a therapeutic milieu committed to bringing stability to psychiatrically disturbed individuals through medication and a structured setting. This reinforces the family's need to have the patient taken care of without their needing to change. The supervisor's task then becomes one of helping the resident to redefine the psychiatric hospitalization as a family crisis requiring the family to accept responsibility for the problems and to discover more functional alternatives to conflict resolution than the selection of a family member to be the symptom bearer.

Impact of Psychiatric Diagnosis within the Family

A further dilemma is the necessity within a system dedicated to differential diagnosis to sensitize the resident diagnostician to the family's tendency to generalize the implications of a psychiatric diagnosis to include every area of social functioning, and the need to reassert the family's potential to provide a context for significant change and growth [27].

The resident has to contend with a plethora of data from various mentors at a stage of training when his level of experience is such that he is most susceptible to conflicting opinions and direction offered by supervisors who play a significant role in his professional development. He will experience cognitive dissonance as well as hierarchical double binds.

The family therapy supervisor is faced with the task of helping the resident to understand his position in the system, to use data selectively, to reconcile conceptual differences, and to come to terms with the hierarchical impasse.

In the case of a hallucinating patient, the individual therapy supervisor recommended delaying active intervention until psychotic symptomatology had diminished; whereas the family therapy supervisor was recommending to the trainee that the family should expect the patient to be active in other areas of competence in spite of his hallucinations. The family therapy supervisor was able to take advantage of systemic realities as to the need for active patient participation in the milieu and the shared concern of the ward attending and staff about a prolonged hospitalization without significant behavioral change. Staff discussion, initiated by the family therapy supervisor (the ward social worker), allowed the trainee to metacommunicate on conflicting supervisory input and to reach the autonomous decision to reinforce the family's expectations of competent functioning. In this instance, the psychotic symptoms subsided and the patient made significant progress.

Reenactment of the Family Drama within the Milieu

Not infrequently, a hospitalized patient and/or family member may elicit support from staff for maintenance of dysfunctional behavior within the family at variance with the trainee's therapeutic goals. The supervisor's task is to teach the trainee the interrelatedness of individual staff transactions with family members and the potential for patient "acting-out."

In one instance, during a live supervisory family session, a once quiet, withdrawn patient began speaking to his mother in a more assertive manner, which was initially encouraged. As the discussion continued, however, the patient went on to confront his mother with the fact that it was a staff member who had interpreted to him that she (mother) was "infantalizing." This pseudo-assertive stance reflected a coalition between staff and patient which conflicted with the positive connotation within which the parents had been engaged in the therapeutic task, and as such, was disruptive to therapy.

Determination of Therapeutic Furlough and Date of Discharge

A further hierarchical issue critical to therapeutic outcome is the necessity for the supervisor, in collaboration with the resident trainee, to be able to determine when and under what conditions a patient needs to spend time away from the hospital with his family (therapeutic furlough) and, more importantly, to determine date of discharge. While it is legally encumbent upon the administrative staff to make such decisions, in practice these are all too often arrived at without sufficient regard for the phase of family therapy and the necessity at times for family and therapist to take a calculated therapeutic risk. The family therapy supervisor is strategically situated to help the resident negotiate a compromise in the best interests of the patient and his family.

Resistance to Systemic Change:
Paradoxical Strategies

In attempting to introduce an ecosystemic model of family therapy into an institution where the medical model prevails we found ourselves unwittingly employing the same linear thinking by seeking to replace one set of primary theoretical constructs for another. As in all systems where homeostasis is threatened and the system seeks to minimize and resist change, the more we tried to convert our colleages to a new epistemology, predictably, the more rigid the resistance. In like institutions such resistance could substantially undermine attempts to establish a family therapy training program of this kind, so that understanding and handling systemic resistance is crucial. In this instance, a major strategy for integrating family therapy training within a traditional psychiatric residency program has been that of "joining with the resistance" and attempting a synthesis of transactional with individual psychodynamic processes. It is the family therapy supervisor's task within such a situation to find ways of aligning with the existing system (of which he is a part) in order to produce change. For instance, instead of imposing concepts and language alien to the prevailing psychodynamic model, the family therapy supervisor needs to join with the resistance by translating the language of systems into such familiar concepts as "secondary gain", "multi-determined behavior" and "personality structure reflecting current familial transactions." Similarly, translating Object-Relations Theory into systemic concepts has also proved helpful. In such ways, the supervisor seeks to ensure that there is consensus about the meaning of what is being described and to incorporate transactional phenomena within the trainee's conceptual repertoire. These issues need to be addressed in order to help the trainee bridge the epistemological gap between family and individual dynamic constructs.

An initial conflict presents itself in that the resident is simultaneously required to perform dual functions of individual and family therapist. An example will serve to illustrate how the family therapy supervisor assists the resident in reconciling this conflict:

A 16-year-old adolescent boy was having difficulty in successfully separating from his family. His mother was overinvolved with him to the exclusion of her husband while the latter overinvolved himself with his work and was isolated from the family. As the adolescent was their major reason for communicating, the family needed to keep him the focus of attention. Mother, father, and the boy all had their own methods for accomplishing this end. Father and, particularly, mother would redefine rebellious adolescent behavior as evidence of a "severe and deeper problem" which was not substantiated by psychiatric examination.

Addressing the role conflict experienced by the resident, the family therapy supervisor, by observing the family's interactions, was able to anticipate possible "transferential" issues that could be expected to emerge in individual psychotherapy. By facilitating the resident's role of individual psychotherapist (i.e., aligning with the prevailing system), the supervisor, paradoxically, aroused the trainee's curiosity about changing family interactions. As the adolescent was, in fact, bringing some of these issues into individual psychotherapy, the trainee became more interested in introducing change into the family structure. This strategy also helped the trainee synthesize his clinical endeavors and emphasized the importance of the adolescent's transactions within the family system.

At the same time, the supervisor must be aware of and able to tolerate subsystem conflict in order that the resident trainee may be protected from excessive systemic pressure and competitiveness. Similar paradoxical techniques familiar to family system therapists will come to mind once the supervisor recognizes and acknowledges the systemic dilemma the situation presents.

Discussion

Central to the inpatient family therapy training program described is the creative opportunity and challenge inherent in the dual roles of ward social worker responsible for after-care planning on an acute care psychiatric unit and primary family therapy supervisor to psychiatric residents assigned to the unit. Many of the systemic issues and dilemmas identified in this section derive from the first hand experience of one of the authors who, for the past several years, has performed that dual function while seeking to maintain a strategic position at the boundaries of the various disciplines which comprise the therapeutic community of an adult inpatient psychiatric ward (Patti M. Seman, M.S.W.). As a full-time member of the ward system, the "primary" family therapy supervisor is in a unique position to implement change by aligning with the system of which she is a member in order to engage nursing staff in a positive, active collaboration with family members and family therapist in treatment planning and process. A first step would be the establishment of collegial alliances with those nursing staff who perform key roles in the decision-making processes affecting patient care. The primary supervisor is then in a position to adopt such relatively basic techniques as sharing with staff at team meetings strategies devised for the family in therapy sessions and inviting active participation outside the therapy sessions in the ongoing change process. Maximal educative use is made of clinical case conferences by highlighting systemic transactions which reinforce symptomatology, while avoiding excessive use of systemic jargon. An example is anticipation of the induction of ward staff into the pathological reenactment of the family drama and pointing out instances where resident, nurse, student, or family therapy supervisor had been so inducted. Conversely, the primary family therapy supervisor is also in a position to sensitize staff to the fact that hierarchical conflicts endemic to the ward system, unless identified and resolved within team meetings, may result in the induction of family members into the conflict.

In her role as family therapy supervisor, the ward social worker can serve as a buffer between neophyte resident trainee and those systemic demands and practices at variance with family involvement in the treatment process, on the one hand, and, academic skepticism and disparagement of the family therapy paradigm, on the other. As a teaching member of the faculty of an academic institution who is at the same time performing a key coordinating function within the mental health care delivery system, the primary supervisor in this setting is in a unique position to further the integration of clinical training and service goals, communicating at the meta level on observed discrepancies between stated philosophical goals and actual clinical practice.

The primary family therapy supervisor is also strategically placed to protect the beginning family therapy resident trainee from the often overwhelming impact of severe family dysfunction at a time when he has not yet developed the basic skills to deal with it. Convinced of the importance of an early success in working with severely troubled families, the primary supervisor uses her position on the ward to assist the resident in the initial selection of family therapy caess. By contrast, the "secondary" family therapy supervisor assigned to the resident is more or less dependent on the trainee's selection of cases for family therapy supervision. Also, the resident trainee is less able to avoid involvement of certain families in the therapeutic process and to rationalize such avoidance, when the supervisor, by virtue of the centrality of her position on the ward, has intimate knowledge of the resident's patients and can confront the avoidance early.

Parenthetically, the primary family therapy supervisor in the program described would appear to be in a much better position to provide a comprehensive and accurate assessment of the resident's abilities as a beginning family therapist than the secondary supervisor whose knowledge of the resident's skills is restricted to observation of the trainee's treatment of a relatively few self-selected cases throughout the training year. Finally, the primary supervisor, as an active participant in the therapeutic system, is in a position to provide the resident with a viable role model for systemic change, demonstrating techniques of joining, enactment, and disengagement analogous to the family therapist's interventions in the family system.

SUMMARY

This chapter describes an intensive one-year exposure to family therapy training on an inpatient psychiatric unit within a mandatory four-year family therapy training program for psychiatric residents at a university hospital. Adopting an ecosystemic frame of reference, basic assumptions regarding choice of supervision/therapy model and predicted resistance to its introduction within a traditional psychodynamically oriented psychiatric institute are identified, and training goals and tasks delineated. Essential components of the supervisor/ supervisee relationship are examined with emphasis on the need to establish mutual trust and respect. From an initial hierarchical structural paradigm, a sequential developmental model of supervision is presented. Live supervision utilizing one-way observation mirror and telephone communication is selected as the supervisory modality of choice on an acute-care inpatient psychiatric facility, and its usefulness and limitations critiqued. Systemic issues and dilemmas intrinsic to family therapy supervision on an inpatient psychiatric facility are also identified and critically appraised, with clinical examples. The centrality of the ward social worker's role as primary family therapy supervisor is highlighted.

While noting Haley's dire admonitions with respect to family therapy training in a psychiatric inpatient setting [23], in the authors' experience, an acute-care inpatient psychiatric unit lends itself to the teaching of brief crisis-oriented family therapy. At the same time, it provides a natural laboratory for the participant-observation of systemic interactional phenomena and hierarchical issues and dilemmas inherent in a "therapeutic milieu" approach to patient care.

What has been presented is a descriptive model of an early, relatively intensive phase of family therapy training for the psychiatric resident which may lend itself to replication in another setting. Assumptions which have dictated the model of treatment and supervision remain to be tested and a valid instrument needs to be developed for measuring the outcome both of supervision and the treatment of patient families on a short-term psychiatric inpatient unit.

Finally, when a family therapy training program has gained acceptance in a department of academic psychiatry, it may be time to raise questions regarding its current form, for example, has transformation given way to accommodation to institutional pressure? Has the ecosystemic perspective reverted to ingrained linear thinking (e.g., viewing the family as "causing" the pathology)? Has the model itself become institutionalized, doctrinaire, and inflexible?

REFERENCES

1. Ackerman, Brian L. "Relational paradox: toward a language of interactional sequences." *Journal of Marital and Family Therapy* 5 (1) : 29–38, 1979.
2. Ackerman, N. "Some considerations for training in family therapy." In: *Career Directions*, Volume II, East Hanover, New Jersey: Sandoz Pharmaceuticals, D. J. Publications, Inc., 1978, p. 206.
3. Andolfi, Maurizio and Menghi, Paola. "A model for training in family therapy." In: M. Andolfi and I. Zwerling (eds.) *Dimensions of Family Therapy*. New York: The Guilford Press, 1980, p. 258.
4. Andolfi, Maurizio. *Family Therapy: An Interactional Approach*. New York: Plenum Press, 1979, pp. 57–58.
5. Ard, B. "Providing clinical supervision for marriage counselors: a model for supervisor and supervisee." *Family Coordinator* 23 : 91–98, 1973.
6. Auerswald, Edgar H. "Interdisciplinary versus ecological approach." Family Process 7 : 204, 1968.
7. Balis, George U. "General systems theory and biosystems: an introduction." In: George U. Balis, Leon Wurmser and Ellen McDaniel (eds.) *Dimensions of Behavior: The Psychiatric Foundations of Medicine*. Boston: Butterworth Publishers, Inc., 1978, pp. 133–179.
8. Bateson, G.; Jackson, D.; Haley, J.; and Weakland, J. "Toward a theory of schizophrenia." *Behavioral Science* 1 : 256–264, 1956.
9. Beckett, J.A. "General systems theory, psychiatry and psychotherapy." *International Journal of Group Psychotherapy* 23 : 296–297, 1973.
10. Bertalanffy, L. *General Systems Theory*. New York: George Braziller, 1969.
11. Bowen, Murray. *Family Therapy in Clinical Practice*. New York: Jason Aronson, 1978, p. 347.
12. Brody, Eugene B. "Psychiatry's continuing identity crisis, confusion or growth?" Psychiatry Digest 30 : 11–17, 1969.
13. Buckley, W. *Modern Systems Research for the Behavioral Scientist*. Chicago: Aldine, 1968, p. xxiv.
14. Caudill, W. *The Psychiatric Hospital as a Small Society*. Cambridge, Massachusetts: Harvard University Press, 1958.
15. Cleghorn, J. and Levin, S. "Training family therapists by setting learning objectives." *American Journal of Orthopsychiatry* 43 : 439–446, 1973.
16. Engel, George L. "The need for a new medical model: a challenge for biochemistry." In: "George .U. Balis, Leon Wurmser and Ellen McDaniel (eds.) *Dimensions of Behavior: The Psychiatric Foundations of Medicine*. Boston: Butterworth Publishers, Inc., 1978, pp. 3–21.
17. Erikson, K.T. Notes on the sociology of deviance. Social Problems 9 : 307–314., 1962.
18. Ferber, A. and Mendelsohn, M. Training for family therapy. Family Process 8 : 25, 32, 1969.
19. Framo, James L. "Chronicle of a struggle to establish a family unit within a community mental health center." In: Philip J. Guerin (ed.) *Family Therapy Theory and Practice*. New York: Gardner Press, Inc., 1976, pp. 23–39.
20. French, Alfred P. *Disturbed Children and Their Families: Innovation in Evaluation*. New York: Human Sciences Press, 1977, pp. 17–31.

21. Germain, Carel B. (ed.) *Social Work Practice: People and Environments, An Ecological Perspective.* New York: Columbia University Press, 1979, p. 7.

22. Guerin, P. and Fogarty, T. Study your own family, Part II. In: Ferber, A.; Mendelsohn, M. and Napier, A. (eds.). The Book of Family Therapy. New York: Science House, 1972, pp. 460–467.

23. Haley, Jay. Why a mental health clinic should avoid family therapy. Journal of Marriage and Family Counseling, 1969, 1 : 3–12.

24. Haley, Jay. *Problem-Solving Therapy: New Strategies for Effective Family Therapy.* San Francisco: Jossey-Bass, 1976, 169–94.

25. Haley, J. "An editor's farewell." Family Process 8 : 149–158, 1969.

26. Haley, Jay. *Leaving Home: The Therapy of Disturbed Young People.* New York: McGraw-Hill, 1980.

27. Harbin, Henry T. "A family oriented psychiatric inpatient unit." Family Process 18 : 281–292, 1979.

28. Johnson, D. *Marriage Counseling.* Englewood Cliffs, New Jersey: Prentice-Hall, Inc., 1961.

29. Kaslow, F. W. et al. *Supervision, Consultation and Staff Training in the Helping Professions.* San Francisco: Jossey-Bass, 1977.

30. Kempster, S.W. and Savitsky, E. "Training family therapists through 'live' supervision." In: N.W. Ackerman; F.L. Bestman; and S.N. Sherman (eds.) *Expanding Theory and Practice in Family Therapy.* New York: Family Service Association of America, 1960.

31. Kniskern, David P. and Gurman, Alan I. "Research on training in marriage and family therapy: status, issues and directors." Journal of Marital and Family Therapy 5 (3) : 82–87, 1979.

32. Kuhn, Thomas S. *The Structure of Scientific Revolutions.* International Encyclopedia of Unified Science, Vol. 2, No. 2. Chicago : University of Chicago Press, 1970.

33. Liddle, Howard Arthur and Halpin, Richard H. "Family therapy training and supervision literature: a comparative review." Journal of Marriage and Family Counseling 4 (4) : 77–80, 1978.

34. Martin, Peter A. "Training of psychiatric residents in marital therapy." Journal of Marital and Family Therapy 5 (3) : 43–52, 1979.

35. Minuchin, Salvador. *Families and Family Therapy.* Cambridge, Massachusetts: Harvard University Press, 1974, p. 156.

36. Montalvo, Braulio. "Aspects of live supervision." Family Process 12 : 343–359, 1978.

37. Ortega, Jose y Gasset. *The Modern Theme.* New York: Harper Torchbooks, 1970, pp. 91–92.

38. Palazzoli, N.S. et al. *Paradox and Counterparadox.* New York: Jason Aronson, 1978.

39. Piaget, J. "Piaget's theory." In: P.H. Mussen (ed.) *Carmichael's Handbook of Child Psychology.* New York: John Wiley and sons, 1970, p. 5.

40. Rickert, Vernon C. and Turner, John E. "Through the looking glass: supervision in family therapy." Social Casework 3 : 132–134, 1978.

41. Rubenstein, D. "Family therapy." In: H. Hoffman (ed.) *Teaching Psychotherapy, International Psychiatry Clinics,* Volume I, Boston: Little Brown and Co., 1964.

42. Shannon, C.E. and Weaver, W. *The Mathematical Theory of Communication.* Urbana: University of Illinois Press, 1949.

43. Sherwood, Michael. "Epistomological formulations for the study of man." In: George U. Balis et al. (eds.) *Dimensions of Behavior: The Psychiatric Foundations of Medicine.* Boston : Butterworth, 1978, pp. 101–113.

44. Stanton, A. and Schwartz, M. *The Mental Hospital.* New York: Basic Books, Inc., 1954, p. 362.

45. Watzlawick, P.; Beavin, J.; and Jackson, D. *Pragmatics of Human Communication.* New York: W.W. Norton, 1967.

46. Watzlawick, Paul. *The Language of Change: Elements of Therapeutic Communication*. New York: Basic Books, 1978, pp. 118–126.
47. Weakland, John H. "The 'double-bind' hypothesis of schizophrenia and third-part interaction." In: D. Jackson (ed.) *The Etiology of Schizophrenia*. New York: Basic Books, 1962.
48. Whitaker, C. "Comment: live supervision in psychotherapy." *Voices* 12 : 24–25, 1976.
49. Wiener, N. *Cybernetics*. New York: Wiley, 1948.

Index

.